NUTRITION ASSESSMENT

A COMPREHENSIVE GUIDE
FOR PLANNING INTERVENTION
SECOND EDITION

Margaret D. Simko, PhD, RD
Clinical Professor of Family Medicine
Department of Family Medicine
University of Medicine and Dentistry of New Jersey
Robert Wood Johnson Medical School
New Brunswick, New Jersey

Catherine Cowell, MS, PhD
Clinical Professor of Public Health
Maternal & Child Health Program
School of Public Health
Columbia University
New York, New York

Judith A. Gilbride, PhD, RD
Associate Professor
Department of Nutrition, Food and Hotel Management
School of Education
New York University
New York, New York

AN ASPEN PUBLICATION®
Aspen Publishers, Inc.
Gaithersburg, Maryland
1995

Library of Congress Cataloging-in-Publication Data

Nutrition assessment : a comprehensive guide for planning intervention
[edited by] Margaret D. Simko, Catherine Cowell, Judith A.
Gilbride. — 2nd ed.
p. cm.
Includes bibliographical references and index.
ISBN 0-8342-0557-2
1. Malnutrition—Diagnosis. 2. Nutrition—Evaluation.
3. Nutrition surveys. I. Simko, Margaret D. II. Cowell, Catherine.
III. Gilbride, Judith A.
[DNLM: 1. Nutrition. 2. Nutrition Assessment. QU 145 N9723 1995]
RC623.N87 1995
616.3'9075—dc20
DNLM/DLC
for Library of Congress 94-3732
CIP

The authors have made every effort to ensure the accuracy of the information herein, particularly with regard to drug selection and dose. However, appropriate information sources should be consulted, especially for new or unfamiliar drugs or procedures. It is the responsibility of every practitioner to evaluate the appropriateness of a particular opinion in the context of actual clinical situations and with due consideration to new developments. Authors, editors, and the publisher cannot be held responsible for any typographical or other errors found in this book.

Editorial Resources: Lenda Hill

Library of Congress Catalog Card Number: 94-3732
ISBN: 0-8342-0557-2

Printed in the United States of America

1 2 3 4 5

To our students and the professionals who have captured the philosophy of comprehensive nutrition assessment, and to the people they serve.

Table of Contents

Contributors

Peter L. Beyer, MS, RD
Associate Professor
Clinical Dietitian Specialist
Department of Dietetics and
  Nutrition
University of Kansas Medical Center
Kansas City, KS

J. Larry Brown, MD
Director
Center on Hunger, Poverty and
  Nutrition Policy
Professor of Nutrition and Health
  Policy
Tufts University School of Nutrition
Medford, MA

Joan Castro, MS, RD
Coordinator Nutritional Research
Sherwood Medical
Philadelphia, PA

Martha T. Conklin, PhD, RD
Associate Professor
College of Health and Human
  Sciences
University of Southern Mississippi
Hattiesburg, MS

Elaine B. Feldman, MD
Professor Emeritus of Medicine
Medical College of Georgia
Augusta, GA

**Charlette R. Gallagher-Allred,
  PhD, RD**
Manager, Organization Services
Ross Products Division
Columbus, OH

Doris Goldberg, MD, MPH
Director, Public Health/Prevention
Medical Residency Training
  Program
New York City Department of
  Health
New York, NY

Helen A. Guthrie, PhD, RD
Professor Nutrition Emerita
The Pennsylvania State University
University Park, PA

**Isabelle A. Hallahan, MA, RD,
  LD, CHE**
Williamsville, NY

Jean H. Hankin, DrPH, RD
Nutrition Researcher
Professor of Public Health
Cancer Research Center of Hawaii
University of Hawaii
Honolulu, HI

Julie O'Sullivan Maillet, PhD, RD
Associate Dean for Academic Affairs
& Research
University of Medicine and Dentistry
of New Jersey
School of Health Related Professions
Newark, NJ

Carla Mariano, EdD, RN
Associate Professor and Director
Advanced Education in Nursing
Science
Master's Degree Program
New York University
New York, NY

Nicholas H.E. Mezitis, MD
Assistant Professor of Clinical
Medicine
Columbia University, College of
Physicians and Surgeons
Director of Clinical Pharmacology
Division of Endocrinology, Diabetes
and Nutrition
St. Luke's/Roosevelt Hospital
Center
New York, NY

Mary Mycek, PhD
Adjunct Professor of
Pharmacology
University of Medicine and Dentistry
of New Jersey
New Jersey Medical School
Newark, NJ

George Owen, MD
Medical Director
Owen Associates
Scottsdale, AZ

F. Xavier Pi-Sunyer, MD, MPH
Chief, Endocrinology, Diabetes and
Nutrition
Director, Obesity Research Center
St. Luke's/Roosevelt Hospital
Center
Professor of Medicine, Columbia
University
College of Physicians &
Surgeons
New York, NY

Gordon E. Robbins, MPH
Associate Director for Program
Operations
National Center for Chronic Disease
Prevention and Health Promotion
Centers for Disease Control and
Prevention
Atlanta, GA

Barbara J. Scott, MPH, RD
Associate Professor
Nutrition Education and Research
Program
School of Medicine
University of Nevada, Reno
Reno, NV

Laura P. Sherman, MS
Project Director
Nutrition-Cognition Initiative
Center on Hunger, Poverty and
Nutrition Policy
Tufts University
Medford, MA

Helen Smiciklas-Wright, PhD, RD
Professor of Nutrition
Nutrition Department
The Pennsylvania State University
University Park, PA

Sachiko T. St. Jeor, PhD, RD
Professor and Director
Nutrition Education and Research Program
School of Medicine
University of Nevada, Reno
Reno, NV

Linda Toohey, RD, RN, BSN
Medical-Surgical Registered Nurse
Clara Maass Health Care Systems
Belleville, NJ

Frederick L. Trowbridge, MD, MSc
Director, Division of Nutrition
National Center for Chronic Disease Prevention and Health Promotion
Centers for Disease Control and Prevention
Atlanta, GA

Marion Feitelson Winkler, MS, RD, LDN, CNSD
Surgical Nutrition Specialist
Department of Surgery and Nutritional Support Service
Rhode Island Hospital
Providence, RI

Catherine E. Woteki, PhD, RD
Senior Policy Analyst
The White House Office of Science and Technology
Executive Office of the President
Washington, DC

EDITORS

Margaret D. Simko, PhD, RD
Clinical Professor of Family Medicine
Department of Family Medicine
University of Medicine and Dentistry of New Jersey
Robert Wood Johnson Medical School
New Brunswick, NJ

Catherine Cowell, BS, MS, PhD
Clinical Professor of Public Health
Maternal & Child Health Program
School of Public Health
Columbia University
New York, NY

Judith A. Gilbride, PhD, RD
Associate Professor
Department of Nutrition, Food and Hotel Management
School of Education
New York University
New York, NY

Foreword

The planning of any successful nutrition intervention program requires expertise in the scientific assessment of the nutrition-related health problems in chronic disease of both individuals and communities and is essential for medical nutrition therapy, primary prevention, and health promotion. Dietitians and nutrition practitioners require up-to-date knowledge concerning the tools of nutrition assessment. They also require, along with the skills in selecting appropriate methods and in interpreting the findings, outcomes of an assessment. This revised publication fulfills these needs for the practice of nutrition in hospitals and communities in the 21st century.

In this edition, experienced researchers, physicians, dietitians, and public health nutritionists describe the appropriate nutrition assessment tools for use among various age groups, from infants to the elderly. Particular attention is given to the identification of individuals and groups in the United States who are at risk of developing nutrition-related health problems.

Knowledge of the tools of nutrition assessment is only the first step. The findings must be interpreted and adapted to meet the needs and lifestyles of the particular patients and groups. Examples of appropriate intervention models for use in hospitals and public health settings are provided. Finally, the importance of program evaluation and quality improvement is emphasized at the level of the individual patient, the medical care institution, and the community.

The current focus on health care reform in the United States makes it imperative that credentialed nutrition professionals be recognized as the "experts" in nutrition assessment and therapy by governmental and private health agencies, allied health professionals, and the public. This publication will provide both future and current nutrition practitioners with the additional knowledge and skills they need to serve as the qualified "experts" in our profession.

Jean H. Hankin, DrPH, RD
Nutrition Researcher
and
Professor of Public Health
Cancer Research Center of Hawaii
University of Hawaii
Honolulu, Hawaii

Preface

The primary goal of a nutrition service is to improve the nutritional status of a patient or client. A defined, systematic, and comprehensive approach is most effective to combat malnutrition. This approach, known as comprehensive nutrition assessment, includes six steps: identification, screening, planning, implementation, evaluation, and monitoring. Because the steps are interrelated, our book presents and addresses them collectively.

The purpose of this second edition is to assist health care team members in understanding the process of nutrition assessment. All chapters have been revised, updated, and expanded. New features include chapters on adult anthropometry, critical care, hunger and food insufficiency, case management, preventive pediatric ambulatory care in the United States, nutrition monitoring and evaluation, and quality improvement.

The text is divided into five parts. Part I provides a comprehensive view of historical perspectives and future expectations and needs. Basic principles and theory about nutrition assessment are presented, including how to profile a population and identify groups at nutritional risk. Part II provides updated information about assessment methodology: physical/clinical signs, anthropometry (pediatric and adult), interactions of drugs with foods and nutrients, dietary intake methods, and laboratory assessment of nutritional status. Part III addresses case management, documentation, and the planning and implementation of nutrition services in ambulatory, acute, critical, and geriatric care settings. Part IV emphasizes nutrition monitoring and evaluation, and the importance of productivity and cost-effectiveness in the provision of nutrition services. Part V offers case models for integrating the material in the book into daily practice. The appendices include pertinent resource materials relevant to the topics discussed in the text.

The 21 chapters are designed to stimulate students and practitioners to create their own systems of intervention by viewing the process as a whole. The contributors have surveyed the literature and shared their experiences, provided valuable insights into traditional methods, and suggested innovative techniques.

Our 18 years of experience with nutrition assessment began with workshops to improve the quantity and quality of assessment through grants from the Department of Health, Education and Welfare (now Department of Health and Human Services) and the Maternal and Child Health Program. Our efforts in subsequent workshops, classes, and publications have culminated in this revised and updated edition. Nutrition assessment is now an accepted concept by dietetic practitioners and other health care professionals. This revised book on nutrition assessment focuses on its use in the management and delivery of nutrition services and patient care. Thus we add another block to the foundation and expansion of nutrition assessment.

Margaret D. Simko
Catherine Cowell
Judith A. Gilbride

Acknowledgments

We want to recognize the colleagues and organizations who helped us establish the framework for the first edition of *Nutrition Assessment: A Comprehensive Guide for Planning Intervention*: the Bureau of Maternal and Child Health, Department of Health and Human Services, especially Ann Prendergast and Mary Egan; the staff of the former Bureau of Nutrition, New York City Department of Health; the Department of Home Economics and Nutrition at New York University; and our students and workshop participants, who helped us demonstrate the applications of comprehensive nutrition assessment. Without their efforts and support, this book would not have become a reality.

Our sincere thanks to those who have assisted with the preparation of this revised edition: the Department of Family Medicine, University of Medicine and Dentistry of New Jersey, Robert Wood Johnson Medical School, for support of this project, especially Jeanne Olsen and several office staff members who revised disks and developed graphics for some of the tables, figures, and exhibits; and the Maternal and Child Health Program at Columbia University, especially Zenobia Ferguson for preparing some of the complex exhibits. We also thank Teresita E. Carrillo, Ratna Kolhatkar, Liane Latkany, and the dietitians at Valley Hospital, Ridgewood, NJ, for providing excellent examples for the case models and making suggestions for the revision of the Profile. Most importantly, we recognize the efforts of all the contributors who have shared their expertise and enabled us to generate this second edition.

Part I

___

Overview of Nutrition Assessment

Chapter 1

The Process of Nutrition Assessment

Judith A. Gilbride, Margaret D. Simko, and Catherine Cowell

OVERVIEW

Nutrition assessment is a dynamic process, ever-changing and evolving. A step-by-step process should be used to assess the nutritional needs of a group and to plan a measurable nutrition intervention program appropriate for a specific health care setting. Dietitians and nutritionists should assume the primary responsibility for nutrition assessment in a variety of settings. As the initiators of assessment, they need to understand the strengths and limitations of various techniques and adapt the procedures to fit the situation. Protocols—based on observation and experience, and developed in concert with physicians, nurses, pharmacists, and other health care professionals—should be used in community, ambulatory, acute, long-term care, and managed care settings.

WHAT IS NUTRITION ASSESSMENT?

The concept of nutrition assessment is more than the evaluation of nutritional status. It is a comprehensive process of identifying individuals and population groups at nutritional risk and of planning, implementing, and evaluating a course of action.[1] For some investigators, *nutrition assessment* means simply the identification of current nutritional status and nutrient requirements.[2] Others interpret it as a systematic method of gathering data on individual patients, classifying the degree of malnutrition, and instituting appropriate treatment and intervention techniques.[3] The American Dietetic Association defined it as "a comprehensive approach, completed by a registered dietitian, to defining nutrition status that uses medical, nutrition, and medication histories; physical examination, anthropometric measurements, and laboratory data." For legislative purposes, the American Dietetic Association (ADA) has defined it as "the evaluation of nutrition needs of individuals based upon appropriate biochemical, anthropometric, physical, and dietary data to determine nutrient needs and recommend appropriate nutrition intake including enteral and parenteral nutrition."[5]

Health care practitioners who do nutrition assessments must first understand the steps involved in providing comprehensive care. This will lead to the correction or prevention of dietary and nutritional problems. The nutrition intervention then proceeds to the correction or prevention of the problem, to follow-up or referral, and finally, as necessary, to evaluation.

The level of implementation and care will depend on an institution's organizational structure, health care practitioners, and available resources. To optimize efforts to meet the needs of individuals and groups, institutional or agency personnel should find creative alternatives to achieve the goal of improving the nutritional status of the population served.

Health care practitioners must see their role as one that involves a commitment to provide comprehensive nutritional care that ensures continuity, quality, and cost-effectiveness. To achieve these goals, they must work closely as a team through a network of communications and collaborate from the first step of nutrition assessment to the point where the patient/client shows improvement and regains health.

DATA COLLECTION

Four types of data are pertinent in determining the nutritional status of a patient or client: dietary, biochemical, anthropometric, and physical. The dietary history provides subjective information from the patient about appetite, weight changes, activity levels, food habits, special diets, bowel functions, medications, food aversions, intolerances, allergies, and symptoms related to the digestion and assimilation of nutrients. This dietary information illuminates and expands documentation in the medical and nursing histories. The diet history reveals data about the energy and nutrient intake of the patient that can be compared to standards. These data often explain and concur with objective laboratory findings that reflect the biochemical levels of nutrients in urine, blood, and tissue stores. Anthropometric measurements—including those of height, weight, skinfold, and body circumference—provide a good index of body protein and calorie reserves. Weight fluctuations over time are often the first indicator of a change in nutritional status. Clinical indicators reveal physical signs present in the patient that serve to detect nutritional deficiencies and excesses. It is recommended that all four types of measurements be employed collectively to obtain the most complete and accurate picture of an individual's nutritional status.

The importance of nutrition assessment has been clearly identified, but various methods will continue to evolve. The parameters to detect and classify the severity of malnutrition should be practical, accurate, and relevant to the goals of therapy. The simplest and least expensive test may not always be warranted in a time when consumers of health care can demand specialized nutritional care or when patients are the ultimate decision makers in selecting their desirable or most appropriate care.

SETTINGS FOR NUTRITIONAL CARE

Dietitians and nutritionists practice in a variety of settings. Some are in education, research, and food service management; others provide direct patient care or participate in managed care in the community, in ambulatory settings, and in health care institutions, principally acute or long-term facilities.

The community nutritionist designs local and federal programs in preventive nutrition and provides surveillance for ongoing treatment and care for the public and target groups at nutritional risk. The community nutritionist plans, organizes, and coordinates nutrition support measures and evaluates the effectiveness of services. In selecting appropriate techniques for population surveys, factors to consider are cost, convenience, time, and invasiveness. Although it is important to use the most convenient method, it is also advisable to preserve accuracy and to correlate findings with clinical, anthropometric, dietary, biochemical, and ecological factors.

Ambulatory care is provided in a noninstitutionalized setting (outpatient clinic, private office, or managed care plan) that obviates hospitalization and provides routine maintenance and treatment of chronic conditions that do not require bed care. The dietitian or nutritionist is responsible for assessing the nutritional needs of the clients served and for organizing and conducting nutrition education programs for clients and staff. Dietetic practitioners in outpatient settings emphasize the preventive aspects of nutrition care and health promotion and disease prevention. In-depth counseling is given to individual clients, along with regularly scheduled nutrition classes. Common procedures for assessment include anthropometric measurements for serial readings, qualitative and quantitative dietary evaluations, observations of physical signs and symptoms, and, when necessary, biochemical tests.

Acute care professionals are identified under such familiar titles as staff dietitian, clinical dietitian, clinical nutrition specialist, and nutrition support dietitian, or by area of practice: renal dietitian, pediatric dietitian, oncology dietitian, and so forth. Whatever the title, the acute care professional is the member of the health care team who is responsible for the nutritional therapy of individuals needing immediate treatment or health maintenance on a short-term basis. The guidelines of the Joint Commission on Accreditation of Healthcare Organizations recommend the writing of routine policies for nutrition assessment procedures.[6] Primary or acute care requires nutrition services that ensure the interaction of the initiator of nutrition assessment techniques with the physician, nurse, pharmacist, and social worker, as well as with the most important member of the team, the patient/client. Nutrition support is provided by a formalized nutrition support service or an informal team of nutritional, nursing, and medical specialists. A wide variety of parameters is available in this setting, provided the costs and benefits can be justified for improving nutritional care. The current standard of care in accredited hospitals mandates the monitoring of the nutritional status of patients. If intensive therapy is indicated—for example, nutrition support of diabetes care—it should be provided under the guidance of a team trained in nutrition support or diabetes.

Long-term care is provided by chronic care hospitals, nursing facilities, and home care services, and by psychiatric, child care, domiciliary, and rehabilitative institutions. In these settings, a part-time or full-time dietitian with clinical and administrative experience is often responsible for the effective functioning of the dietary department—from nutritional care policies to food-purchasing procedures. Special problems exist for the elderly, since aging occurs at different rates in different individuals. In addition, the variance of nutritional indicators is greater among older adults than it is among younger adults. Monitoring weight loss and gain is very important, as are dietary analysis and changes in physical and functional status. There is a need to define "abnormality" in the aged for various parameters and to either concur on appropriate standards or create new ones. Biochemical tests are extremely variable, particularly for those patients on long-term drug therapy. In individual workups, anthropometric measurements may not be the most sensitive indicators to use.

A MODEL FOR PLANNING NUTRITION INTERVENTION PROGRAMS

Nutrition intervention in a health care setting should maximize the use of existing resources to provide nutrition support measures and program effectiveness. To make the process work, the following six goals must be met:

1. identifying those who need nutritional care
2. assessing the kinds of care that are needed
3. determining the available and accessible resources
4. developing strategies for extending the resources to provide the highest quality of nutritional care possible that will lead to the prevention or correction of the nutritional problems
5. evaluating progress and measuring the outcomes of the nutrition support and intervention
6. monitoring the process over time to ensure continuity of care and identifying any emerging needs of the group

Identifying who needs nutritional care is the first goal of a system for nutrition intervention. In assessing the nutritional needs of any population group—whether in a hospital, extended care facility, or community health care agency—it is essential to determine who most urgently needs nutrition services. Since it is generally not possible or necessary to provide the same level of nutritional care to everyone, the first question is, Which patients/clients are at greatest nutritional risk?

Figure 1–1 illustrates a model for nutrition intervention. The circle diagram includes the six steps of the system covering the input and process. Completion of these steps provides the output to meet the goals of the system.

Step 1: Identification

The first step is to establish the need for nutrition intervention and to determine the population that may be at greatest nutritional risk. To accomplish this step, consider the patients or clients to be served and identify:

- What nutrition problems exist in the selected population?
- Who constitutes the target group of people (most) frequently affected by these problems?
- What are the demographic characteristics?
- Where are the resources for providing nutritional care?
- How can the target group be "screened" to establish who needs nutrition intervention, to what extent, and to what level of intensity?

The Nutrition Profile, presented in Chapter 5, is a tool that can assist in finding out background information about the clients, the facility, and the community environment. Information organized in this manner is very useful, since program

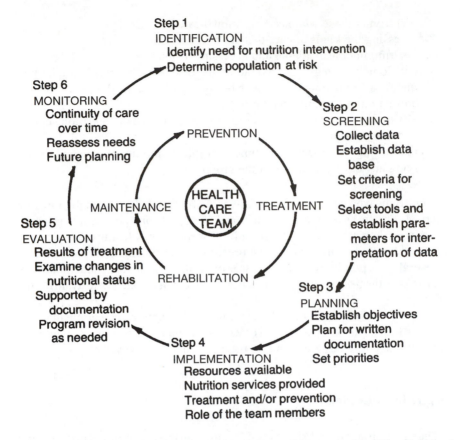

Figure 1–1 A Systems Model for Nutrition Intervention—The Process of Providing Nutritional Care. *Source:* Reprinted with permission from the Department of Home Economics and Nutrition, New York: New York University, © 1979.

planning is affected by the problems and the extent of resources that exist in the community and in its institutions or community agencies.

Step 2: Screening

In this step, the kinds of care needed are assessed. Baseline data are gathered to screen or "sort out" those population groups at greatest nutritional risk. The instrument to screen all patients entering a facility should be brief so that the information can be compiled in five to ten minutes. A broad-based tool of this type usually screens for basic information such as height, weight, weight change, serum albumin, total lymphocyte count, hemoglobin, and changes in appetite or food tolerance. Specialized patient populations require the accumulation of additional data or test results. In fact, some nutrition support units incorporate an initial screen and then a follow-up tool. Others use a computer for analyzing and comparing several parameters with standards or preset criteria. Some tools are designed so that the clients are able to provide the information themselves; in others, the answers are noted on the form by supportive health care personnel.

The screening tool should be developed or adapted specifically for each situation so that it is appropriate for the setting. A simple screening tool can be used to screen quickly those clients who need follow-up, nutrition therapy, nutrition education, or diet counseling. Criteria are established to evaluate the information obtained from the screening tool and to set priorities for the nutritional needs of patients or clients.

Laboratory data, diet histories, and clinical and biochemical information serve as means of assessing or measuring the nutritional status of the client. By comparing individual assessment data against preestablished parameters or standards, one can classify the client in terms of the level of nutritional risk. For example, if underweight children are identified as a population at risk, the heights and weights of those children can be compared to a standard height/weight chart or growth chart to screen out those with weights less than the norm or standard. See Chapter 7 for preestablished criteria that can determine who is at greatest risk by percentage weight loss (<15% of standard) or weight gain (>50% of standard) or <5th or >95th percentile on the growth charts.

Step 3: Planning

A realistic goal for the nutritional care of the group should be identified. Priorities should be set to meet the most urgent objectives. Selected resources can assist in program planning. For example, laboratory data will reflect the biochemical levels of nutrients in the blood, urine, and tissues. Often it is possible to use information that is already being collected by the facility, such as diet histories that provide information about individual eating habits, lifestyles, and nutritional problems. Clinical assessment reveals physical signs that can help detect nutritional deficiencies or excesses. Information such as height and weight data is most useful for routine application in a screening protocol. Forms and questionnaires and the Nutrition Profile in Chapter 5 are useful tools in planning nutrition services. Human resources, such as assistance from other health care personnel and support staff, can also be used. The incorporation of information already collected by someone else saves time and extends care.

The major objective of the plan is to improve the nutritional status of the target or at-risk group, as well as to improve or maintain the nutritional status of the entire population. The plan should consider the levels of care needed and the most effective way to provide the care. Specific objectives should be set within a time frame, since all objectives may not be immediately attainable. It is recommended that the plan or protocol be written and stored in a central place for the health care team to review and revise.

Step 4: Implementation

Implementation means carrying out the plan, using available resources, facilities, and staff. It involves the development of strategies for maximizing resources to provide the highest-quality nutritional care that will lead to the prevention or correction of nutritional problems.

Management techniques should be designed to ensure that the plans will be carried out with the greatest efficiency. In the situation of underweight children cited in Step 2, a system of serial assessment of heights and weights of the population could be established. Intervention could be implemented by designated team members who would routinely review the data and compare them with a standard. The system could be extended further by initiating "routine" care for those who place above the standard and of specific care for those at risk who fall below the standard.

Step 5: Evaluation

Ongoing evaluation is needed to measure the progress and success of the program or to reveal areas for improvement. Using the database established during the screening process, data are gathered at sequential times and compared with the baseline data to determine if the health status of the population has changed. In our example of underweight children, those at risk who received nutrition intervention should show improvement in weight status as a result. If no improvements are found, the reasons for failure should be sought, and the program should be reexamined to ascertain if changes are warranted.

Step 6: Monitoring

To monitor is to check the system over a period of time to ensure continuation of quality care and to identify new nutritional needs, if any, of the population. Even when all goals of the system have been met, it is essential to continue to monitor changes that occur in the nutritional and/or health status of the group.

The model suggested in Figure 1–1 as a systems approach to planning nutrition intervention programs is designed in a circle to illustrate that the process of providing nutrition care is ongoing and that the system is repeated as new needs emerge. Although the overall goal of the system is to assess nutritional needs, provide intervention, and improve the nutritional status of a group, important aspects of the system are that the nutrition care is measurable and that program effectiveness can be readily determined.

REFERENCES

1. Simko MD, Cowell C, Gilbride JA. *Assessing the Nutritional Needs of Groups: A Handbook for the Health Care Team.* New York, NY: New York University, New York University Department of Home Economics and Nutrition; 1980:3–8. Support for this work was provided by HSA-79-118(p), BCHS/HSA, HSA, Rockville, Md.

2. Mason M, Wenberg G, Welsch PK. *The Dynamics of Clinical Dietetics.* 2nd ed. New York, NY: John Wiley & Sons; 1982:10–11.

3. Blackburn GL, Bistrian BR, Maini BS, Schlamm BA, Smith MF. Nutritional and metabolic assessment of the hospitalized patient. *J Paren Enter Nutr.* 1977;1:11.

4. American Dietetic Association. ADA's definition for nutrition screening and nutrition assessment. *JA Diet Assoc.* 1994;94:__.

5. American Dietetic Association. *Economic Benefits of Nutrition Services.* Unpublished paper, Health Care Reform Legislative Platform, March 18, 1993:7.

6. *Accreditation Manual for Hospitals.* Chicago, Ill: Joint Commission on Accreditation of Healthcare Organizations; 1993.

Chapter 2

Nutrition Assessment in the 21st Century

Catherine Cowell, Judith A. Gilbride, and Margaret D. Simko

OVERVIEW

Nutrition assessment is the first step in developing nutrition goals for a population, a community such as a state, region, county, or city, or an individual. Newer scientific knowledge about the relationship of diet to the incidence of chronic disease has helped to create a more health-conscious society. There is greater awareness by Americans of the responsibility that they have for their health. Communities across the country are facing the social and health issues of a growing population of vulnerable individuals and families. During a period of rising unemployment and a general downturn in the economy, we have seen growing numbers of the homeless, the hungry, those infected with the human immunodeficiency virus (HIV) and AIDS, those with drug-resistant tuberculosis, and those with elevated levels of lead. These issues are so critical that they require communities to assess the magnitude of the problem and identify those who are at risk. All of these health issues are heightened by the number of infants who are born of substance-abusing women, some of whom enter school with developmental and behavioral lags. To address these problems, several health and medical reform plans and strategies have been developed to meet societal needs for vulnerable groups.

THE CHANGING ENVIRONMENT

Emerging nutrition problems were the catalysts for identifying indi-viduals and groups at high risk for malnutrition. Advocates, including social scientists,

13

dietitians and nutritionists, health providers, and others, were among the first to be concerned about the poor, especially mothers, infants, children, and the elderly, because they are among the most vulnerable. Poor individuals and families most likely are unable to purchase adequate amounts of nourishing food, pay for decent housing and basic utilities, and be covered by health insurance.

Repeatedly the problem of hunger generates a groundswell of surveys that is accompanied by renewed interest in community and individual assessments. An example was the "war on hunger," a national effort in the 1960s that generated a renewed focus on hunger among individuals and the communities where they lived.[1] At the same time, Jelliffe[2] was identifying four forms of malnutrition as

- undernutrition, caused by a chronic lack of sufficient food
- overnutrition, caused by an excess of food over time
- specific deficiency states caused by a lack of individual nutrients
- diets with nutrient imbalance

These are the basic forms of malnutrition that are recognized today at a time of high technology in medicine and pharmacy. Initial screening of the poor provides data that give early indications of probable risk of malnutrition. This information can be used as baseline data for monitoring purposes, and can identify those needing further evaluation and follow-up.

As the relationship between nutrition and health status was emphasized, newer techniques of nutrition assessment, an increase in the number of surveys and studies, and monitoring activities emerged. Growing interest in evaluating the impact of nutrition programs created a climate to target intervention strategies used to meet the needs of patients. Children in a well baby clinic, patients in a hospital, clients/residents in a nursing home, and mothers (prenatal and postpartum), infants, or young children in a WIC (Supplemental Food Program for Women, Infants and Children) clinic—are all part of an expanding network of nutrition assessment, monitoring, and follow-up.

ROLE OF DISCIPLINES AND SPECIALISTS

Disciplines, other than nutrition/dietary and medicine, have been engaged in expanding the knowledge base of the relationship between nutrition and health. Epidemiology, anthropology (medical and physical), social and behavioral sciences, economics, and agriculture were among those disciplines that took interest in assessment and began to explore a range of topics. Topics covered such varied areas as risk factors associated with chronic diseases, health and nutrition beliefs, knowledge and practices, body composition, growth and development, and nutrition and learning.

Within the medical and dietary professions, hospital clinicians and others began to take a lead alongside the dietary staff in developing nutrition support teams to prevent malnutrition in the hospital setting.[3] These activities were occurring at a time when new specialized areas surfaced. Specialists in cardiovascular diseases, renal disease, sports medicine, children with special needs, behavior modification, weight control, women's health, and aerospace medicine have been making inroads in nutrition assessment.

DEVELOPMENT OF PUBLIC POLICY

While newer disciplines and specialists emerged, health policies and programs were implemented that formed the framework in this changing environment. The Early and Periodic Screening, Diagnosis and Treatment Program, known as EPSDT, a Medicaid-sponsored program of reimbursement for nutrition screening, assessment, and counseling of low-income children up to age 21 years, was introduced.[4] Nutrition assessment of preschool age children is one part of the Head Start Performance Standards.[5] Height, weight, and hemoglobin/hematocrit are the measurements obtained for each child enrolled, whether in a half- or full-day program. The Standards provide guidance for specific diagnoses and follow-up. The Child Health Record, another example of a tool used in Head Start programs, is designed to obtain general health information, family health history, physical examination/screening/assessment, immunization history, dental health, nutrition, serial growth indicators, and psychological and social development.[6] The topics of food, eating, growth, and development are woven throughout this questionnaire, which is comprehensive and provides significant data about a vulnerable group of low-income children.

The U.S. Department of Agriculture established two federal programs to address hunger and malnutrition—Food Stamps and WIC.[7] Both assessment of the community and assessment of the individual are components of the WIC program. The eligibility criteria (income and nutritional risk), the number of women, infants, and children up to age five eligible for WIC and the actual number enrolled are three indicators of the magnitude of the problem in a community. Each state agency responsible for WIC has a defined set of nutrition and health screening standards consisting of dietary risk, anthropometric, and laboratory values.

The importance of contemporary activities of nutrition assessment of communities and population groups is better appreciated through knowledge of the past. Numerous researchers, scientists, and practitioners were pioneers in exploring, developing, and testing the process of assessing individuals and populations to allow for making realistic decisions, including those of public policy. By persevering and using a range of tools from history taking—medical, social, and dietary—to data collection and analyses, health providers are able to address local community nutrition needs, especially the needs of those at risk of malnutrition.

HISTORICAL MILESTONES OF NUTRITION ASSESSMENT

In 1932 in Berlin the first conference was held to discuss the physical, clinical, and physiological aspects of nutrition assessment. This conference, sponsored by the Health Organization of the League of Nations, promoted the publication of a monograph detailing procedures for conducting nutrition surveys.[8] This monograph, published by the Technical Commission of Nutrition of the Health Organization, was the first organized attempt to develop dietary standards. At the same time, Bigwood's *Guiding Principles for Studies on the Nutrition of Populations* appeared.[9] This work has become a classic reference for detailing the procedures for conducting nutrition surveys. Although these initial methods have been revised and expanded, the basic approach and philosophy have remained the same for over 60 years.

In the late 1940s, the Food and Agriculture Organization (FAO) and the World Health Organization (WHO) were established under the aegis of the United Nations, and a Joint Expert Committee on Nutrition was formed with representatives from both organizations. These representatives met for the first time in 1949 and, after compiling information on nutritional status and dietary patterns of particular populations and on food supplies and economics, recommended the establishment of nutrition policies for each nation. The Joint Committee of WHO published another report in 1951 that highlighted anthropometric, clinical, and dietary data but did not make recommendations or standards. The committee has since published a succession of reports that recommend and encourage work on assessment, nutritional status, requirements of nutrients, protein-energy malnutrition, nutritional anemia, food technology, and toxicology.[10]

The International Committee on Nutrition for National Defense (ICNND), with representatives from nine departments of the U.S. government, was organized with the major objectives of providing technical assistance to developing countries in assessing the nutritional status of their populations, defining problems of malnutrition, and establishing plans for action and for extending the use of local resources. One of the founders of ICNND and its first executive director was Harold R. Sandstead.

The ICNND produced a *Manual for Nutrition Surveys* based on the studies done with military personnel in the Near and Far East. A second edition of the manual,[11,12] published in 1963, was expanded to emphasize uniformity in methods, techniques, procedures, and guidelines; identification of team member responsibilities; interpretative guidelines for dietary, biochemical, and clinical data; and training procedures for personnel.

The WHO Report of the Expert Committee on Medical Assessment of Nutritional Status has recommended a standardization of methods to conduct nutrition surveys and report results.[10]

In 1966, Derrick B. Jelliffe completed a noteworthy publication entitled *The Assessment of the Nutritional Status of the Community.*[2] This work, prepared with the advice from 25 specialists in various countries, became the foundation for subsequent publications on assessment of population groups in developed countries. Jelliffe stressed the value of prevalence and incidence surveys and the practical use of direct and indirect methods for identifying malnutrition. The major emphasis was given to the nutritional problems of "vulnerable" groups in developing areas of the world. In a second publication, Jelliffe focused on simple, affordable methodologies for assessing the health and nutritional status, and the ecological factors—economic, cultural, physiological—of vulnerable groups.[13] This book is an important publication for professional health and nutrition providers, especially for those training students interested in both domestic and international community health programs.

A newer and more detailed source of information about anthropometric, laboratory, and dietary assessment indicators is the work reported by George Christakis.[14] This publication is another notable one that describes a number of assessment methods and tools depending on the level of resources available at the community level (Table 2–1).

GROWING NATIONAL INTEREST

The recognition that malnutrition is a health problem in the United States has been relatively recent. Before the 1960s, little attention was paid to the nutritional health in this country, and malnutrition went undetected. The 1972 Ten State Nutrition Survey and the National Health and Nutrition Examination Survey (NHANES–Phase I), conducted by the National Center for Health Statistics, revealed vulnerable groups and individuals in different areas of the country, with evidence of clinical and subclinical malnutrition.[15] Population

Table 2–1 Selected Milestones of Nutrition Assessment for Populations

1930–1959	1960–1970	1970s	1980s	1990–2000
	1968–1970 Ten State Nutrition Survey & Preschool Nutrition Survey		1989 *Diet and Health National Research Council*	
1950s Joint Commission of FAO & WHO report				
1950s International Committee on Nutrition for National Defense (ICNND) organized	1969 White House Conference on Food, Nutrition, & Health		1988 Surgeon General's Report on *Nutrition and Health*	Surgeon General's Report— *Healthy People 2000*
	1966 Derrick B. Jelliffe's publication	1976–1980 Phase II— National Health & Nutrition Examination Survey (NHANES–II)	1988–1994 Phase III initiated → National Health & Nutrition Examination Survey (NHANES III)	1990s DHHS/USDA Publication— *Nutrition & Your Health*
1940s FAO & WHO Joint Expert Committee on Nutrition founded	WHO Report of Recommended Standards for Nutrition Surveys			
		1971–1974 Phase I— National Health & Nutrition Examination Survey (NHANES–I)	1988 *The Future of Public Health* National Research Council—Institute of Medicine	National Nutrition Monitoring & Related Research Program (NNMRRP)
1932 Berlin Conference & Bigwood's *Guiding Principles*		1973 George Christakis' publication	1982–1984 Hispanic Health & Nutrition Examination Survey (HHANES)	1990 *Nutrition During Pregnancy Nutrition During Lactation* National Research Council—Institute of Medicine
			1980 Surgeon General's Report— *Promoting Health/Preventing Disease*	
			1980 DHHS/USDA publication— *Nutrition & Your Health*	

groups that were deprived socially, economically, educationally, or medically were found to be at nutritional risk. Undernutrition was associated with growth cessation and developmental handicaps, poor outcomes of pregnancy, susceptibility to infectious diseases, delayed recovery from illness, and shortened life expectancy.

The Ten State Nutrition Survey of 1968–1970 examined the prevalence of malnutrition and other hunger-related problems among low-socioeconomic-level populations in Texas, Florida, and New York.[16] The first phase of NHANES followed in 1971–1974. This was the first attempt to assess persons at all socioeconomic levels. The survey determined nutritional status on a representative sample of the U.S. population. Using a sample of 30,000 persons aged 1 to 74, NHANES–I data included biochemical analyses of urine and blood, physical and dental examinations, dietary interviews, and body measurements (1971–1974).[17] The second phase of NHANES, 1976–1980, was followed by the Hispanic Health and Nutrition Examination Survey (HHANES), 1982–1984.[18]

These surveys have developed a foundation for applied domestic programs. Response to NHANES–I enhanced methods for monitoring and surveillance in the U.S. population. Monitoring, as set up as a mandate from Congress in 1977, established a system to evaluate and reevaluate the nutritional status of Americans in order to measure the effectiveness of programs. Federal, state, and local agencies carried out a surveillance system that was comprehensive in the areas of diet and nutrition assessment for the evaluation of large populations to identify potential problems and at-risk groups.

The 1969 White House Conference on Food, Nutrition, and Health further stimulated interest in nutrition.[18] Consumers, practitioners, and researchers viewed a range of nutrition-related topics that included methods for identifying nutritionally vulnerable groups, the nation's food supply, food assistance policies and programs, and nutrition education and training. The nutritional status of Americans at that time was the basis for formulating corrective programs for those who were malnourished or at nutritional risk.

Since that conference, there has been expansion of some nutrition programs, greater efforts in surveillance and monitoring, and evidence of action directed at reducing malnutrition (Table 2–1). There has also been considerable renewed interest in methods of nutrition intervention and preventive health care. Medical, health, and dietary elements have increased efforts to evaluate critically the benefits of nutrition in the setting of corrective therapy and the teaching of preventive measures. One outcome of this attention is that nutrition assessment has emerged as one of several strategies for combating nutritional abnormalities and misinformation. The concept of nutrition assessment has expanded from its original meaning of simply identifying those needing nutritional help. Currently, nutrition assessment encompasses some of the well-known multiple factors that affect nutritional status and eventually the quality of life. Nutrition assessment efforts are crucial during a period of changing lifestyles in our society. If nutrition assessment is one of the keys in achieving a better quality of life, it must become a priority effort, supported by knowledgeable professionals who are committed to providing quality care.

By 1980 the role of diet in disease prevention continued to gain national support. First was the release of the Department of Health and Human Services' publication *Promoting Health/Preventing Disease: Objectives for the Nation.*[19] Of the 300 objectives, 17 related to nutrition in the three broadly grouped areas of prevention services, health protection, and health promotion. Each of the nutrition objectives is quantifiable, allowing interim comparisons and evaluation in the year 2000, the target date proposed in the report.

To further support this national effort was the release, in 1980, of the first edition of *Nutrition and Your Health: Dietary Guidelines for Americans.*[20] This publication was the result of a joint effort between the U.S. Department of Agriculture and the U.S. Department of Health and Human Services. A revised edition of these guidelines was published in 1985 and was used for implementing national nutrition education activities.

YEAR 2000 AND BEYOND

Healthy People 2000 objectives in the Surgeon General's National Health Promotion and Disease Prevention publication set the stage for establishing a national strategy to improve the health status of the population and improve the potential for a better quality of life.[21] This Surgeon General's report emphasized behavioral and environmental changes needed to reduce the risks of diseases that are the leading causes of disabilities and death, such as cancer, coronary heart disease, stroke, and diabetes. Nutrition and diet were among the priorities addressed on this national health agenda.

For example, one of the risk reduction objectives is to "increase to at least 50 percent the proportion of overweight people aged 12 and older who have adopted sound dietary practices combined with regular physical activity to attain an appropriate body weight." This objective, which appears in both the chapter on nutrition and the chapter on physical fitness, reinforces the potential health benefits of weight loss in overweight persons. Using baseline data reported from the National Health Interview Survey, the goal promotes weight loss with diets lower in fat and higher in dietary fiber (vegetables, fruits, and grains) concurrently with increased physical activity.

Clearly this objective points to the need for comprehensive nutrition assessment that integrates anthropometric, biochemical, dietary, and physical data on a client/patient. Even before there is a problem of overweight, prevention can be addressed early on in life through encounters of the child and parent at child health clinics or programs with a health component like day care/Head Start and schools. Once there is the problem of overweight, anthropometric measurements such as height, weight, skinfold, and body circumference data provide an index of body proteins and calorie reserves. A reliable diet history indicates important data about food habits, including cultural foods, food likes, dislikes and intolerances, appetite, supplements and medications, special diets, weight loss/gain, bowel functions, and physical activity. These data are valuable in planning with the client/patient meals and snacks that are lower in fat, especially saturated fat, and higher in dietary fiber. Intervention of increased activity can also be addressed as a part of the dietary counseling or by a specialist in sports medicine or physical fitness. Through a physical examination and laboratory analyses of specimens of blood, urine, and tissue, data are provided about nutrient excesses and biochemical levels of nutrients. A critical review of all four types of nutrition assessment data simultaneously provides a comprehensive picture of the nutritional status of the client/patient before intervening with a weight control and physical fitness program. There should be periodic and continuous monitoring of the client/patient if the goals of weight loss (based on the principles of a sensible and nourishing diet) and physical fitness are to be achieved.

It was the defining of nutritional status by the Joint Nutrition Monitoring Evaluation Committee that reinforced the process of nutrition assessment as comprehensive and as an integral part of health care and health delivery systems.[22] Their definition states that "the nutritional status of an individual is the condition of his or her health as influenced by the intake and utilization of nutrients. Because nutritional status cannot be measured directly by any single test, assessment is dependent on the collective interpretation of relevant dietary and health data."[22(p35)] It is apparent that no one measurement or value from such tools as anthropometric, laboratory, clinical, or dietary assessment can be used alone to identify a nutrition-related health problem. Effectively using a combination of tools, along with emerging concepts of risk factors and the assessment of physical and mental health functioning, providers of care can achieve the highest level of nutrition assessment.

In the future a major thrust will be putting *Healthy People 2000* into practice across the country. It is critical that there be national policy and continuing support to improve the health of all children and adults. Paramount is the integration of nutrition assessment from the federal, state, and local government levels along with public and private agencies and organizations. Nutrition assessment efforts will increasingly meet these new challenges:

- the range of nutrition problems presented by the increase in the number of medically, socially, and emotionally at-risk subpopulation groups
- reform of the health care system, such as managed care or managed competition, which assures quality health and nutrition services that are available, affordable, and accessible

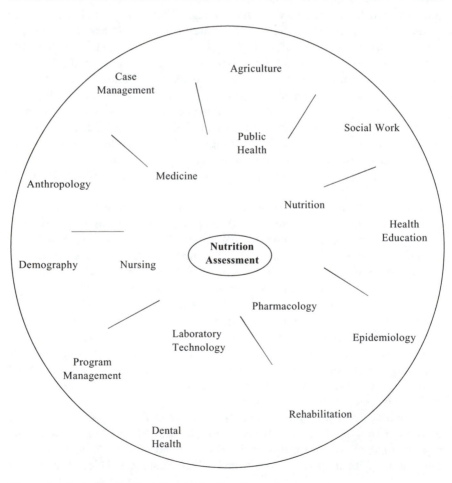

Figure 2–1 Expansion of Disciplines in Nutrition Assessment

- positioning and promoting preventive health services in the public health arena, which incorporates nutrition assessment and policy development, and assures quality care

To meet these challenges, uniquely trained and qualified nutrition/dietary personnel are needed to provide dynamic leadership and serve as professional role models for those in training programs. These leaders need to perform nutrition assessment in a variety of health care settings that utilize newer interdisciplinary and transdisciplinary teams, and the latest technology, methods, and equipment. There is an expanding interdisciplinary team of representatives from surgery, medicine, pharmacy, therapists, and others (see Figure 2–1). It is incumbent that nutrition assessment team members fully understand the role of each member and are committed to providing the highest quality of care. In a changing environment, those who are training nutrition providers must recognize the complexity of assessment and provide the skills that will allow them to function at all levels of work, from entry level to administration, management, and research. A recent report prepared by a consortium of concerned organizations of dietitians and nutritionists documented that nutrition programs and services are the cornerstone of cost-effective prevention to health care.[23]

The discipline of nutrition continues to evolve over the years as research has expanded our knowledge base, and the same is true of the process of nutrition assessment. Reexamination of what is known and exploration of the unknown will affect the practical application of nutrition assessment. Those specializing in providing nutritional care must adapt the principles of nutrition assessment to meet the needs of individuals and families in an ever-changing environment. Our prediction is that the next century will be more challenging for nutrition assessment than this one.

REFERENCES

1. Caliendo MA. *Nutrition and the Food Crisis.* New York, NY: Macmillan Publishing Co; 1979:53.

2. Jelliffe DB. *The Assessment of the Nutritional Status of the Community.* Geneva, Switzerland: World Health Organization; 1966.

3. Blackburn GL, et al. Nutritional and metabolic assessment of the hospitalized patient. *J Paren Enter Nutr.* 1977;1:11.

4. American Academy of Pediatrics Committee on Child Health Financing. Medicaid's EPSDT Program: a pediatrician's handbook for action. Elk Grove Village, Ill: *American Academy of Pediatrics.* 1987;1:4–6.

5. *Head Start Program Performance Standards.* Rockville, Md: Administration for Children and Families, Head Start Bureau; 1984:39–52. U.S. Department of Health and Human Services publication 45-CFR 1304.

6. *Child Health Record.* Washington, DC: US Government Printing Office 425, 81 (1986): 150–679.

7. Kaufman M. *Nutrition in Public Health.* Gaithersburg, Md: Aspen Publishers, Inc; 1990: 110–111.

8. Owen AY, Frankle RT. *Nutrition in the Community.* 2nd ed. St. Louis, Mo: CV Mosby Co.; 1986:392.

9. Bigwood EJ. *Guiding Principles for Studies on the Nutrition of Populations.* Geneva, Switzerland: League of Nations Health Organizations; 1979.

10. FAO/WHO Joint Expert Committee on Nutrition. *Food and Nutrition Strategies in National Development.* Rome, Italy: Food and Nutrition Organization of the United Nations; 1976.

11. Interdepartmental Committee on Nutrition for National Defense. *Manual for Nutrition Surveys.* Washington, DC: US Government Printing Office; 1957.

12. Interdepartmental Committee on Nutrition for National Defense. *Manual for Nutrition Surveys.* 2nd ed. Washington, DC: US Government Printing Office; 1963.

13. Jelliffe DB, Jelliffe EFP. *Community Nutritional Assessment.* New York, NY: Oxford University Press; 1990.

14. Christakis G, ed. *Nutrition Assessment in Health Programs.* Washington, DC: American Public Health Association; 1973.

15. *Plan and Operation of the Health and Nutrition Examination Survey.* Rockville, Md: National Center for Health Statistics; 1975.

16. US Dept of Health, Education, and Welfare. *Ten-State Nutrition Survey in the United States 1968–1970.* Atlanta, Ga: Centers for Disease Control; 1972.

17. Lowenstein FW. Preliminary clinical and anthropometric findings from the first Health and Nutrition Examination Survey. *Am J Clin Nutr.* 1976;29:918.

18. Shils ME, et al. *Modern Nutrition in Health and Disease.* Philadelphia, Pa: Lea & Febiger, 1994;2:1634.

19. *Promoting Health, Preventing Disease: Objectives for the Nation.* Washington, DC: US Dept of Health and Human Services; 1980.

20. *Nutrition and Your Health: Dietary Guidelines for Americans.* Washington, DC: US Government Printing Office; 1980, 1985, and 1990.

21. *Healthy People 2000: National Health Promotion and Disease Prevention Objectives.* Washington, DC: US Dept of Health and Human Services, Public Health Service; 1990.

22. *Nutrition Monitoring in the United States.* Washington, DC: US Government Printing Office; 1989:35.

23. *Economic Benefits of Nutrition Services: Health Care Reform Legislative Platform of the American Dietetic Association, Associated Faculties of Graduate Programs in Public Health, Associated State and Territorial Public Health Directors, and the Society for Nutrition Education.* March 18, 1993.

Chapter 3

Malnutrition in the Hospital

Judith A. Gilbride and Joan Castro

OVERVIEW

For two decades accurate assessment of nutritional status in hospitals has intrigued clinicians. Malnutrition was first reported among medical and surgical patients in the 1970s. Failure to recognize and treat malnutrition still seems to be a problem, although less so. The art of assessing is an appraisal of subjective and objective information to allow decisions to be made. Data are derived from dietary, medical, and social histories and range from an initial screen to a complex set of actions involving several nutritional/metabolic variables. Distinctions are made between starvation and malnutrition in stressed patients, but controversy exists on the most effective approach of diagnosing, evaluating, and monitoring the nutritional status of patients. High-risk patients who are not identified as malnourished and treated early have longer hospital stays, slower recovery from infections and complications, increased rates of morbidity and mortality, and higher cost associated with medical intervention and rehabilitation.

RECOGNIZING THE IMPORTANCE OF NUTRITION STATUS ASSESSMENT

Interest in nutrition assessment in the clinical setting was first sparked by Sandstead in 1967.[1] Sandstead advised family physicians, internists, and pediatricians to treat the whole patient. Attention to food intake and nutritional status was recommended as an important component of the routine physical examination. In 1974, Butterworth hinted that doctors, nurses, and dietitians were disregarding the presence of malnutrition symptoms in hospitalized patients.[2] He asserted that malnutrition affected hospitalization by causing longer stays, higher costs, and increased mortality rates. This brought to light the important role of the medical team in identifying, treating, and preventing malnutrition. A Boston survey of hospital charts found inadequate assessment of nutritional status and little of the necessary documentation to make a diagnosis.[3]

The rate of malnutrition in hospitals has been reported at 30 to 50 percent in medical and surgical patients and 30 to 60 percent in nursing home patients. However, detecting malnutrition differs from institution to institution. A single parameter with a specific cutoff has not been found to be a reliable indicator of nutritional status. A combination of clinical judgments and objective measurements is more valid and reproducible in documenting malnourished patients. Early recognition and treatment has been shown to decrease morbidity and mortality, reduce lengths of stay, and lower costs of aggressive medical care and nutrition intervention incurred by malnourished patients.

A reevaluation and comparison of malnutrition rates in general medical patients were conducted in 1976 and 1988[4] to determine changes in malnutrition prevalence. An aggregate score, called likelihood of malnutrition (LOM), was used with a chart review of the following parameters: plasma folate, plasma ascorbate, triceps skinfold, arm muscle circumference, total lymphocyte count, serum albumin, and hematocrit. High LOM scores predicted longer lengths of stay and showed a trend to increased mortality. The length of stay was about the same in 1988 as in 1976, 30 and 31 days respectively. Length of stay, however, paired from admission to follow-up, indicated an improvement in 1988 compared to 1976, suggesting that the identification of malnutrition has improved by 16 percent since 1976.[4] Vigilance is essential in detecting malnutrition by dietitians and other health professionals. Other researchers continue to document high incidence of malnutrition in health care institutions (see Table 3–1).

The dental profession also plays a role in recognizing signs of malnourishment. The oral cavity is an area that can provide early signs of malnutrition. Dentists incorporate assessment techniques in their routine checkups, and some have designed elaborate screening models.[11]

WHAT IS MALNUTRITION?

Several approaches have been used to define malnutrition, beginning with Jelliffe's categories of undernutrition, overnutrition, deficiency states, and nutrient imbalance.[12] These classifications still serve as a broad framework for interpreting alterations in dietary intake. Advances in medicine and the under-

Table 3–1 Summary of Selected Malnutrition Surveys in Health Care Institutions

Researchers/Year	Population	Parameters	Results
Mowe et al, 1994[5]	311 elderly subjects admitted to a hospital medical service	albumin, BMI, TSF, AMC, dietary intake	52.9% males, 60.6% females with under-nutrition present on admission; 65% males, 69% females with insufficient intake prior to admission
Abbasi and Rudman, 1993[6]	2,811 skilled VA nursing home residents	albumin, weight	11.8% were underweight, 27.5% were hypoalbuminemic
Coates et al, 1993[4]	228 medical patients admitted to an acute care facility	albumin, TLC, HCT/Hgb, weight/height, TSF, folate, ascorbate = likelihood of malnutrition score (LOM)	38% had a high LOM score that predicted longer lengths of stay and increased mortality; 46% had high LOM at the 2-week follow-up
Mowe and Bohmer, 1991[7]	121 elderly patients admitted to an acute care facility	albumin, weight, TSF, AMC, MAC	54.5% were undernourished
Thomas et al, 1991[8]	61 patients admitted to a nursing/home rehabilitation facility	albumin, weight, BMI, TSF, MAMC, Hgb, TLC, Index score of ≥4 defined malnutrition	54% of new admittants were malnourished, 37% remained malnourished after 2 months
Pinchofsky and Kaminski, 1987[9]	227 nursing home residents from two facilities	albumin, weight, TSF, MAMC, AMC, prealbumin, retinol binding protein, TLC, HCT/Hgb, DHS	52% incidence of PCM, 24% adult kwashiorkor-like, 19% kwashiorkor-marasmus mix, 9% marasmus
Chen et al, 1985[10]	373 hospitalized medical and surgical patients	albumin, weight/height, weight loss, AMC, TSF, CHI, TLC, Hgb	30–57% were malnourished

Note: BMI = body mass index, TSF = triceps skinfold, AMC = arm muscle circumference, VA = Veterans Administration, HCT = hematocrit, Hgb = hemoglobin, DHS = delayed hypersensitivity skin testing, TLC = total lymphocyte count, CHI = creatinine height index.

standing of disease-related malnutrition as well as malnutrition resulting from chronic failure to ingest an adequate diet have encouraged classifications of less-than-ideal nutrition states. Shils outlined the etiologies of disease-related malnutrition as follows[13]:

- conditions causing malabsorption
- anorexia caused by systemic disease
- hypermetabolism
- metabolic dysfunction
- iatrogenic or treatment-induced causes

The effects of these conditions in the clinical environment are manifested as weight loss, delayed wound healing, electrolyte and fluid imbalance, depressed cellular immunity, and, in acute states, progressive weakness, skin breakdown, and endocrine abnormalities.

In hospitals today, causes of malnutrition are often referred to as primary and secondary. *Primary malnutrition* refers to inadequacies and imbalances in the diet, with respect to either the quality or the quantity of food consumed. This condition could result from any of the following factors: poor access to food as a result of poverty, environmental factors that affect food availability, ignorance of how to budget funds or select a balanced diet, or self-induced starvation for appearance. *Secondary malnutrition* refers to the increased risk of malnutrition due to a disease or disability that alters nutrient requirements, utilization, or excretion. Common conditions that cause secondary malnutrition are chronic diseases such as cardiovascular or renal impairment, neoplastic disorders, congenital disease, infectious disease, physical impairment, dental problems, and addiction to alcohol or drugs.

Failure in nutritional health can be categorized further by inadequate intake, inadequate absorption, defective utilization, increased losses or excretion, increased requirements, and metabolic alterations.[14] Exhibit 3–1 summarizes these conditions.

PROTEIN CALORIE MALNUTRITION

Severe and distinct forms of protein calorie malnutrition (PCM) are known as marasmus, kwashiorkor, and marasmus-kwashiorkor mix. These conditions can be identified according to dietary, anthropometric, clinical, and biochemical signs.

Marasmus, caused by a chronic protein and energy deficit, is characterized by a metabolic adaptive decrease in energy expenditure. Manifestations include

- cachectic nonedematous appearance with depressed anthropometric measurements such as loss of skeletal muscle, decreased adiposity, growth retardation (weight and height for age less than 60 percent of standard)

Exhibit 3–1 Conditions That Affect Nutritional Status

Inadequate Intake

- inadequate energy and protein intake
- anorexia or systemic disease
- inability to feed self
- food allergies
- iatrogenic

Inadequate Absorption

- chronic gastrointestinal disorders (celiac, Crohn's)
- side effects of drug therapy
- regional enteritis
- gastrointestinal pathology (parasites, malignancy)
- surgical removal of bowel

Defective Utilization

- metabolic dysfunction (organ failure)
- inborn errors of metabolism
- electrolyte imbalances
- drug/nutrient interactions

Increased Excretion

- vomiting
- diarrhea
- draining of fistulas/abscesses, or GI fluids
- dialysis, blood loss

Increased Requirements

- fever/infections
- trauma/sepsis/stress/burns
- pregnancy, growth
- hyperthyroidism
- malignancy
- surgery

Metabolic Alterations

- ebb-flow phase
- cytokine production
- increased hormonal and biochemical systems
- altered nutrient utilization (futile cycles)

- physically, an emaciated appearance with sparse, thin, dry, and dull hair; depressed heart rate, blood pressure, and body temperature; and a decrease in activity
- endocrine changes such as elevated levels of epinephrine, corticosteroid, and cortisol, and reduced levels of insulin and thyroid hormone; serum protein levels are preserved in the early stages due to marked recycling of amino acids and a decrease in urea synthesis, but when starvation is prolonged they will become marginal or slightly depressed, and the viscera are usually small[15,16]

Kwashiorkor, caused by an acute protein deficiency, is characterized by pitting, painless edema that extends into the extremities. This disorder is often referred to as hypoalbuminemic malnutrition and is diagnosed by a serum albumin level of less than 3.0 g/dl. Manifestations include

- less dramatic wasting of skeletal muscle mass and weight status than in patients with marasmus
- physically, notable skin lesions and epidermal peeling, easily pluckable discolored hair, distended abdomen, enlarged fatty liver, and cold extremities, with decreased cardiac output and tachycardia
- endocrine changes such as an increase in renin-aldosterone and growth hormone, a decrease in somatomedin and insulin levels, severely depressed serum protein levels, leading to an edematous appearance and an altered electrolyte state, impaired protein absorption and metabolism, and reduced peristalsis[15,16]

Marasmus-Kwashiorkor Mix is defined as an advanced protein and energy deficit superimposed by increased protein requirements or losses.[14,16] This leads to a rapid depression in both anthropometric and visceral protein measurements, with notable edema, wasting, and deterioration of organ mass.

These forms of PCM were defined by investigators in developing regions of the world who looked primarily at their occurrence in the pediatric population. The different forms were observed and reported to predominate in distinct areas, often where drought or inadequate food supplies existed. Subsequent investigations have led to the realization that the etiology of these forms of malnutrition is multifactorial, involving macronutrient, micronutrient, and environmental factors.[17,18]

Jelliffe formulated a nutritional pyramid (Figure 3–1) that demonstrated the different forms of PCM for children and their interrelationships. The levels were identified in Figure 3–1 as follows[19,20]:

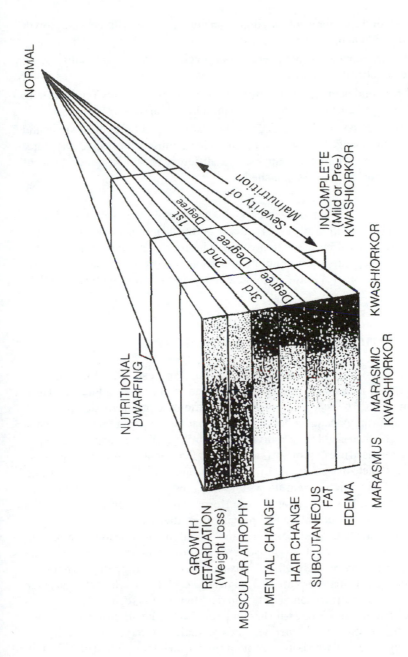

Figure 3–1 Nutritional Pyramid, Showing Tentative Interrelationships between Various Forms of Protein-Calorie Malnutrition in Tropical Preschool Children. *Source:* Reprinted from Jelliffe, D.B., Protein-calorie Malnutrition in Tropical Preschool Children. *J Pediatrics*, Vol. 54, p. 244, the American Academy of Pediatrics, © 1959.

- The top or peak represents adequate nutritional status with normal growth and development.
- In the first degree, growth retardation occurs, with weight status being affected more than stature.
- In the second degree, biochemical changes are noted, with a reduction in transport proteins in the later stage (mild kwashiorkor).
- The third or severe degree of PCM is characterized by clinical signs and functional changes, with wasting of somatic muscle stores, edema, fatty liver, and psychomotor changes. The different features of each form of malnutrition can be distinguished.

Rao hypothesized that marasmus and kwashiorkor are the same disease occurring in two different stages.[21] He described an adaptive process that occurs in marasmus, caused by the action of the adrenal cortex, and suggested that failure of this adaption system or failure of the adrenal cortex to produce adequate amounts of cortisol leads to the biochemical and clinical picture found in kwashiorkor.

MALNUTRITION IN THE ACUTE CARE SETTING

Clinicians now recognize that the PCM found in hospitalized patients, although similar, is distinct from the PCM found in starving children in Third World countries.[22] Classical forms of malnutrition are primarily due to undernutrition and an inadequate food supply, leading to metabolic and endocrine changes that enable the individual to survive. These adaptive changes include a decreased use of protein as a precursor for glucose and an increased use of fat stores (ketosis) as the main source of energy. This nitrogen-sparing, alternate fuel utilization system allows for some preservation of visceral proteins and increased utilization of fat stores. Hormonal regulation allows for the decrease in energy expenditure and provision of alternate fuel substrates by a decrease in insulin, thyroid hormone, and somatomedins production and an increase in glucagon, growth hormone, and corticosteroid production.[16,23] In the pediatric population, poor growth velocity and development, apathy, irritability, and psychological alterations are early signs of PCM. It is unclear at what stage the impact of malnutrition on growth and development is reversible.

A stressed individual is one who has undergone an acute physiological burden such as a significant trauma, thermal damage, major surgery, perfusion injury, or a septic episode, and who is usually monitored in an intensive care unit. Protein calorie malnutrition in stressed individuals develops in response to this physiological stress and/or injury. PCM modifies the body's metabolic profile, altering nutritional requirements and intake and utilization of nutrients, and can quickly lead to severe body protein depletion. The disease state, immobility, medications, and treatment modalities alter commonly used nutritional assessment parameters such as serum albumin, weight, and physical appearance.

Under stress, the body experiences an ebb and flow phase.[24,25] The ebb phase is the initial response to injury or trauma and lasts for 24 to 48 hours. This phase is characterized by a stage of low oxygen consumption and decreased plasma insulin levels, with a drop in blood pressure and metabolic demands. In the flow phase, hypermetabolism is prominent, with an increase in oxygen consumption, carbon dioxide production, hyperglycemia, and gluconeogenesis lasting three to four days. However, patients may go through multiple ebb and flow phases. This persistent hypermetabolic state can result when complications such as infection/sepsis or anastomotic disruption occur and can lead to multiple organ dysfunction and even death. Furthermore, the metabolic response to trauma can differ from that of sepsis. In sepsis the body first goes through a "high flow" period that, if not controlled, will lead to a low flow (ebb) or septic shock.

The metabolic response to stress is regulated by hormonal and inflammatory mediators.[26,27] The hormonal response occurs with elevated serum concentrations of cortisol, catecholamine, glucagon, growth hormone, aldosterone, and antidiuretic hormone.[28] These hormones produce a state of hypermetabolism and hypercatabolism, which leads to an elevated resting energy expenditure rate, hyperglycemia, altered substrate use, and increased oxygen consumption, lipolysis, and sodium and water retention. The inflammatory mediators, cytokines (protein hormones), are responsible for the onset of fever, gluconeogenesis, increased leukocyte count, hepatic production of acute phase proteins, proteolysis, altered lipid metabolism, and pronounced anorexia.[29] In the hypermetabolic state, critical reduction of lean body mass (LBM) due to uncontrolled protein catabolism can occur in as little as 14 days as compared with 60 to 90 days in starvation. This difference between starvation and hypermetabolism has been well outlined by Cerra (Table 3–2).

MALNUTRITION IN THE INTENSIVE CARE UNIT

It has been hypothesized that malnutrition is one of the contributing causes of organ failure in the intensive care unit.[26,27,30] Malnutrition can alter the gut's integrity, and in the presence of injury this may facilitate the passage of enteric flora or endotoxins into portal circulation.[31] In animals bacterial translocation has been demonstrated and is thought to contribute to morbidity and mortality.[32] A decrease in respiratory muscle mass secondary to starvation will decrease contractility and alter the ability to cough; impair lung function, gas exchange, ventilatory response to hypoxia, and the pulmonary defense system; and prolong

Table 3–2 Hypermetabolism versus Starvation

Characteristic	Starvation	Stress
Cardiac output	–	++
Systemic vascular resistance	NC	–––
Oxygen consumption	–	++
Resting energy expenditure	–	+++
Mediator activation	NC	++
Regulatory responsiveness	++++	+
Regulatory quotient	0.75	0.85
Primary fuels	fat	mixed
Proteolysis	+	+++
Protein oxidation	+	+++
Branched-chain oxidation	+	+++
Hepatic protein syntheses	+	+++
Ureagenesis	+	+++
Glycogenolysis	+	+++
Gluconeogenesis	+	+++
Lipolysis	++	+++
Ketone body production	++++	+
Rate of development of malnutrition	+	++++

Note: NC, no change; –, decrease; +, increase.

Source: Reprinted from Cerra, F.B., The Hypermetabolism Organ Failure Complex, *World Journal of Surgery*, Vol. 11, pp. 173–181, with permission of the International Society of Surgery, © 1987.

---

mechanical ventilation.[33] Malnutrition appears to be a contributing factor in the hepatic and kidney failure of the multiple system organ dysfunction that occurs in intensive care patients.

The cost of treatment in the ICU has risen substantially along with the cost of rehabilitation, if these patients survive. Nutritional support to prevent the occurrence of malnutrition during hypermetabolism is different from the treatment of traditional malnutrition and is critical to a patient's improvement. The goal is not repletion but maintenance and preservation, which is described by the team as metabolic support. A lower calorie-to-nitrogen ratio is indicated, as well as a mixed fuel source while limiting fluid administration. We have learned in nutrition support that more is not always better. Overfeeding, in view of the decrease in nutrient clearance, can further impair organ function, alter the immune system, and lead to respiratory and hepatic dysfunction, and glucose intolerance.[26,30,34] Nutrition support requires timely and ongoing nutrition assessment and close monitoring.

Although the malnutrition that develops in hospitalized individuals resembles marasmus and kwashiorkor, it is referred to by a variety of terms.[35,36] Bistrian uses the term *hypoalbuminemic malnutrition* or *syndrome*, and Hill refers to it as *adult marasmus* and *kwashiorkor*; others refer to it in the general terms of *protein calorie* or *protein energy malnutrition* and attempt to categorize it as mild, moderate, or severe. The search for an appropriate term stems from the need to differentiate its specific causes, signs/symptoms, and rationale for treatment. A uniformly accepted definition will eventually lead to ease of identification, resolution, and prevention. An accepted classification of malnutrition in the hospital is crucial to understanding its influence on patient outcomes and cost of treatment.[35,36] Dietitians must take the leadership role in recognizing, treating, and monitoring the outcomes of malnourished patients.

NUTRITION SUPPORT TEAMS

Data demonstrating not only the presence of malnutrition in hospitalized patients but also the relationship between malnutrition and morbidity and mortality has led to the development of nutrition support teams (NST). These interdisciplinary teams consist of personnel from the medical staff, nutrition, nursing, and pharmacy.[37] Some teams have a coordinator; others are coordinated by a member of the team. Depending on the facility, the expertise of disciplines and the services available will determine whether the team is part of each individual departmental budget, has a separate cost center, or has an independent budget.

Nutrition support teams, also called *hyperalimentation teams* in some institutions, may work as an independent service and assume total responsibility for carrying out nutrition intervention, including the use of elaborate computer-assisted nutritional procedures and research. Some teams, however, function on a consultation basis and use already established procedures and personnel to follow up on recommended nutrition prescriptions. Such teams have been shown to be more cost-effective.[37,38] The primary responsibilities of NSTs are to identify patients who have been shown to benefit from nutrition support, select the appropriate nutrition modality, establish enteral and parenteral formularies, and reduce complications of nutrition intervention. In addition, they review the literature on nutrition support, educate patients and staff, establish policy and procedures, and implement a quality assurance monitoring program.[37,39] Regardless of the team design, NSTs should adhere to established policy and procedures, practice guidelines, and the guidelines of a larger reference group and of any state or other governing regulatory bodies.

SCREENING FOR MALNUTRITION

Over the last decade the roles of the dietitian and support staff have evolved to optimize the quality of nutrition care, maximize the reimbursement rate, and control cost. Nutrition screening and assessment are essential documentation systems that promote early identification and appropriate treatment of patients requiring nutrition intervention. The 1994 Joint Commission on Accreditation of Healthcare Organizations *Accreditation Manual for Hospitals* mandates that an initial assessment/screening of each patient be completed to determine the need for care, the type of care to be provided, and the need for further assessment.[40] Each hospital must develop a screening program that is designed to meet the needs of the population it serves and accommodate staff resources.

Nutrition screening is the gathering of baseline data that will help identify patients at risk for malnutrition and the level of care required. It is usually a 5- to 15-minute procedure that is completed during the first 24 to 72 hours after hospital admittance. The screening instrument often focuses on dietary parameters: prior diet and current diet order, appetite, food allergies and intolerances, oral health problems, and bowel function. Clinical, biochemical, and anthropometric parameters are also included: medical condition, serum albumin, weight and height, and weight history. A subjective global assessment was developed by Detsky and is used by medical personnel, going beyond a simple screen.[41] All screening instruments should have a rating or scoring system to identify level of risk for malnutrition.

The methods selected should agree with current knowledge in the nutrition field, provide sufficient information to make a valid recommendation, favor false positive conclusions, and be reproducible. The screening form must be part of the patient's permanent medical record. It should also comply with established protocols included in the policy and procedure manual and be routinely reviewed to assure that it meets established goals and objectives. The hospital's medical staff and medical records department need to know how to interpret the screening form in order to identify the code for malnutrition under the payment system.[42–45]

BEYOND SCREENING

The high cost of medical care in the United States contributed, in 1983, to the implementation of a prospective payment system based on diagnosis.[43–45] Under Medicare and third-party payment systems, rates for reimbursement are based on principal diagnosis, principal procedure, comorbidity and complicating (CC) factors, sex, age, and status at discharge. The International Classification of Disease (ICD-9-CM) includes codes for nutritional deficiencies[46]:

- No. 260, *kwashiorkor*, is defined as nutritional edema with dyspigmentation of skin and hair.
- No. 261, *nutritional marasmus*, is defined as nutritional atrophy with severe calorie deficiency.
- No. 262, *severe nonspecific protein calorie malnutrition*, is defined as nutritional edema without mention of dyspigmentation of skin and hair.

Nutrition services are required to document their cost-effectiveness and revenue-generating capacity, and careful coding for malnutrition is important to this effort.

Although it is well documented that malnutrition exists in the hospital setting, many institutions continue to view dietetics as a nonreimbursable service. Early identification, treatment, and documentation of malnutrition, prior to development of malnutrition-related CC, can affect a patient's length of hospital stay and increase hospital reimbursement. A malnutrition CC has shown to increase reimbursement by 50 to 60%. Trimble found, in an acute care community hospital, that coding for malnutrition as a major CC increased revenue by $103,000 per year.[47,48] However, if malnutrition is one of several CCs, it will not affect the reimbursement rate.[46–51]

With staff limitations, the need to optimize resources and avoid duplication of activities has forced institutions to optimize the assessment process. As a result, an initial assessment or nutrition screen can be performed by a nutrition technician, a nutrition or nursing aide, a nurse, admitting personnel, or the patient.[45] This cost-effective approach allows the dietitian and diet technician the time to work with high-risk patients, improve nutrition outcomes, and perhaps decrease length of stay for patients.

For the dietitian as nutrition assessor, practice guidelines exist (see appendices) for establishing protocols and procedures for routine and comprehensive care. Outcome-oriented measures and clinical indicators assist in ensuring that patients have high-quality, cost-effective care.[52]

REFERENCES

1. Sandstead HH, Carter JP, Darby WJ. How to diagnose nutritional disorders in daily practice. *Nutr Today*. 1969, Summer;19–25.
2. Butterworth CE. The skeleton in the hospital closet. *Nutr Today*. 1974, March/April;4–8.
3. Butterworth CE, Blackburn GL. Hospital malnutrition. *Nutr Today*. 1975, March/April;8–17.

4. Coats KG, Morgan SL, Bartolucci AA, Weinsier RL. Hospital-associated malnutrition: a reevaluation 12 years later. *J Am Diet Assoc.* 1993;93:27–33.

5. Mowe M, Bohmer T, Kindt E. Reduced nutritional status in an elderly population is probable before disease and possibly contributes to the development of disease. *Am J Clin Nutr.* 1994;59:317–324.

6. Abbasi AA, Rudman D. Observations on the prevalence of protein-calorie undernutrition in VA nursing homes. *J Am Geriatr Soc.* 1993;41:117–121.

7. Mowe M, Bohmer T. The prevalence of under diagnosed protein-calorie undernutrition in a population of hospitalized elderly patients. *J Am Geriatr Soc.* 1991;39:1089–1092.

8. Thomas DR, Verdery RB, Gardner L, Kant A, Lindsay J. A prospective study of outcome from protein-energy malnutrition in nursing home residents. *J Paren Enter Nutr.* 1991;15:400–404.

9. Pinchofsky DGD, Kaminski MV. Incidence of protein calorie malnutrition in the nursing home population. *J Am Coll Nutr.* 1987;6:109–112.

10. Chen WJ, Vu LJ, Mo ST, Chen KM. Prevalence of protein-calorie malnutrition in hospitalized patients. *J Formosan Med Assoc.* 1985;84:228–237.

11. Nizel AE, Pappas A. *Nutrition and Clinical Dentistry.* Philadelphia, Pa: WB Saunders; 1989.

12. Jelliffe DB. *The Assessment of the Nutritional Status of the Community.* Geneva, Switzerland: World Health Organization; 1966.

13. Shils M. Lecture at a nutrition assessment workshop: "Nutrition Support." Presented at the Manhattan Veterans Administration Hospital; January 25, 1978; New York, NY.

14. Wellman NS. The evaluation of nutritional status. In: Howard RB, Herbold NH, eds. *Nutrition in Clinical Care.* New York, NY: McGraw-Hill Book Co; 1978:290–301.

15. Coward WA, Lunn PG. The biochemistry and physiology of kwashiorkor and marasmus. *Brit Med Bull.* 1981;37:19–24.

16. Torun B, Chew F. Protein-energy malnutrition. In: Shils ME, Olon JA, Shike M, eds. *Modern Nutrition.* 8th ed. Malvern, Pa: Lea & Febiger; 1994:950–973.

17. Jelliffe DB, Jelliffe EFP. Causation of kwashiorkor: toward a multifactorial consensus. *Pediatrics.* 1992;90:110–113.

18. Jackson AA, Golden MHN. Protein energy malnutrition: kwashiorkor and marasmic kwashiorkor physiopathology. In: Brunser O, Carrazza FR, Gracey M, Nichols BL, Senterre J, eds. *Clin Nutr Young Child.* New York, NY: Raven Press Ltd; 1991;133–153.

19. Jelliffe DB. Protein-calories malnutrition in tropical preschool children. *J Pediatr.* 1959;54:227–256.

20. McLaren DS. A fresh look at protein-energy in the hospitalized patient. *Nutrition.* 1988;4:1–6.

21. Rao KSJ. Evolution of kwashiorkor and marasmus. *Lancet.* 1974:709–711.

22. Craig RM. Criteria for the diagnosis of malnutrition. *JAMA.* 1986;256:866–867.

23. McMahon M, Bistrian B. The physiology of nutritional assessment and therapy in protein-calorie malnutrition. *Dis Month.* 1990;36:375–417.

24. Cuthbertson DP. Post-shock metabolic response. *Lancet.* 1942;1433–1437.

25. Nelson KM, Long CL. Physiological basis for nutrition in sepsis. *Nutr Clin Prac.* 1989;4:6–14.

26. Bower RH. Nutritional and metabolic support of critically ill patients. *J Paren Enter Nutr.* 1990;14:257S–259S.

27. McMahon MM, Farnell MB, Murray MJ. Nutritional support of critically ill patients. *Mayo Clin Proc.* 1993;68:911–920.

28. Wilmore DW, Aulick LH. Metabolic changes in burned patients. *Surg Clin North Am.* 1978;58:1173–1188.

29. Hardin TC. Cytokine mediators of malnutrition: clinical implications. *Nutr Clin Prac.* 1993;8: 55–59.

30. Cerra FB. How nutrition intervention changes what getting sick means. *J Paren Enter Nutr.* 1990;14:164S–168S.

31. Henken-Langkamp B, Glezer JA, Kudsk KA. Immunologic structure and function of the gastrointestinal tract. *Nutr Clin Prac.* 1992;7:100–106.

32. Deitch EA, Xu D, Qi L, Specian RD, Berg RD. Protein malnutrition alone and in combination with endotoxin impairs systemic and gut-associated immunity. *J Paren Enter Nutr.* 1992;16:25–31.

33. Rochester DF, Esau SA. Malnutrition and the respiratory system. *Chest.* 1984;3:411–414.

34. Alexander JW, Gonce SJ, Miskell PW, Peck MD, Sax H. A new model for studying nutrition in peritonitis: the adverse effect of overfeeding. *Ann Surg.* 1989;209:334–340.

35. Hill Gl. Body composition research: implications for the practice of clinical nutrition. *J Paren Enter Nutr.* 1992;16:197–217.

36. McClave SA, Mitoraj TE, Thielmeier KA, Greenburg RA. Differentiating subtypes (hypoalbuminemia vs marasmic) of protein calorie malnutrition: incidence and clinical significance in a university hospital setting. *J Paren Enter Nutr.* 1992;16:337–341.

37. McMahon MM. Development of the nutrition support service. Presented at conference at New England Deaconess Hospital, Boston, Mass. Hyperalimentation: A practical approach; Sept 12–14, 1990.

38. Nehme AE. Nutritional support of the hospitalized patient. *JAMA.* 1980;243:1906–1908.

39. Bank RC. Nutrition support in the community hospital. Presented at the American Society for Parenteral and Enteral Nutrition (ASPEN), Orlando, Fla; Jan 19–22, 1992.

40. *Accreditation Manual for Hospitals.* Chicago, Ill: Joint Commission on Accreditation of Healthcare Organizations; 1994.

41. Detsky AS, Smalley PS, Chang J. Is this patient malnourished? *JAMA.* 1994;271:54–58.

42. Hunt DR, Maslovity A, Rowlands BJ, Brooks G. A simple nutrition screening procedure for hospital patients. *J Am Diet Assoc.* 1995;85:332–335.

43. Nagel MR. Nutrition screening: identifying patients at risk for malnutrition. *Nutr Clin Pract.* 1993;8:171–175.

44. Fatzinger P, Kammer A, Garrett M. Development and use of preprinted forms and adhesive labels in medical record charting. *J Am Diet Assoc.* 1992;92:982–985.

45. Foltz MB, Schiller R, Ryan AS. Nutrition screening and assessment: current practices and dietitians' leadership roles. *J Am Diet Assoc.* 1993;93:1388–1395.

46. *International Classification of Diseases. Clinical Modification Tabular List.* 9th ed. Washington, DC: US Dept of Health and Human Services; 1989.

47. Trimble JM. Reimbursement enhancement in a New Jersey hospital: coding for malnutrition in prospective payment systems. *J Am Diet Assoc.* 1992;92:737–738.

48. Sayarath VG. Nutrition screening for malnutrition: potential economic impact at a community hospital. *J Am Diet Assoc.* 1993;93:1440–1442.

49. Ford DA, Fairchild MM. Managing inpatient clinical nutrition services: a comprehensive program assures accountability and success. *J Am Diet Assoc.* 1990;90:695–702.

50. Delhey DM, Anderson EJ, Laramee SH. Implications of malnutrition and diagnosis-related groups (DRGs). *J Am Diet Assoc.* 1989;89:1448–1451.

51. Bernstein LH, Shaw-Stiffel TA, Schorow M, Brouillette R. Financial implications of malnutrition. *Clin Lab Med*. 1993;13:491–507.

52. Queen PM, Caldwell M, Balogun L. Clinical indicators for oncology, cardiovascular and surgical patients: reports of the ADA Council on Practice Quality Assurance Committee. *J Am Diet Assoc*. 1993;3:338–344.

Chapter 4

Hunger as a Public Health Issue

J. Larry Brown and Laura P. Sherman

OVERVIEW

Hunger, as the chronic underconsumption of nutrients needed for physical growth and maintenance of health, has reemerged and is spreading across the United States. Among those who are particularly susceptible to the ravages of hunger are pregnant women, infants and children, and the elderly. Because hunger, even in a mild form, affects the health status and functioning level of those who experience it, health professionals must address this issue within the comprehensive context it requires. Hunger goes beyond the unique technical expertise of the nutrition assessment team to the political and social arena to address the development and implementation of appropriate public and social policies.

INTRODUCTION

Recent analyses suggest that 30 million people suffer from hunger in the United States.[1] This number represents a 50 percent increase in hunger since 1985, when the Physician Task Force on Hunger in America alerted the nation that hunger was once again a significant public health problem.[2] The existence and continuing growth of hunger is disturbing since hunger was dramatically reduced in the United States during the 1970s.

The health effects of chronic undernutrition, and the social sequelae of those health effects, make hunger a critical public health problem. To understand what is at stake, we must consider the general impact of diet on health, and the risks faced by individuals who are ill-nourished at different stages in the life cycle. Given this information, one can determine the extent to which those risks are manifest in the United States today, creating, in effect, an epidemiology of hunger.

Food is used by the body as energy to fuel all activities; it provides the building blocks for growth and development, and the substances used to promote health and prevent or combat disease. Undernutrition, in terms of quantity or quality of diet, may compromise any of these functions. Specific effects of an inadequate diet vary according to the age, sex, and biological status of the individual affected. The human organism is particularly vulnerable to hunger in periods of rapid growth, such as infancy and adolescence, and in old age, due to characteristics of the aging organism.

IMPACT OF HUNGER DURING PREGNANCY

The period of greatest risk is gestation: the pregnant woman needs extra nutrients to meet the needs of the developing fetus. When nutrition is inadequate during pregnancy, both mother and child are at risk.[3] Stores of maternal nutrients may be depleted to provide for the baby. Maternal anemia is one possible consequence of this depletion. Toxemia of pregnancy, a life-threatening condition involving rapid weight gain and a sharp increase in blood pressure due to excessive retention of fluid, is also thought to reflect inadequate nutrition, especially inadequate protein.

The greatest risk from poor nutrition during pregnancy, however, is borne by the infant. Risks include prematurity, defined as birth at less than 37 weeks gestation, and low birth weight, defined as less than 2,500 grams. The infant born too early or too small is poorly equipped to adapt to extrauterine life. Sequelae may include respiratory distress syndrome, weak immune response, and long-term growth and development problems.[4] At the most extreme, low birth weight results in infant death. Low birth weight is now the third leading cause of death among infants.[5]

IMPACT OF HUNGER ON CHILD HEALTH

The rapid growth years of early childhood comprise a second period of high risk. A critical locus of vulnerability is the central nervous system, since the human brain grows most rapidly from the first trimester of pregnancy through early childhood. After the preschool years, brain growth slows sharply until maturity, when it stops. Before maturity, especially in early infancy, nutritional deprivation may lead to permanent developmental deficit.[6]

Poor nutrition may result in functional impairment of the child.[7] Research suggests that before easily measured changes in growth occur, a child's body may adapt to inadequate food consumption by curtailing energy use.[8] Since energy use is necessary for all the activities associated with normal development—play, learning, social interaction—the underfed child is placed at risk of developmental delay.

Both long- and short-term hunger adversely affect children's cognitive and behavioral functioning. Formal studies as well as observational evidence show that when children miss breakfast their behavior and academic performance suffer. A recent study of the effect of the School Breakfast Program on school performance of low-income children showed that children who participated in the program performed better on standardized tests, and were late and absent less often, than children who did not participate. These academic improvements may be due to the effects of a morning meal or to the more long-term benefit related to improved 24-hour dietary intake.[9]

The various risks entailed by poor childhood nutrition interact multiplicatively. The victim does not, typically, experience a clear-cut single effect of hunger. Rather, the low birth-weight child who receives inadequate postnatal nutrition may then be more vulnerable to infections such as otitis and colds, which in turn may curtail dietary intake.[10] The result, as seen by clinicians, may be growth failure, characterized by sharply delayed growth and development, requiring medical intervention and sometimes hospitalization.[11]

IMPACT OF HUNGER ON ADULT HEALTH

After the childhood years, functional impairment may be the most significant effect of hunger in the United States. Adults of all ages who are poorly nourished, like children, are vulnerable to infections and various deficiency diseases.

In old age the risks of malnutrition also are heightened further. During these years the impact of food on the maintenance of health and the prevention of disease is particularly crucial. The majority of elderly suffer at least one chronic condition, such as hypertension or diabetes, that require special diets.[12] Potential deficiency diseases increase the requirements for certain essential nutrients, for example, calcium intake to prevent osteoporosis.[13] Some conditions of old age may impair digestion or the absorption of nutrients, making the choice of nutrient-dense foods critical.[14] At the same time, old age often entails a number of obstacles to an adequate diet. Difficulties in such activities as shopping and cooking, trouble in chewing some foods, and a lack of appetite due to social isolation and resulting in depression can all interfere with food and nutrition in old age. Moreover, it is especially difficult to address these problems if resources are limited. For the low-income elderly person, adequate nutrition often constitutes an insurmountable problem.[12]

HEALTH IMPACT OF HUNGER IN THE UNITED STATES

Having outlined the extent of hunger and its link to health status, the important issue to address is the health effects of hunger in the United States today. Unfortunately, the data available to address this question are limited. Malnutrition, even in extreme forms, is not a reportable condition in the United States. Currently this country is lacking a timely, consistent, and scientifically designed nutrition monitoring system to capture the extent and severity of hunger.

SOURCES OF DATA

The most comprehensive information available on the relationships among income, diet, and health of Americans is derived from the National Health and Nutrition Examination Survey (NHANES). This survey, conducted periodically by the National Center for Health Statistics, gathers a wide range of health and nutrition information from a representative sample of the American population. A national survey, conducted between 1976 and 1980, indicated that poor Americans were more likely than nonpoor to consume inadequate calories, Vitamin C, iron, and a number of other nutrients.[15]

NHANES, though an important source of information over the long term, is neither collected nor analyzed with sufficient rapidity to serve as a surveillance system to shed light on the impact of current policy. The relevant information available and accessible is from vital statistics, local and state studies on health status and nutrition, and information from a national system of surveillance of a large (although not representative) sample of low-income children. These sources comprise material for hunger epidemiology.

Birth outcome data are revealing indicators of the nutritional status, as well as the general health status, of any population. The infant mortality rate (IMR) is the number of deaths that occur before the age of one year for every 1,000 live births in a given population. This measure is used internationally as an index of nutritional well-being. Because it is available for many countries, IMR also provides a basis for international comparisons.

In comparison with other countries, the United States ranks 22nd in IMR.[16] Countries that do better include those in Scandinavia; Western European nations including England, France, and Germany; and Japan and Australia.

There is no system for calculating an infant mortality rate specifically for poor women in the United States. Such a statistic would shed light on the impact of poverty on health and thus get more directly at the effects of hunger. Birth certificates do not, however, ascertain income status. The evidence that is available on differences in IMR for different socioeconomic groups is compelling nonetheless. Race is often used as proxy for class since African Americans are, on average, much less well off than white Americans. In 1991, the latest year for which key data are available, the African-American infant mortality rate in the United States was 17.6 per thousand. That figure is comparable to figures for developing countries and more than twice the rate for whites. A Children's Defense Fund analysis of federal data shows that while the overall infant mortality rate dipped from 10.0 deaths per thousand in 1988 to 8.9 deaths per thousand in 1991, the rate for African-American babies was no better than 20 years ago.[16]

It is not only these single-year IMR figures that are of concern but IMR trends over time as well. This is particularly true in the United States since new technology has become available in recent years that makes it possible, albeit at enormous cost with some risk of long-term impairment, to save many low birth-weight infants. Given the dissemination of this technology, one would expect to observe a notable decrease in IMR. Instead, the data show the position of the United States to be deteriorating relative to other countries.

Infant mortality is not the only birth outcome that reveals poor maternal health and nutrition. The records on low birth weight show that it, like infant mortality, is unevenly distributed. Nationally, in 1991, African-American babies were more than twice as likely as white babies to be born low birth weight.[16]

Similar socioeconomic variation is reflected in the data on the growth of children. Of various indicators that characterize the health and nutrition status of American children, anthropometric data (measurements of height, weight, and other body dimensions) are most widely used. Height and weight are routinely measured in medical examinations. The existence of nationally developed and accepted norms makes it possible to compare the growth of any one child to standardized growth curves, or of any subpopulation group to the population as a whole. When these comparisons are made, a pattern of socioeconomic differences is revealed.

Nutrition monitoring of low-income children in the United States shows that these children fall behind their peers in height. The Pediatric Nutrition Surveillance System (PedNSS) continuously monitors the nutritional status of high-risk groups of low-income infants and children in various states who participate in selected health service delivery programs including Maternal and Child Health; Early and Periodic Screening, Diagnosis, and Treatment (EPSDT); the WIC program; and Head Start. Data compiled between 1973 and 1987 have consistently shown that 9 to 11 percent of children fall below the fifth percentile for height for age.[17]

The fifth percentile is the national norm below which one would expect to find only 5 percent of children of a given age group. A range of 9 to 11 percent of children below the fifth percentile indicates that among poor children nearly twice the expected proportion are falling below this point. This suggests that poor children in America are subject to what is called *stunting*, defined as height-for-age below expected levels. It is important to note that the PedNSS system is not representative of all poor children in the United States, since PedNSS includes data only on children enrolled in programs, and thus is biased in an optimistic direction. Children enrolled in reporting programs are those most likely to be receiving a range of health and nutrition services that other poor children lack, suggesting that a significantly larger proportion of all poor children may be experiencing growth stunting.

Increasing evidence in this country points to the impact of nutrition on function even in the earliest stages of life. One study found poor maternal nutrition and weight gain to be associated with poor performance on several components of the Brazelton Neonatal Assessment Scale (a widely used scale for evaluation of infants).[18] Another study that examined the impact of Vitamin B_6 deficiency, common among pregnant women in America, found an association with low Apgar scores even in normal birth-weight babies.[19]

Current research on the effects of iron deficiency anemia on learning, attention, and memory clearly shows that anemia has an adverse effect on a child's performance. This is a significant finding since iron deficiency anemia is one of the most prevalent nutritional disorders in the world, especially among poor children.[20]

Although the exploration of functional impairment due to low-level nutritional deficiency is a relatively new field, studies are suggestive. Complemented by additional work done on children in this country and by a somewhat richer body of research on children and adults in developing countries, studies on the relationship between nutrition and cognition indicate the high price paid by poor Americans for the kind of undernutrition prevalent in the United States.[21]

The most extreme expressions of malnutrition, in contrast to the more subtle indicators discussed above, are disease and mortality. Data on morbidity and mortality also indicate differences among Americans based on socioeconomic status. In general, studies have shown that poor children experience more illness, and are more affected by illness, than other children. For conditions particularly linked to nutritional status, data show distinct differences based on income.

The health condition that most starkly reveals the impact of poverty on nutritional status and health is *failure to thrive*, a syndrome involving significant growth and developmental delay. Nonorganic failure to thrive (NOFT) refers to growth faltering due to nonorganic causes. The causes of NOFT are complex—in some cases the cause is restricted to poverty and lack of food, whereas other cases involve interactions between socioenvironmental conditions and problems in mother-child interaction, including abuse and neglect. In 1985 a prospective study showed that 5.5 percent of low-income infants were diagnosed with

NOFT.[22] Unfortunately, current data systems do not distinguish well between failure to thrive caused by poverty and lack of food versus other factors.

Data on morbidity and mortality suggest the impact of poor nutrition among low-income adults as well. Hypertension, diabetes, and cardiovascular disease are more common among poor American adults and endemic within some population groups. Each of these conditions can reflect lifetime nutritional inadequacy, and each affects the poor disproportionately.[23]

Since very few illnesses are reportable, researchers generally depend on mortality statistics to provide information about prevalence. As with infant mortality, we have no precise way to characterize death certificates by income in order to see how different socioeconomic groups compare. Race is used again as a proxy for socioeconomic class. For nutrition-related causes of death, the African-American to white ratios are cardiovascular disease, 1:43; pneumonia and influenza, 1:52; and diabetes, 2:30.[24] Thus race, the best available indicator for income, serves to illustrate the higher risk that disadvantaged populations face of dying from nutrition-related disease.

These data on poverty, malnutrition, and illness are not always clear or easy to assess. There are gaps and relationships that require approximation. In some cases we are hampered by lack of baseline data, a lack that makes pinpointing trends over time difficult. In other instances we lack prevalence data for socioeconomic groups and must use race as a proxy. Nonetheless, certain findings are clear:

1. Infants of poor mothers die more frequently due to maternal undernutrition.
2. When they live, they are at greater risk of low birth weight and associated health impairments.
3. Poor children are less likely than their better-off peers to be adequately nourished and are more likely to suffer growth deficits and cognitive deficiencies associated with undernutrition.
4. Poor children are at higher risk of nutrition-related illness, even including illnesses associated with extreme malnutrition in developing countries.
5. Poor adults are at greater risk and die younger of nutrition-related disease than other Americans.

In short, hunger is tied directly to poverty, and both hunger and poverty are associated with adverse health outcomes.

HUNGER AND PUBLIC POLICY

The clear association between poverty and nutritional status suggests that to understand the phenomenon of increasing domestic hunger one must examine the status of low-income households. In this sense hunger is like any infectious disease: it has a cause. Three factors appear to account for the "disease" of hunger. One is the condition of the nation's "safety net," the array of programs to assist people at or below the official poverty level. Another is public nutrition policy. The third factor is the rise in unemployment and in economic jeopardy stemming from recession.

The American safety net is weak compared with other industrialized nations. For example, the United States is one of only two industrialized nations that have no program of national health insurance. In many states poor families are denied public assistance if the father remains in the home, no matter how destitute the family may be.[25] The federal Aid to Families with Dependent Children program (AFDC), designed to protect children and families during difficult times, comes into play in the majority of states only if the family first breaks apart. Additionally, AFDC benefits for families and children have fallen sharply in recent years. After adjusting for inflation, benefits for a family of three with no other income were 23 percent lower in constant dollars in the typical state in 1991 than they had been in 1980.[26]

The inadequacy of the unemployment insurance program is another example of the failing safety net. The proportion of unemployed people receiving unemployment insurance benefits set a record low for five of the six years from 1984 to 1989. In an average month in each of these years, no more than 34 percent of the unemployed received benefits. In 1990, some 37 percent of the unemployed received benefits, but this was a record: it represented the lowest proportion of the unemployed to receive benefits in any year that included the start of a recession.[27]

The effectiveness of the Food Stamp program is constrained by both its limited reach and the inadequacy of its benefits. Although all impoverished people are not eligible for Food Stamps due to asset limits, the ratio of poor to monthly Food Stamp recipients serves as a barometer to gauge Food Stamp availability among the poor. During the past decade or so, this ratio has varied as much as from 59:100 (59 recipients for every hundred people in poverty) to 68:100.[28]

Although it is the most extensive of the nation's means-tested food assistance programs, the Food and Nutrition Service recently estimated that only 59 percent of those eligible for Food Stamps receive them.[28] Those who do receive assistance get an average of $0.76 per meal.[29] It is not surprising that survey data repeatedly show that Food Stamp households run out of food in the last week to ten days of each month.[2,30,31]

Moreover, Food Stamp benefits are not high enough to allow recipients to meet the Recommended Dietary Allowances (RDAs) for all basic nutrients. The U.S. Department of Agriculture (USDA) bases benefits on the Thrifty Food Plan. This meal plan was devised initially as a model for basic nutrition in periods of economic hardship. When the plan was first developed, USDA nutritionists warned that families buying food at this expenditure level on a protracted basis would not receive adequate nutrition. Research shows their concern to be justified; 88 percent of individuals whose food expenditures equal the Thrifty Food Plan fail to receive the RDAs.[32] This plan serves as the norm for determination of Food Stamp benefits today.

In 1991 the number of Americans living in poverty grew to 35.7 million, the highest level shown in more than 20 years. With a poverty rate of 14.2 percent, one in every seven Americans lived in poverty. The 1991 poverty rate repre-

---

Exhibit 4–1 Recent National Response to Hunger

USDA National Hunger Forum, June 1993

The Department of Agriculture sponsors the largest federal anti-hunger forum since the 1960s. Secretary of Agriculture Mike Espy states "We can and we must do better as we address the hunger needs of Americans all across the country. President Clinton and I are committed to reforming our nutrition programs to better reach those who are in need and to promote self-sufficiency . . . a study showing that 12 million American children are going hungry is further evidence that alleviating hunger must be a high priority."[33]

Mickey Leland Childhood Hunger Relief Act 1990–1993

The most important domestic anti-hunger legislation since 1977. The bill improves the Food Stamp Program for families with children by increasing access and benefits as well as reducing barriers.

1990:   House of Representatives approves the bill by a vote of 336–83. During the Budget Summit agreement between the President and Congress, the bill fails.

1991:   Senate Agriculture Committee approves the Leland bill (14–1) and the House Agriculture Committee approves it unanimously.

1992:   Leland bill passes the House with a 256–163 vote as part of the Children's Initiative.

1993:   Leland bill passes Congress as part of the 1993 Omnibus Budget Reconciliation Act (OBRA).

Medford Declaration to End Hunger in the United States, May, 1992

A bipartisan document signed by more than three thousand national leaders, describing the economic costs and unacceptability of domestic hunger, that outlines how the problems could be ended.

Table 4–1 Recent Studies to Document Hunger in the United States

Year	Sponsor	Findings
1994	Second Harvest	Based on the results of a national survey of its client agencies. Second Harvest estimated that 26 million Americans received emergency food services. This estimate included only those Americans seeking emergency food at Second Harvest facilities, and did not include all Americans experiencing hunger.[34]
1993	Urban Institute	Study of hunger among the elderly estimated that between 2.5 million and 4.9 million Americans age 65 and older were hungry.[35]
1993	Center on Hunger, Poverty and Nutrition Policy, Tufts University	Analysis of all hungry Americans revealed that of the 30 million hungry, 12 million were children and 3.2 million were elderly.[36]
1993	U.S. Conference of Mayors (annual)	Survey of 29 major cities reported increase in hunger coinciding with inability of emergency food assistance programs to respond to need.[31,38]
1992	National Board of Emergency Food and Shelter (United Way)	Survey of member agencies showed that over three-quarters experienced a 30% increase in demand over previous year with accompanying inability to meet demand.[39]
1992	Breglio poll: Research/ Strategy/Management Inc.	National poll of registered voters indicated that more than 30 million people were hungry. It also revealed that 93% of respondents said hunger was a serious national problem. Two-thirds said it was solvable and were willing to pay $100 more in taxes to solve it.[41,42]
1992	Center on Hunger, Poverty and Nutrition Policy, Tufts University	At the request of Congressman Tony Hall (Chairman, House Select Committee on Hunger) the Center used separate analyses of existing data to conclude that 30 million Americans were hungry. This estimate coincides with Breglio estimate.[1,43,44]
1991	Food Research and Action Center (FRAC)	Community Childhood Hunger Identification Project (CCHIP) estimated that over 5.5 million children under age 12 were hungry and another 5.5 were at risk of hunger.[44]
1985	Harvard Physician Task Force on Hunger	Epidemiological model estimated that 20 million Americans were hungry.[2]

sented an increase over the previous years and was higher than the rate in any year of the 1970s or 1980s except for 1982 through 1984, when unemployment was at especially high levels.[26]

The steady increase in poverty is in part attributable to a change in the distribution of income. Throughout the 1980s people at lower income were unfavorably affected by such changes. During this time, income shifted out of the lowest and middle three quintiles of the population and into the highest quintile. In other words, the rich got richer, and the poor got poorer. Another factor contributing to the rise in poverty levels is the decline in wages. More than ever before, full-time workers are earning wages too low to enable them to climb out of poverty through work. In 1990, 18 percent of full-time workers were paid wages too low to lift a family of four out of poverty, an increase of about 50 percent since 1979.[37]

Exhibit 4–1 illustrates federal responses to hunger. Table 4–1 outlines studies to document hunger in the United States.

The renewed national commitment to end hunger points to possibilities for positive changes in our nation. A commitment to guarantee food security or sufficiency would impact on the negative effects of hunger. Food security would assure that individuals and families can receive an adequate supply of nourishing and safe food.[45]

The larger question—the truly challenging one—is how to eliminate the cause of hunger: poverty. The country pays a high price for poverty, and hunger is only one part of it. From a public health perspective, it is the height of folly to permit such a significant risk factor for illness and premature mortality to persist. From a moral perspective, the prevalence of poverty in the world's wealthiest nation is yet another matter.

REFERENCES

1. Brown JL. Letter to Tony Hall, Chairman, House Select Committee on Hunger. Washington, DC: US House of Representatives; September 8, 1992.

2. Physician Task Force on Hunger in America. *Hunger in America: The Growing Epidemic.* Middletown, Conn: Wesleyan University Press; 1985.

3. Hack M, Breslau N, Weissman B, et al. Effect of very low birth weight and subnormal head size on cognitive abilities at school age. *N Engl J Med.* 1991;325:231–237.

4. Hoekelman RA, Blatman S, Burnell P, Friedman S, Sidel H. *Principles of Pediatrics: Health Care for the Young.* New York, NY: McGraw-Hill Book Co; 1978.

5. *Health of America's Children.* Washington, DC: Children's Defense Fund; 1992.

6. Brazelton TB. Nutritional factors affecting mother–child relationship during infancy. In Suskind R., ed. *Textbook of Pediatric Nutrition.* New York, NY: Raven Press; 1981.

7. Liebel RL, Pollitt I, Kim I, Viteri F. Studies regarding the impact of micronutrient status on behavior in man: iron deficiency as a model. *Am J Clin Nutr.* 1982;35:1211–1221.

8. Barrett D, Radke-Yarrow M, Klein RE. Chronic malnutrition and child behavior: effects of early caloric supplementation on social and emotional functioning at school age. *Dev Psychol.* 1982;18:541–556.

9. Meyers AF, Sampson AE, Weitzman M, et al. School Breakfast Program and school performance. *AJDC.* 1989;143:1234–1238.

10. Chandra RK. Interactions of nutrition, infection, and immune response. *Acta Paediatr Scand.* 1979;68:137.

11. Frank D, Allen D, Brown JL. Primary prevention of failure to thrive: social policy implications. In Drotar D, ed. *New Directions in Failure to Thrive.* New York, NY: Plenum Press; 1985:337–357.

12. Posner BM. *Nutrition and the Elderly.* Lexington, Mass: Lexington Books; 1979.

13. Franz M. Nutritional requirements of the elderly. *J Nutr Elderly.* 1981;1(2):39–56.

14. Albanese AA, Wein EH. Nutritional problems in the elderly. In Administration on Aging, US Dept of Health and Human Services, ed. *Aging: Nutrition and the Elderly.* Washington, DC: US Government Printing Office; 1980:7–13.

15. National Center for Health Statistics, Department of Health and Human Services. Hematological and nutritional biochemistry reference data for persons 6 months–74 years of age: United States 1976–80. *Vital Health Statistics* 1983;Ser.2(232).

16. *State of America's Children.* Washington, DC: Children's Defense Fund; 1991.

17. *Nutrition Monitoring in the United States: An Update Report on Nutrition Monitoring.* Washington, DC: Public Health Service, Dept of Health and Human Services; 1989: publication 89-1255.

18. Picone TA, Allen LH, Olsen PN, Ferris ME. Pregnancy outcome in North American women: effects of diet, cigarette smoking, stress and weight gain on neonatal, physical and behavioral characteristics. *Am J Clin Nutr.* 1982;36:1214–1224.

19. Roepke JLB, Kirkssey A. Vitamin B$_6$ nutriture during pregnancy and lactation. *Am J Clin Nutr.* 1982;32:1211–1221.

20. Pollitt E, Idjradinata P. Reversal of developmental delays in iron deficient-anemic infants treated with iron. *Lancet.* 1993;341:1–4.

21. Pollitt E. Developmental impact of nutrition on pregnancy, infancy, and childhood: public health issues in the United States. *Int Rev Res Mental Retardation.* 1988;15:33–80.

22. Drotar D, Strum L. Prediction of intellectual development in young children with early histories of nonorganic failure to thrive. *J Pediatr Psychol.* 1988;13:281–296.

23. Kitagawa EM, Hauser PM. *Differential Mortality in the U.S.: A Study in Socioeconomic Epidemiology.* Cambridge, Mass: Harvard University Press; 1973.

24. National Center for Health Statistics, US Dept of Health and Human Services. *Monthly Vital Statistics Report.* 1992;40(8).

25. US House of Representatives, Committee on Ways and Means. *Children in Poverty.* Washington, DC: US Government Printing Office, 1985.

26. *Number on Poverty Hits 20-Year High as Recession Adds 20 Million More Poor, Analysis Finds.* Washington, DC: Center on Budget and Policy Priorities; 1992.

27. Greenstein R. Testimony before the House Committee on Ways and Means. Washington, DC: US House of Representatives; March 13, 1991.

28. Trippe C, Doyle P. *Food Stamp Program Participation Rates.* Alexandria, Va: US Dept Agriculture, Food and Nutrition Service; 1992.

29. *Food Stamp Statistical Summary of Project Areas Operations Report, January 1992.* Washington, DC: US Dept Agriculture, Food and Nutrition Service; 1993.

30. *Community Childhood Identification Project: A Survey of Childhood Hunger in the United States.* Washington, DC: Food Research Action Center; 1991.

31. US Conference on Mayors. *Human Services FY82.* Washington, DC: 1982.

32. US House of Representatives, Subcommittee on Domestic Marketing, Consumer Relations, and Nutrition of the Committee on Agriculture. *A Review of the Thrifty Food Plan and Its Use in the Food Stamp Program.* Washington, DC: US Government Printing Office; 1985.

33. US Dept Agriculture. Office of Public Affairs. *USDA National Hunger Forum.* Release no. 0458.93. Washington, DC: USDA; June 8, 1993.

34. VanAmburg Group. *Second Harvest 1993 National Hunger Survey.* Chicago, Ill: VanAmburg Group; 1994.

35. Burt MR. *Hunger Among the Elderly: Local and National Comparisons.* Washington, DC: Urban Institute; 1993.

36. Center on Hunger, Poverty and Nutrition Policy. *Childhood and Elderly Hunger Estimates.* Medford, Mass: Center on Hunger Poverty and Nutrition Policy; 1993.

37. US Bureau of the Census. *Workers with Low Earnings: 1964 to 1990.* Washington, DC: US Dept of Commerce; 1992.

38. US Conference on Mayors. *A Status Report on Hunger and Homelessness in America's Cities: 1992: A 29-City Survey.* Washington, DC: 1992.

39. *Emergency Food and Shelter National Board Program Survey Results.* Alexandria, Va: Emergency Food and Shelter National Board Program; 1992.

40. Frank DA, Napoleone M, Roos N, Peterson K, Cupples LA. Seasonal changes in weight for age in a pediatric emergency room: a heat or eat effect? Abstract presented at the National Conference of the American Public Health Association; 1991; Boston, Mass.

41. Breglio VJ. *Hunger in America: The Voters' Perspective.* Lanham, Md: Research/Strategy/Management Inc.; 1992.

42. Breglio VJ. Testimony to the House Select Committee on Hunger. Washington, DC: US House of Representatives; April 30, 1994.

43. Brown JL, Gershoff SN, Cook JT. The politics of hunger: when science and ideology clash. *Int J Health Services.* 1992;22:221–237.

44. *Poverty in the United States: 1988 and 1989.* Washington, DC: US Bureau of the Census, 1992. Current Population Reports.

45. Frankle RT, Owen AY. *Nutrition in the Community.* 3rd ed. St. Louis, Mo: CV Mosby; 1993:29.

Chapter 5

The Tools of Nutrition Assessment

Margaret D. Simko, Judith A. Gilbride, and Catherine Cowell

OVERVIEW: WHAT IS AN ASSESSMENT TOOL?

A tool is "any device used for doing or facilitating work."[1] It has also been defined as "a means to an end, as an instrument or implement used to accomplish a purpose."[2] Thus, it may be a form to assess or provide insight into the client's/ patient's nutritional background or needs. It can also be the information gathered and recorded for this purpose. Tools are generally adapted or individualized to take and give only those data of interest in a specific situation. Generally, a series of tools will be selected to strengthen the validity of data collection and implementation of nutrition intervention.

Data Collection Instruments as Assessment Tools or Forms

Nutrition assessment tools include many forms or instruments for gathering data to assess the nutritional status of the patient/client. Examples are:

- *Screening forms.* "Nutrition screening is the process of discovering characteristics or risk factors known to be associated with dietary nutritional problems. Its main purpose is to identify individuals who are potentially at high risk, that is, who have complex and involved problems that touch upon nutrition."[3] Screening forms are used to assess the kinds of care or level of care needed in order to provide health care interventions to individuals or groups and to identify those most vulnerable or at greatest risk. In nutrition, the screening form is used to screen or "sort out" those populations at

55

greatest nutritional risk. A screening tool may be simple or complex depending on its intended use; the data may be gathered by one practitioner or by a number of health care professionals. Exhibits 15–1 and 15–2 illustrate screening tools that provide a section for the initial screening of the patient and then allow for more in-depth assessment of the same patient. See Chapter 1 for additional information about screening.

- *Dietary intake forms.* Dietary intake forms are tools used to collect information about an individual's food intake. These instruments include 24-hour recall forms, food frequency checklists, food records, and dietary history questionnaires. The formats for these forms will be similar, but usually they are individualized for a particular institution or situation. Chapter 10 provides an in-depth discussion of the methods employed for using each of these forms and examples of forms.

- *The Nutrition Profile form.* The Nutrition Profile is a broad needs assessment form (or set of forms) that can be used to collect or organize information about the population served and available resources. The primary purpose is to help identify the nutrition-related problems of a population. As a diagnostic tool, it provides a systematic method of compiling descriptive information that can be used to meet the nutrition or health-related needs and to expand resources within a demographic area. It can serve as a basis for planning nutrition intervention programs.[4]

Objective Data as Assessment Tools

Objective data can be quantified and can serve as assessment tools. These tools provide specific, quantifiable data to assess individual patients or groups, and to monitor nutrition intervention outcomes. If correct techniques and reliable instruments are used to provide these data, they are generally accurate and reveal good, comparable measures. Laboratory data and anthropometric measurements are two tools frequently utilized in nutrition assessment.

- *Laboratory values.* Laboratory data offer a large number of measurements to select for nutrition assessment. Selection of the number of measurements is based on the complexity of the assessment. Laboratory data provide baseline information that can be sequentially compared and interpreted. Because laboratory values include a "normal range," assessments can be made that are very specific. Chapter 11 provides a full discussion of the use of laboratory data as a component of assessment.

- *Anthropometric measures.* Anthropometric measurements can be simple, such as height and weight, or more complex, such as measurement of body density and body fat. The most readily available tools are for measurement of height and weight. These techniques are inexpensive in terms of time and equipment required and can be repeated and compared serially. However, recording of height and weight can be inaccurate and misleading if the equipment is poor or if improper techniques are used. Chapters 7 and 8 provide detailed discussions regarding techniques for using this assessment tool as well as guidelines for interpretation of data.

Subjective Data As Assessment Tools

Subjective data require the collection of information that is then evaluated by sets of standards that are qualitative and less specific than those for quantitative data. Although these tools are extremely important in the nutrition assessment process, caution is advised in the use of subjective assessment data, and they are usually compared with objective data from the same individual or group. Clinical judgment and experience are important factors in evaluating subjective data.

- *Physical signs.* Physical or clinical signs provide important assessment data. Visual examination of hair, face, eyes, skin, lips, nails, and musculoskeletal, cardiovascular, and gastrointestinal status can be revealing in identifying the presence of malnutrition. Examination of gums, teeth, and tongue should not be overlooked and can reveal abnormal nutritional status—especially in children. Sensory perception is important because inability to smell can lead to decreased food intake. Descriptive standards have been set for "normal" appearance, and lists, charts, and photographs of signs of malnutrition have been developed to assist in this assessment (see Chapter 6).[5,6]

- *Food intake information.* Food intake and diet patterns collected on any of the assessment tools are also qualitative. These data are compared with a set of standards such as the RDA, food groups, dietary guidelines, or the USDA pyramid. A judgment is made about the quality of the food intake. As discussed in Chapter 10, errors can be made in reporting and collecting these data, and they are generally only one of the tools used in the total nutrition assessment of the patient/client.

- *Environmental and functional information.* Environmental and functional information are other tools that play an important role in assessing nutritional status.[7] Is the client physically able to purchase adequate food? Are finances sufficient to buy food? Who shops for food? Is there adequate and safe storage for food products? Is someone able to prepare meals? Is he or she eating alone? Social isolation can lead to inadequate and improper food intake. Can clients feed themselves? These questions are pertinent in determining who is at risk for inadequate or improper food intake.

- *Subjective global assessment (SGA).* This is an alternative method of nutrition assessment that collects and evaluates subjective data for identification of patients at nutritional risk. It includes only data from a physical examination and medical history.[8] Anthropometric measurements and laboratory data are not included. The medical history focuses on weight change, dietary intake changes, gastrointestinal symptoms (nausea, vomiting, diarrhea, anorexia), functional capacity (walking, ambulatory, bedridden), and metabolic (stress) demands of disease. The physical examination focuses on subcutaneous fat, muscle wasting, presence of edema in the ankles or sacral region, and ascites. Data are rated by a SGA system that ranks the patient as well nourished, moderately or possibly malnourished, or severely malnourished.

HOW ASSESSMENT TOOLS ARE USED

The tools of nutrition assessment provide information for a number of different purposes. First and foremost, they document baseline data about the nutritional status of an individual or group. These data are then referred to at sequential intervals when follow-up assessments are completed to monitor nutritional progress of patients or groups. Monitoring provides documentation of the effectiveness of nutrition intervention and an opportunity to evaluate the advisability of changing the intervention when needed. Last, the tools of nutrition assessment provide documentation to conduct cost-effective analysis (see Chapter 20).

Specifically, each tool might be used in the following way.

How Screening Tools Are Used

A screening tool is not used for nutrition assessment per se. Rather, it provides a small amount of nutritional information to divide groups of people quickly into categories and make decisions about appropriate nutrition interventions and levels of care. Screening is usually the first step in an algorithm outlining levels of care with an appropriate monitoring system. See Figure 17–1 for an example of a screening tool recommended for screening elderly individuals living in the community. Figure 15–1 illustrates an algorithm screening tool used in one hospital.

How Dietary Assessment Tools Are Used

Dietary assessment is usually the first step in nutrition assessment, and is used to evaluate the food intake in greater depth than a screening process can.

Generally, screening will have indicated that the client needs a more extensive dietary evaluation. The tool or combination of tools selected depends on the depth necessary and should be appropriate for appraising each situation.

How Laboratory Assessment Tools Are Used

Laboratory data are usually collected upon admission to hospitals. Physicians order those tests that they deem most appropriate for diagnosis. Laboratory data are valuable adjuncts to the dietary assessment of the patient. A full discussion of the use of laboratory data appears in Chapter 11.

How Physical Assessment Tools Are Used

Physical signs observed during the clinical examination of the patient provide an overall impression of nutritional status. Examination of the body observing obvious obesity, wasting, pallor, robustness, or apathy will provide important information about the potential general nutritional status of the patient. Physical assessment is more evident and of greater value in children. However, physical signs of disease are not always evident in early stages. Physical assessment provides a general impression, and this information will usually be followed by the use of other tools to complete the nutrition assessment. See Chapter 6 for a complete discussion of the use of physical signs as tools to evaluate nutritional status.

How Anthropometric Assessment Tools Are Used

The most common anthropometric tool is documentation of height and weight. Care should be taken so that the individuals responsible for measuring height and weight have training in how to perform and record measurements accurately. Patient reporting about height and weight should not be substituted for actual measurements since the validity of patient reports is questionable. Depending on the goals and need, other forms of anthropometric assessment may be employed. For example, research centers and rehabilitation services employ calipers and measuring tapes for measuring skinfold and body circumference.[9]

HOW THE NUTRITION PROFILE IS USED

The Nutrition Profile is a written document or set of forms that provides a total picture of the nutritional problems and resources of a defined population. The various forms are presented in Appendixes 5–A, 5–B, and 5–C. The process of collecting demographic and nutritional data acts as a guide to evaluate the population and to plan nutrition support systems and intervention programs.

The profile provides a global view of the community to be served and identifies specific characteristics of a facility and client or patient population. It allows one to

- identify those who may be in need of nutritional care
- review the availability and utilization of existing supportive health personnel
- indicate where to implement or upgrade nutrition support services
- expand opportunities for nutrition intervention strategies
- plan procedures for evaluation and monitoring

The most important consideration in the process of data collection involves the development of a group profile as the basis for identifying groups at nutritional risk and planning intervention. Thus the data collection must be systematic, giving a description of nutrition-related problems of various subgroups in the client population in the facility or the community served. Since institutions and community organizational structures vary, the collection of a database or profile is based on the availability of staff or organizational requirements. The key to effective utilization of the profile may be to adapt the tool to meet the needs and individual characteristics of a specific health care setting.

If a tool is "any device used for doing or facilitating work," then the Nutrition Profile is a tool because it facilitates and identifies background information about clients, institutions, and the community. Descriptive indicators identified by the profile include a description of the population served, demographic and socio-economic factors, and the presence of nutrition-related diseases.

How Information Is Organized in the Profile

The information in the Nutrition Profile is organized in three sections. The first section encompasses the entire community serving the people in a defined area, such as a city, township, or county. A "community assessment paints a picture of the health of the community, its ecology, and the factors influencing the way its people live."[5] Subgroups in that community receive health care from a variety of facilities, such as hospitals, nursing homes, and neighborhood clinics.

The profile then focuses on the characteristics of the specific population subgroup that receives services from each identified facility. Within a community there usually are a number of facilities that provide health care to a variety of patients and clients. One use of the profile is the sharing of information across facilities within a community, since some clients might be served simultaneously or at different times by more than one facility. Table 5–1 summarizes the content for the Nutrition Profile in each of its three sections—community, facility, and client. Data can be collected by an individual or a team. A team is more efficient because they pool information, shorten time, and provide greater awareness.

Procedures for Completing the Nutrition Profile

Prior to the collection of the relevant data for the profile, some basic questions must be addressed:

- What is the purpose of the data?
- What time period are the data to cover?
- Who has primary responsibility for collecting and recording the data?
- How will these data be shared and utilized for program and development?

Each of these questions is important. Unless their answers are developed by the team working together, the whole purpose of the profile will be lost. The greater the input by all members of the team, the more likely there will be improved communications within the team, leading to quality care for the patients/clients.

Once the procedures for data collection are agreed upon, the process moves into the implementation phase, based on how the process of the data collection is designed. At all times there should be feedback to the team about progress, problems, and plans, since even long-term care facilities exist in dynamic environments that change as a result of external and internal forces. Open and continuous sharing of information enables the team to resolve problems and modify plans for completing the profile.

Accurate data are the keystone of the profile. Incorrect data will increase errors and mislead program planners. Facility census data should reflect the patient/client population being served as accurately as possible. Medical records and computer systems are reliable sources of information. When team members understand the importance of these data, their commitment to the collection of quality data is ensured. Figure 5–1 shows the flow of communication among team members that will facilitate the process of obtaining a profile. Exhibit 5–1 suggests some sources of information for the Nutrition Profile.

Table 5–1 Summary of Content of the Nutrition Profile

Community	Facility	Client
1. Geographical or other boundaries	1. Name, location, and type (acute, chronic, long-term)	1. Population distribution (a) total (b) age
2. Population within boundaries (a) total (b) age (c) gender	2. Patients served last calendar/fiscal year	2. Length of stay distributions
3. Socioeconomic status of population	3. Staffing patterns	3. Patient/client mobility
4. Ethnic composition	4. Patterns of staff conferences	4. Current primary medical diagnosis
5. Housing characteristics	5. Record keeping	5. Census of diets
6. Food marketing facilities	6. Program evaluation and review	6. Other pertinent data (unique to the patient/ client group)
7. Health status indicators	7. Nutrition assessment data collection	
8. Health resources	8. Dietary services	
9. Community health care programs	9. Supplemental feedings	
10. Food and nutrition assistance programs	10. Nutrition education	
11. Education programs	11. Other pertinent data (unique to the institution)	
12. Nutrition education programs		
13. Nutrition training programs		
14. Other pertinent data (unique to the community)		

Identify need for specific data units

Interdisciplinary team conference
- formulate plan for data collection
- determine responsibilities of team members/groups in collection

↕

Collect data from internal sources
- medical/dietary
- business and other records

↕

Continue data collection from external sources

Official agencies—local health/hospital departments
Local community social service agencies
Local school board—school food service
Library
Colleges and universities—public administration or public health, health education, home economics, and nutrition

↕

Analyze recorded data—statistical analysis, summary of data, visuals (charts, graphs)

↕

Identify population at risk

Interdisciplinary team conference
- describe population at-risk problems, gaps in services, manpower utilization

↕

Determine program priorities

↕

Implement revised plans and programs

↕

Evaluate programs and review programs

Interdisciplinary team
- meet as needed for periodic review of programs and services

Figure 5–1 Flowchart for Collecting Data for the Nutrition Profile.

Exhibit 5–1 Some Sources of Information for the Nutrition Profile

---

The Community Profile:

Population:
Census Bureau (most recent data)
Health departments
Social service departments
Universities and colleges—programs in nutrition, medicine,
    urban health, allied health, community health, nursing
Offices of congressional, state, and local representatives;
    federal, state, and local bureaus of labor, statistics, or commerce
Department of aging
Board of education
City/county government offices

Housing:
Same as above, and in addition: departments of housing,
Department of Housing and Urban Development

Food marketing facilities:
Local offices for supermarket chains
Local office of consumer affairs or markets
Local association of food stores or farmers' markets
Local newspapers and advertisements

Health statistics:
Regional, state, and municipal health/hospital departments
State and local health agencies
State health planning agencies
State and local universities and colleges, community medicine,
    population studies, health planning
Health systems agencies
Data from the National Center for Health Statistics and the
    Health and Nutrition Examination Survey

Community and mental health care programs:
Local hospitals, nursing homes, home health care agencies
Local health and social services departments
Local prepaid health care groups
Local programs for the elderly, handicapped, and special groups
Community health centers
Migrant health centers
Indian health clinics
School health services for data on pregnant teenagers

Community agencies:
Local United Fund or equivalent
Local telephone directory
Local health, social services department, and education agencies
Local March of Dimes
Local community action and/or legal services organizations
Local Cooperative Extension service
Local community colleges, universities, and professional schools
Local home health care agencies
Local Heart, Cancer, and similar associations
Local courthouse

---

continues

Exhibit 5–1 continued

Food and nutrition programs:	State and local health departments, social services State or local board of education Local community action groups
Nutrition education programs:	County, city health departments Board of education Social services departments Local Cooperative Extension office Local office of the Heart, Cancer, Dairy and Diabetes Associations
Educational facilities:	Local board of education State commissioner of education
Nutrition training programs:	Local educational institutions, universities, and colleges Community colleges and vocational (trade) schools National, state, and local organizations of dietitians and nutritionists Local school food service office

The Facility Profile:

Clients served:	Professional Standards or Utilization Review Agencies Computerized data banks Department of medical administration Admitting department Daily admission and discharge bulletin or report
Staff:	Chief or director of each department Administrator's records of staffing patterns Tables of organization Volunteer department
Routine team meetings:	Directors of each department Department of medical records Utilization review Committee reports Medical/patient care unit
Nutrition assessment tools:	Dietary department Laboratory director Patients' charts
Dietary services:	Director of dietetic services Nourishment unit Nursing cardex
Nutrition education and training programs:	In-service training records Dietary department Administration

continues

Exhibit 5–1 continued

The Client Profile:

Population distribution:	Medical records Census data Statistics division
Length of stay:	Administration Medical records Utilization review Accounting department Self-auditing reports
Patient mobility:	Nursing records Patients' charts Social services
Diagnosis:	Statistical reports Nursing cardex Patients' charts Medical records
Diets:	Diet manual Diet cardex Diet and meal census records
Feeding skills:	Nursing cardex Diet cardex

Source: Adapted from Margaret D. Simko, Catherine Cowell, and Judith A. Gilbride, *Assessing the Nutritional Needs of Groups: A Handbook for the Health Care Team* (New York: New York University, Department of Home Economics and Nutrition, 1980).

Advantages of Using the Profile

An obvious positive outcome of using the Nutrition Profile is the increased communication among the team members involved in the process. A free flow of communications cuts across both horizontal and vertical structures of management. Lower, middle, and executive/administrative staff are directly or indirectly a part of the profile process. Yet regardless of the level of management, those on the team who have direct responsibility for a service or unit or who are assigned representatives have the ultimate role of guiding the process. Interaction by team members for a common goal may be the catalyst for stimulating innovative interagency efforts beyond everyday activities. Subsequently this could develop a stronger team commitment to fulfill the mission of the institution.

The purpose of the profile pinpoints the challenge to professional dietitians and nutritionists to provide dynamic leadership in the nutrition assessment process. The profile provides the practitioner with a database for describing the state of the art for dietary/nutritional services. It can enable quality nutrition services to be planned around stated goals and objectives. Several strategies are available to the resourceful and innovative professional who wants to maximize the potential of existing personnel or acquire additional staff. Finally, the early formulation of short- and long-term goals based on the profiles should include ways of measuring performance and outcomes.

Because cost-effectiveness is of great concern, all or part of the profile can be used to determine costs of providing minimal, medium-level, or maximal care, based on staffing resources and patterns. In addition, the cost of service based on particular billing systems can be determined. Such an overview of cost and billing fees provides the basis for the financial structure that is necessary to prepare short- and long-range projections.

WHY NUTRITION ASSESSMENT TOOLS ARE USED

1. Nutrition assessment tools are used to determine baseline data in order to identify who needs nutritional care and to plan nutrition intervention. To assess the nutritional needs of any population group—whether in a hospital, extended care facility, or community health care agency—it is essential to determine who most urgently needs nutrition services. Since it is generally not possible or necessary to provide the same level of nutritional care to everyone, the first question is, which clients are at greatest nutritional risk?

2. Nutrition assessment tools provide data for planning nutrition instruction for individuals or groups. A realistic goal for nutritional care should be identified. Priorities should be set to meet the most urgent objectives. Selected tools can assist in planning. For example, laboratory data will reflect the biochemical levels of nutrients in the blood, urine, and tissues. Dietary histories provide information about individual eating habits, lifestyles, and nutritional problems. Clinical assessment reveals physical signs that can help detect nutritional deficiencies or excesses. Information such as height and weight data is most useful for routine application in an assessment protocol.

The major objective of the plan is to improve the nutritional status of the individual or group, as well as to improve or maintain the nutritional status of the entire population. The plan should consider the levels of care needed and the most effective way to provide the care. Specific objectives should be set within a time frame, since all objectives may not be immediately attainable. It is recommended that the plan be written and stored in a central place for the health care team to review and revise.

3. Nutrition assessment tools provide data to monitor patient or program progress. Monitoring is the checking of progress over a period of time to ensure continuation of quality care and to identify the new nutritional needs. Even when all goals of the nutrition intervention plan have been met, it is essential to continue to monitor changes that occur in the nutritional and/or health status of individuals or groups. An in-depth discussion of monitoring appears in Chapter 18.

4. Nutrition assessment tools provide data to evaluate outcomes of nutrition assessment in individuals or groups. Positive outcomes are needed to determine the effectiveness of the plan or program. Monetary decisions are often made comparing program cost to the rate of positive outcomes (see Chapter 20). Ongoing evaluation is needed to measure the progress and success of the program. Data are gathered at sequential times and compared with the baseline data to determine if health status or specific outcome measures have changed.

The following questions, among others, are relevant in evaluating an intervention program:

- Has the nutritional status of the clients changed?
- Were the procedures and standards appropriate to the population?
- Were the goals of the program met within the time frame?
- Did members of the health care team fulfill their responsibilities in carrying out the program?
- Would a different intervention program produce greater improvement, be more cost-effective, be less time consuming, or affect a larger group of individuals?

If the answers are not appropriate, the program goals and resources must be reevaluated and perhaps redesigned toward more realistic results. Figure 1–1 illustrates a system or model for nutrition care that can incorporate many of the tools described. The circle diagram includes the six steps of the system illustrating the input and process of providing nutritional care. Completion of these steps provides the output to meet the goals of the system.

CONCLUSION

A wide variety of tools are available that are essential in the comprehensive nutrition assessment of individuals and groups. Usually no one tool can be used as a definitive indicator of nutritional status; rather, it must be combined with data obtained through other assessment tools. In practice, the tools will need to be selected and adapted to the needs of each facility, community, or agency.

REFERENCES

1. Simko MD, Cowell C, Gilbride JA. *Nutrition Assessment: A Comprehensive Guide for Planning Intervention.* Gaithersburg, Md: Aspen Publishers, Inc; 1984:30.

2. Mason M, Wenberg BG, Welsh PI. *The Dynamics of Clinical Dietetics.* 2nd ed. New York, NY: John Wiley & Sons; 1982:347.

3. Dwyer JT. *Screening Older Americans' Nutritional Health: Current Practices and Future Possibilities.* Washington, DC: The Nutrition Screen Initiative; 1991.

4. Simko MD, Cowell C, Gilbride JA. *Assessing the Nutritional Needs of Groups: A Handbook for the Health Care Team.* New York, NY: New York University Department of Home Economics and Nutrition; 1980:13. Support for this work was provided by HSA-79-118 (p), BCHSI/HSA, HHS, Rockville, Md.

5. Christakis G, ed. *Nutritional Assessment in Health Programs.* Washington, DC: American Public Health Association, Inc; 1973:1.

6. Shils ME, Olson JA, Shike M, eds. *Modern Nutrition in Health and Disease.* 8th ed. Philadelphia, Pa: Lea & Febiger; 1994:909–923.

7. Austin A. Environmental assessment of the elderly. In: Simko MD, Cowell C, Hreha MS, eds. *Practical Nutrition: A Quick Reference for the Health Care Practitioner.* Gaithersburg, Md: Aspen Publishers, Inc; 1989:245–254.

8. Detsky AS, McLaughlin JR, Baker JP, et al. What is subjective global assessment of nutritional status? *J Paren Enter Nutr.* 1987;11:8–13.

9. Coats KG, Morgan SL, Bartolucci AA, Weinsier RL. Hospital-associated malnutrition: a reevaluation 12 years later. *J Am Diet Assoc.* 1993;93:27–33.

Appendix 5-A

The Nutrition Profile:
Level 1—Community Profile

I.   POPULATION DESCRIPTION *(Describe the Characteristics of the Population Served)*

Total Population in Area Served	Gender		As of (Date)		
	Male	Female			

Age Distribution	Number	Percent	Ethnic Racial Composition	Number	Percent
Under 1 Year			American Indian .		
1–14 Years			Asian/Pacific		
15–24 Years			Islander		
25–44 Years			Black		
45–64 Years			Hispanic/Latino ..		
65–79 Years			White		
80 Years and Over .			Other (Specify): ..		

(Check One)		(Check One)	
☐ **Actual Count/Data** ☐ **Best Estimate**		☐ **Actual Count/Data** ☐ **Best Estimate**	

Socioeconomic Data	Number	Housing Characteristics	Number	No. of Tenants
No. of Persons Employed ____%		Low-Income		
No. of Persons Unemployed ___%		Projects		
Food Stamp Program (Annual) ...		Middle-Income		
Living at the Poverty Index		Housing Projects .		
Elderly Living at the Poverty		Rooming Houses ..		
Index		Residential Hotels .		
Public Assistance Cases (Annual)		Shelters		
Aid to Fam. & Dep. Children		Senior Houses		
(AFDC)		No. of Individuals		
Supplementary Security Income		Households		
(SSI)		Other:		
Estimate of Avg Per Capita Income $		Avg Size of Family		

Food Marketing Facilities	Approximate No.
Supermarkets	
Food Co-ops	
Farmers' Markets	
Small Neighborhood Stores	
Other (Specify):	

Source: © 1984 ® 1994 Margaret D. Simko, PhD, RD, Catherine Cowell, PhD, Judith A. Gilbride, PhD, RD.

II. HEALTH STATISTICS INDICATORS FOR THE LAST YEAR 19___

Birthrate		Infants of Low Birth Weight (2,500 Grams and Under)	
Mother's Age	**No.**	**Mother's Age**	**No.**
15 Years and Under		15 Years and Under	
16–17 Years		16–17 Years	
18–19 Years		18–19 Years	
20–29 Years		20–29 Years	
30–39 Years		30–39 Years	
40 Years and Older		40 Years and Older	
Total		Total	
Causes of Deaths	**No. of Deaths**	**Morbidity and Mortality**		
Alcoholism		**Reported Incidences**	**Cases**	**Deaths**
Cancer		AIDS		
Diabetes		Drug and Substance Abuse		
Heart Disease		Lead Poisoning		
Other:		Tuberculosis		
		Other Significant Diseases:		

III. HEALTH RESOURCES

Residential Institutions and Programs for Children			Community and Mental Health Programs		
Kind	**No.**	**No. of Residents**	**Hospitals**	**No.**	**Total Beds**
Group Homes			Municipal		
Foster Care Program			Voluntary		
Other (Specify):			Proprietary		
Food Assistance Programs			Governmental		
Program	**No.**	**No. of Partic- ipants**	Teaching Hospitals		
Adult Day Care			Other:		
Child Care Food Programs			HMOs/Clinics		
			Continuing Care Communities		

Food Assistance Programs (Continued)	Number	No. Served	Community & Mental Health Programs (Continued)	Number	No. Served
School Breakfast ...			Nursing Facilities		
School Lunch			Official Public Health Agency		
Special Summer Feeding			Voluntary Health Agency		
Elderly Feeding Programs			Other (Specify):		
Under Title (III) Congregate					
Meals on Wheels ...					
Other (Specify):					
Supplemental Feeding Programs:					
WIC—Women					
Infants					
Children					
Commodities Distribution Program					
Soup Kitchens					
Food Pantries					
Other (Specify):					

IV. EDUCATIONAL PROGRAMS

Educational Facilities			
Schools		**Number**	**Enrollment**
PUBLIC SCHOOLS	Elementary		
	Middle		
	Secondary		
	Vocational		
PRIVATE SCHOOLS	Elementary		
	Middle		
	Secondary		
COLLEGES	Public—2 Year		
	Privately Owned—2 Year		
	Public—4 Year		
	Privately Owned—4 Year		

Adult Vocational Training		
Nutrition Education Programs	**Yes**	**No**
City or County Health Department		
Local Board of Education (NET)		
Community Health Center		
Health Maintenance Organizations (HMOs/PPOs)		
City/County Welfare Social Services Agency		
Maternal and Infant Care Projects (MIC)		
Private Wellness/Health Promotion Programs		
Head Start		
Cooperative Extension		
Supplemental Feeding Program for Women, Infants & Children (WIC) . . .		
Industry-Sponsored		
Tel Med Centers		
Home Care Agency		
Other:		
Nutrition Training Programs			
---	---	---	---
UNDERGRADUATE/PRACTICE	Location	Number	Enrollment
Dietetic Internship			
Coordinated Programs			
Specialty Practice			
UNDERGRADUATE PROGRAMS	Location	Number	Enrollment
Dietitians (ADA approved)			
Dietetic Technicians (AAS)			
Dietary Managers (DMA)			
GRADUATE PROGRAMS IN DIETETICS-NUTRITION	Location	Number	Enrollment
FOOD SERVICE TRAINING	Location	Number	Enrollment

Appendix 5-B

The Nutrition Profile:
Level 2—Facility Profile

(Describe the Characteristics of Your Health Care Facility or Center)

Name of Facility	Date(s)	
Location (City) Type (e.g., Prenatal Clinic, Nursing Facility, Hospital)		

I. CLIENTS SERVED LAST CALENDAR OR FISCAL YEAR 19__	Number
A. Inpatients	
B. Ambulatory Clients (Outpatients)	
C. Home Care	
D. Beds..	
E. Cribs	
F. Other (Specify):	

II. STAFF	Total	Number Contributing to Nutrition Assessment
A. MEDICAL		
1. House Staff		
2. Private Staff		
3. Physicians' Assistants		
4. Residents		
B. NURSING		
1. Nurse Clinicians/Practitioners		
2. Registered Nurses		
3. Midwives		
4. Licensed Practical Nurses		
5. Certified Nursing Assistants		
C. OTHER PROFESSIONALS		
1. Pharmacists		
2. Dentists		
3. Dental Hygienists		
4. Social Workers		
5. Podiatrists		

Source: © 1984 ® 1994 Margaret D. Simko, PhD, RD, Catherine Cowell, PhD, Judith A. Gilbride, PhD, RD.

II.	STAFF C. OTHER PROFESSIONALS (Continued)	Total	Number Contributing to Nutrition Assessment
	6. Psychologists		
	7. Therapists (Specify):		
	....		
	8. Health Educators		
	9. Speech Pathologists		
	10. Others (Specify):		
	D. VOLUNTEERS ☐ Yes ☐ No 1. If yes, number of volunteers available to assist dietary 2. Director ☐ Yes ☐ No		

		CHECK ATTENDANCE FOR		
III.	ROUTINE TEAM MEETINGS	Admissions	Care Planning	Discharge
	A. Physicians			
	B. Physicians' Assistant(s)			
	C. Pediatric Nurse Associate(s)			
	D. Nurse Clinician(s)			
	E. Registered Nurse(s)			
	F. Licensed Practical Nurse(s)			
	G. Other Nursing Staff			
	H. Dietitian/Nutritionist(s)			
	I. Dietetic Technician(s)			
	J. Dietary Manager(s) or Food Service Supervisor(s)			
	K. Pharmacist(s)			
	L. Health Administrator(s)			
	M. Health Educator(s)			
	N. Social Worker(s)			
	O. Case Manager			
	P. Home Care Representative			
	Q. Other (Specify):			

IV. RECORD-KEEPING SYSTEM
    A. Source-Oriented Medical Records   ☐ Yes ☐ No
    B. Problem-Oriented Medical Records ☐ Yes ☐ No
        1. SOAP   ☐ Yes ☐ No
        2. PIE   ☐ Yes ☐ No
    C. Computerized Medical Records   ☐ Yes ☐ No
    D. Other (Specify):

V. PROGRAM EVALUATION AND REVIEW TECHNIQUES
  A. Quality Management/
     Continuous Quality Improvement/CQI   ☐ Yes   ☐ No
  B. Retrospective Audits   ☐ Yes   ☐ No
  C. Concurrent Audits   ☐ Yes   ☐ No
  D. Utilization Review Committee   ☐ Yes   ☐ No
  E. Program Evaluation Procedures   ☐ Yes   ☐ No
  F. Other Committee: ☐ Yes   ☐ No
     CQI Team members include _____
     _____

  G. Number audits per department per year
     1. Nutrition care _____
     2. Food service _____
  H. Other: _____
     _____
     _____

VI. NUTRITION ASSESSMENT	(Check)	
	Screening	Post Screening
A. DIETARY		
1. Nutrition History		
2. 24-Hour Recall		
3. Food Frequency Questionnaire		
4. Food Records		
5. Intake Study		
6. Other (Specify):		
B. LABORATORY		
1. Urinalysis		
2. Complete Blood Count		
3. Complete Lipid Profile		
4. SMA-16		
5. SMA-12		
6. SMA-24		
7. SMA-36		
8. Hemoglobin		
9. Hematocrit		
10. Blood Lead Level		
11. Serum Albumin		
12. TIBC or Serum Transferrin		
13. Creatinine Height Index		
14. Nitrogen Balance		
15. Total Lymphocyte Count		
16. Prealbumin		
17. Hemoglobin Alc		
18. Others:		

	(Check)	
C. CLINICAL	Screening	Post Screening
1. Heights		
2. Weights		
3. Body Circumferences		
4. Skinfolds		
5. Bioelectrical Impedance		
6. Other (Specify):		

D. SCREENING TOOLS	Yes	No
1. Initial		
2. Follow-up		

E. NUTRITION CARE TEAMS		
1. Nutrition Support		
2. Dysphagia		
3. Ethics		
4. Rehabilitation		
5. Other Nutrition Committee (Specify): _____		
6. _____		
7. _____		

VII. DIETARY SERVICES

A. TYPE OF FOOD SERVICE FOR PATIENTS

	Yes No		Yes No		Yes No
1. Centralized	☐ ☐	3. Tray Service	☐ ☐	5. Contracted Vendor	☐ ☐
2. Decentralized	☐ ☐	4. Cafeteria/ Dining Rm.	☐ ☐	6. Other (Specify)	☐ ☐

B. SUPPLEMENTARY FEEDINGS			Avg. No. Day
1. Nourishments/Snacks	Yes ☐	No ☐	
2. Tube Feedings Daily	Yes ☐	No ☐	
3. Oral Enteral Supplements	Yes ☐	No ☐	
4. Peripheral Parenteral Nutrition	Yes ☐	No ☐	
5. Total Parenteral Nutrition	Yes ☐	No ☐	
6. Other (Specify):			

C. DIET MANUAL	Yes	No
1. Developed by Facility		
2. Adapted from Another Facility or Agency/ National Resource		
3. Revised Yearly		
4. Updated Every 2–3 Years		
5. Other Resources (Specify):		

D. STAFFING PATTERNS	Numbers	
1. Registered/Licensed Dietitians		
2. Clinical Nutrition Specialists		
3. Dietitians (Non-RD)		
4. Nutritionists		
5. Consultants (Per Diem FTEs)		
6. Dietetic Technicians		
7. Dietary Managers or Food Service Supervisors .		
8. Kitchen Workers		
9. Cafeteria/Coffee Shop Workers		
10. Other (specify, e.g., clerks)		

E. CLIENT EDUCATION

   1. NUTRITION CLASSES

      a. Taught by Whom _____

      b. How Often _____ Number Usually Present _____

      c. Use of (check) ☐ Lesson Plan ☐ Printed Handouts ☐ Evaluations

   2. DIET COUNSELING

      a. Taught by Whom _____

      b. Length of Average Session _____

      c. Group Sessions: How Often _____ Number Usually Present _____

         Length of Average Session _____

      e. Use of (check) ☐ Lesson Plan ☐ Printed Handouts ☐ Evaluations

3. PROVISION FOR EVALUATION	Yes	No
a. Follow-up by Nutrition Educator		
b. Follow-up by Diet Counselor		
c. Referred to an Outside Agency		
d. Evidence of Client Adherence (Compliance) .		

F. NUTRITION TRAINING FOR STAFF

   1. Dietary   Yes ☐ No ☐ Other (Specify): _____

   2. Interdisciplinary Orientation   Yes ☐ No ☐   Inservice Yes ☐ No ☐

   3. How Often _____;   Length of Training Session(s) _____

Appendix 5-C

The Nutrition Profile:
Level 3—Client/Patient Profile

(Describe the Characteristics of Your Service Population (Clients)

		Number	Percent
I.	POPULATION DISTRIBUTION		
	A. DISTRIBUTION		
	1. Female		
	2. Male		
	Total		
	B. AGE DISTRIBUTION (Check One) ☐ Actual Count/Data ☐ Best Estimate		
	1. Under 1 Year		
	2. 1–14 Years		
	3. 15–24 Years		
	4. 25–44 Years		
	5. 45–64 Years		
	6. 65–79 Years		
	7. 80 Years and Over		
	Total		
II.	LENGTH OF STAY (Check One) ☐ Actual Count/Data ☐ Best Estimate		
	A. FOR SHORT-TERM FACILITY; AVERAGE LENGTH OF STAY _____ DAYS		
	1. Less than 3 Months		
	2. 3 Months to Less Than 6 Months		
	3. 6 Months to Less Than 12 Months		
	4. 1 Year and Over		
	Total		
III.	PATIENT MOBILITY (Check One) ☐ Actual Count/Data ☐ Best Estimate		
	A. Full Ambulatory		
	B. Ambulatory (With Cane, Walker)		
	C. Wheelchair (Self-Managed)		
	D. Room-Bound		
	E. Bed-Fast		

Source: © 1984 ® 1994 Margaret D. Simko, PhD, RD, Catherine Cowell, PhD, Judith A. Gilbride, PhD, RD.

	Number	Percent
F. Other (Specify)		
G. Feeding Skills		
1. Feeds Self		
2. Needs Assistance (Cutting)		
3. Needs Feeding		
4. Tube-Fed		
5. Other (Specify)...............................		

IV. DIAGNOSIS ☐ Actual Count/Data ☐ Best Estimate	Major Diagnosis at Admission	
	Number	Percent
A. AIDS		
B. Cancer		
C. Cardiac Diseases		
D. Diabetes		
E. Gastrointestinal Diseases		
F. Inherited Diseases		
G. Pulmonary		
H. Renal		
I. Stroke		
J. Substance Abuse		
K. Trauma/Accident		
L. Psychiatric		
M. Other (Specify): 1		
2		
3		
Total		
V. DIET PRESCRIPTIONS ☐ Actual Count/Data ☐ Best Estimate		
A. DIETS REPORTED FOR ONE DAY		
1. Regular/House		
2. Texture—Modified		
3. Pediatric		
4. Kosher		
5. Vegetarian		
6. Liquid		
7. Modified/Therapeutic:		
Allergy		

	Number	Percent
7. Modified/Therapeutic (Continued):		
Restricted Residue		
Diabetic		
Fat/Cholesterol Controlled		
High Calorie/High Protein		
Fiber Controlled		
Renal		
Sodium Controlled		
8. Weight Reduction		
9. NPO on Survey Day		
10. Other (Specify):		
B. SPECIAL DIETARY NEEDS FOR ONE DAY		
1. Total Parenteral Nutrition		
2. Peripheral Parenteral Nutrition		
3. Enteral Formula (only)		
4. Other (Specify):		
Grand Total		

Time Frame to Complete Profile _____

Sections 5–1   5–2   5–3

Part II

Assessment Methodology

Chapter 6

Physical Examination As an Assessment Tool

George M. Owen

OVERVIEW

Observation, inspection, and measurement are the major tools of the examiner; they generally provide the clues to the possibility of a nutritional disorder. The clues are then synthesized with the history and with more specific, sensitive testing. The initial observation is most important. Is the individual alert? Robust or feeble? Mobile or confined? Talkative, quiet, or tearful? Pale? The observation alerts the examiner to look for other factors. It is essential to remember that individual variations do not necessarily represent disease; general habitus and appearance (the physical condition) are subject to much normal variation.

THE MEDICAL HISTORY

It is frequently said that the medical-social history of a patient provides 90 percent of the information necessary to arrive at a presumptive diagnosis of a medical condition; the physical examination yields the remaining 10 percent. In considering the physical examination as a tool of nutrition assessment, one must keep in mind that many factors influence food intake and nutrient utilization. Factors that influence food intake include:

- socioeconomic circumstances: income, location, housing, family size
- sources, accessibility, and selection of foods
- dietary patterns, eating habits
- health and physical activity

Factors that influence nutrient utilization include:

- disease (absence of health)
- medicines (drugs)
- alcohol

Several important features of the medical history that help to identify persons who are malnourished or who are significantly at risk of becoming malnourished are outlined in Exhibit 6–1.

PHYSICAL ASSESSMENT

Physical assessment is to be emphasized in cases of suspected malnutrition in both children and adults. Measurements of body length and weight are relatively

---

Exhibit 6–1 Features of a Medical History That Suggest Malnutrition

1. Recent loss of 10 percent or more of usual body weight (adults) or failure to gain weight (infant or young child)
2. Restricted intake of food or nutrients
3. Chronic disease
4. Protracted loss of nutrients
   - vomiting, diarrhea
   - short gut, malabsorption
   - renal dialysis
   - burns, draining wounds
5. Increased metabolic needs
   - burns, trauma
   - fever
6. Use of antinutrient or catabolic drugs
   - anticancer drugs
   - corticosteroids
   - antibiotics, anticonvulsants

Table 6–1 Physical Signs of Value in the Clinical Assessment of Malnutrition

Organ System	Group 1	Group 2
Hair	lack of luster thin, sparse dyspigmentation easy pluckability	
Face	diffuse depigmentation nasolabial dyssebacea	
Eyes	pale conjunctivae conjunctival xerosis Bitot's spots corneal xerosis keratomalacia	corneal vascularization conjunctival injection conjunctival and scleral pigmentation
Lips	angular stomatitis angular scars cheilosis	
Tongue	edema scarlet color purple color atrophic papillae	hypertrophy of papillae fissures geographic tongue
Gums	spongy bleeding	recession
Skin	xerosis follicular hyperkeratosis petechiae pellagrous dermatosis flaky-paint dermatosis edema (subcutaneous)	
Nails	koilonychia	transverse ridging
Musculoskeletal	muscle wasting craniotabes frontal or parietal bossing epiphyseal enlargement beading of ribs	
Gastroenteric	hepatomegaly	
Nervous	psychomotor changes mental confusion	
Cardiovascular	cardiac enlargement	

Source: Adapted from *WHO Expert Committee on Medical Assessment of Nutritional States* (1963) World Health Organization Technical Report #258.

Table 6–2 Selected Physical Signs of Malnutrition

Organ System	Sign
Hair	*Lack of luster.*[P] The hair is dull and dry. Effects of scalp diseases, use of oil and other substances on the hair, and exposure to salt water and hot sun must be taken into account.
	Thin and sparse.[P] The hair may become fine and silky in texture and cover the scalp less abundantly or completely than usual. In some ethnic groups with normally curly hair, malnutrition may produce pathological straightness.
	Dyspigmentation.[P] The hair shows a distinct lightening of the normal color (black to dark brown to light brown to red-brown, etc.). Local practices, such as dyeing the hair, as well as effects of salt water, sunshine, and the use of oil and other substances should be considered.
	Easy pluckability.[P, Z, F] A small tuft or clump of hair can be easily and painlessly pulled out of the scalp. Other changes, such as those listed above, are commonly present.
Face	*Diffuse depigmentation.*[P] This occurs in dark-skinned individuals in severe protein-calorie malnutrition. Pallor associated with anemia may exaggerate the appearance of this condition.
	Nasolabial dyssebacea.[B] This yellow, greasy appearance is produced by plugging of the ducts of enlarged sebaceous glands by sebum.
Eyes	*Conjunctival xerosis.*[A] Dryness, thickening, and lack of luster of the bulbar conjunctiva of the exposed part of the eyeball.
	Bitot's spots.[A] Well-demarcated, superficially dry, white-grey foamy plaques usually located lateral to the cornea in both eyes.
	Corneal xerosis.[A] Hazy or opaque appearance of cornea.
	Keratomalacia.[A] Softening of cornea.
	Corneal vascularization.[R] Invasion of periphery of cornea with fine capillary blood vessels. Usually secondary to chronic irritative or inflammatory process.
Lips	*Angular stomatitis.*[R] Excoriated lesions and fissuring at angles of mouth.
	Cheilosis.[B] Reddening, swelling, ulceration of lips.
Tongue	*Atrophic papillae.*[I] Atrophy at filiform papillae (tastebuds), leaving tongue with smooth or slick appearance.
Gums	*Spongy, bleeding.*[C] Swelling of gingival tissue between teeth, which may bleed on slight pressure.

continues

Table 6–2 continued

Organ System	Sign
Skin	*Xerosis.*(Z, F) Generalized dryness with desquamation of superficial layers.
	Follicular hyperkeratosis.(A) Hypertrophy of the corneous layer of skin surrounding the hair follicles, with formation of plaques.
	Petechiae.(C, K) Small hemorrhagic spots in skin or mucous membranes.
	Pellagrous dermatosis.(N) Symmetrical, clearly demarcated, hyperpigmented areas of skin most commonly located on body regions exposed to sunlight.
	Flaky-paint dermatosis.(P) Symmetrical hyperpigmented patches of skin that desquamate, leaving hypopigmented skin.
Nails	*Koilonychia.*(I) Spoon-shaped deformity of finger nails of both hands in older children and adults.
Musculoskeletal	*Frontal or parietal bossing.*(D) Localized thickening of these bones in skull.
	Epiphyseal enlargement.(C, D) Enlargement of ends of long bones, especially noted in radius and ulna at the wrist.
	Beading of ribs.(D) Symmetrical nodular enlargement of costochondral junctions in ribs. Comparable to epiphyseal enlargement noted in wrists.

Note: Letters in parentheses refer to deficiencies in the following nutrients: *A* = Vitamin A, *B* = B Vitamin Complex, *C* = Vitamin C, *D* = Vitamin D, *F* = Essential Fatty Acids, *I* = Iron, *K* = Vitamin K, *N* = Niacin, *P* = Protein, *R* = Riboflavin, *T* = Thiamine, *Z* = Zinc.

easy to obtain and, if proper equipment and techniques are used, are quite reliable, especially over time. Measurements of skinfold thickness and selected circumferences and lengths of the body allow indirect and noninvasive estimates of body composition that can be very useful in assessing the individual patient (see Chapter 7).

Physical signs and symptoms that have been associated with malnutrition may be categorized in two groups:

- *Group 1:* Signs that are often *associated* with nutritional deficiencies and, in fact, appear to be *caused* by deficiencies. Some signs are unique or specific manifestations of deficiency of a single nutrient; most reflect deficiencies of two or more nutrients.
- *Group 2:* Signs that *may be related* to malnutrition and that need further investigation.

Any physical finding that suggests a nutritional abnormality should be considered a clue, not a diagnosis. It should alert the examiner to search carefully for other signs and to undertake additional studies—for example, biochemical analysis—to elucidate the significance of physical signs. In evaluating cutaneous signs, environmental factors, such as excessive heat or sun, wind or cold, or lack of personal hygiene must be taken into account, along with ethnicity, age, and sex of the patient.

In Table 6–1, physical signs of malnutrition in Groups 1 and 2 cited above are categorized according to organ system. A more detailed description of various physical signs is provided in Table 6–2.

CONCLUSION

As noted by Figueroa-Colon[1] (Figure 6–1), easily recognizable clinical signs and symptoms are detected only in advanced stages of nutritional depletion.

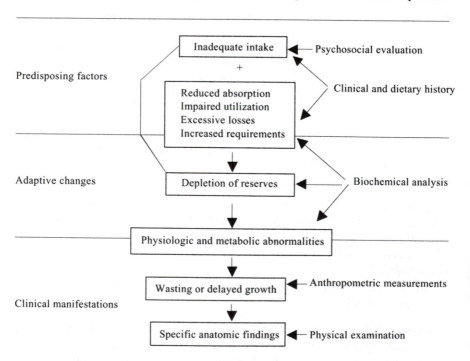

Figure 6–1 Levels of Nutritional Assessment in Relationship to the Natural History of Disease. *Source:* Reprinted from Figueroa-Colon, R., Clinical and Laboratory Assessment of the Malnourished Child, in *Textbook of Pediatric Nutrition*, R.M. Suskind and L. Lewinter-Suskind, eds., p. 192, with permission of Raven Press, © 1993.

Amalgamation of information obtained from social, dietary, and medical histories, anthropometric measurements, observations from physical examination, and selected laboratory determinations will allow earlier assessment of nutritional status.

REFERENCE

1. Figueroa-Colon R. Clinical and laboratory assessment of the malnourished child. In: Suskind RM, Lewinter-Suskind L, eds. *Textbook of Pediatric Nutrition*. 2nd ed. New York, NY: Raven Press, Ltd; 1993.

Chapter 7

Pediatric Anthropometric Techniques and Their Application

Gordon E. Robbins and Frederick L. Trowbridge

OVERVIEW

Healthy People 2000 set a national health agenda for making significant reductions in preventable death and disability concurrently while reducing the disparities in health status of subpopulation groups in our society and promoting an improved quality of life. To continue the progress made in the health status, of children, vigorous monitoring of growth should be one of the priorities of pediatric health providers. One health objective is to reduce growth retardation, especially among low-income children. Accurate anthropometric techniques and their interpretation for all pediatric populations served will help achieve this objective. Early identification of nutrition-related problems and early intervention strategies will reduce health problems and promote health.

INTRODUCTION

Anthropometric measurements, that is, measurements of size, weight, and proportions of the human body, are frequently the first step in assessing nutritional status. In children, physical growth is one of the best indicators of nutritional status; hence careful measurement is essential. Of the many measures of growth, those of length/stature and weight are most frequently obtained and provide the most useful information. Scientists continue to debate whether environmental influences, especially nutrition, are more important in determin-

93

ing body size than is genetics or other biological factors. However, nobody disputes the fact that the physical dimensions of the body are influenced by nutrition, especially during childhood. Therefore anthropometric measurements are highly useful in identifying certain types of malnutrition that affect body size and composition.

ANTHROPOMETRIC INDICATORS

Anthropometric indicators have long been used to identify individuals, particularly children, who are either "normal" or "malnourished" and who need preventive and/or therapeutic services.

Weight-for-Height Index

Weight-for-height is an anthropometric index that relates body mass to stature. Acute undernutrition, generally characterized by low weight-for-height, has been termed *wasting*. Conversely, overnutrition or *obesity* is characterized by high weight-for-height.

Height-for-Age Index

The height-for-age index is a measure of linear growth. Frequent periods of acute food deprivation or infection or a prolonged period of inadequate food intake—especially during the first two years of life when growth is most rapid—may cause measurable growth retardation. The result is a child who is low in height-for-age. This condition is called *stunting*. Although improved diet may result in an increase in height, some permanent growth retardation may occur, particularly if the period of stress or nutritional deprivation is prolonged. Whereas weight-for-height is generally interpreted as an indicator of present nutritional status, height-for-age is considered an indicator of long-term nutritional adequacy.[1,2]

Weight-for-Age Index

For many years, the weight-for-age index has been a basic tool for evaluating health and nutritional status in children. However, this index does not distinguish between present and long-term malnutrition. On the other hand, weight-for-age and height-for-age are both useful indexes when used in serial measurements of children under five years of age in clinic settings. Weight-for-age is particularly useful in regard to infants under one year of age, especially if length measurements cannot be performed accurately. In such cases, weight-for-age may be the most valid index of nutritional status.

An individual's height and weight values need to be expressed in relation both to each other and to reference population values. Thus height-for-age is the relationship of observed height to expected height for a specific age and sex; weight-for-age is the relationship of observed weight to expected weight for a specific age and sex; and weight-for-height is the relationship of observed weight to expected weight for a specific height and sex.

Head Circumference Index

Head circumference is usually assessed in determining the nutritional status of children, but it is not as useful as body length or weight in detecting malnutrition. Nevertheless, it is an important method of screening for variations in head size due to non-nutritional abnormalities, such as microcephaly and macrocephaly in children younger than two years of age. For selected centiles of head circumference for the first year of life see Appendix A.

Mid-Upper-Arm Circumference Index

Measurement of mid-upper-arm circumference, although recommended by the World Health Organization for use in developing countries and used in major surveys in the United States, has received little attention from clinicians.[3] However, this measurement can provide an estimate of arm soft tissue and, more specifically, of nutritional wasting. When arm circumference is used in conjunction with triceps skinfold thickness, an estimate of arm muscle area can be made that appears to correlate well with estimates of the body's muscle mass.[4] Some studies conducted in developing countries suggest that mid-upper-arm circumference may be almost as sensitive as height and weight in detecting children at high risk for morbidity and mortality.[5]

Triceps Skinfold Thickness Index

Triceps skinfold thickness is an anthropometric index that provides an estimate of body fat. This index is useful in determining whether an individual's heaviness is caused by excess body fat. Unlike the weight-for-height index, triceps skinfold thickness can be used to differentiate between an individual who is heavy because of muscle mass and one who is simply obese. This index requires attention to detail and considerable practice; even then, reproducible results are difficult to obtain. Its use should be limited to follow-up of individuals who have been found by other means to be overweight. Triceps skinfold thickness seldom proves to be practical as a routine screening measurement.

SELECTION OF ANTHROPOMETRIC METHODS

Recommendations on procedures and techniques for performing selected measurements (described below) are quite straightforward and vary little from procedural guidelines presented elsewhere.[6-8] Difficulties of considerable complexity emerge, however, when one is deciding which measurements to obtain for which age groups and in determining how to interpret the data. The selection of specific measurements and their interpretation will depend on whether the assessment is for routine monitoring or for diagnostic purposes and on the nature of any suspected nutritional abnormality.

Anthropometric indicators are most sensitive when applied to young children. For infants, routine measurements should always include weight and length of the child (when recumbent). Measurements of triceps skinfold thickness and arm circumference are useful when a nutritional abnormality, for example, obesity or wasting, is suspected. For older children and adults, height and weight are the most important measurements, although triceps skinfold thickness and arm circumference are useful as additional measures of overnutrition.

The proper interpretation of an anthropometric measurement may be obscured if it has not been made with sufficient accuracy or precision. *Accuracy* is the degree to which a measurement corresponds to a true value. *Precision* is the degree to which successive measurements of the same individual agree within specified limits. Thus it is possible to have precise measurements that are decidedly inaccurate.

MEASUREMENT PROCEDURES

There is a deceptive simplicity about obtaining measurements of the body, especially height and weight measurements. Sometimes, in fact, these measurements are regarded as so simple to obtain that they are done with little care or attention to detail. However, careful attention to proper equipment and procedures is imperative if measurement results are to be reliable.

Preparing the Patient

In general, before any measurements are obtained, the patient should be prepared as follows:

- Any physical handicaps or deformities that may prevent accurate measurements need to be identified and noted in the patient's record. Measurement of handicapped patients requires special techniques (not discussed in the present context).
- Only minimal indoor clothing, such as underwear or a clinic gown, should be worn. Coats, shoes, and head coverings must be removed. If an infant's diaper is not removed, allowance should be made for its weight.
- The patient's age must be determined and recorded. For children, it is important to calculate age to the nearest month. Children less than 24 months of age must be supine when their length is measured; children 24 to 36 months of age who are able to stand by themselves can be either supine or standing when they are measured. Children 36 months of age and older are always measured while they stand. An assistant is required for the proper measurements of children, especially those less than 24 months of age.
- If a child is unmanageable, the measurements should be obtained later when the child may be more cooperative. If the measurements must be made when the child is unmanageable, a note should be made that the measurements may be inaccurate.

Length Measurement

Equipment

For length measurement, measuring boards, such as that shown in Figure 7–1 can be used. These devices have a movable footboard and an immovable headboard, both of which are perpendicular to the measurement surface. The "0" mark on the measuring tape is at the fixed headboard. The footboard must slide easily and yet not be so loose as to cause inaccurate readings.

Technique

The child is placed on the measuring device parallel to the tape, with the crown of the head against the immovable headboard. The head should be facing directly

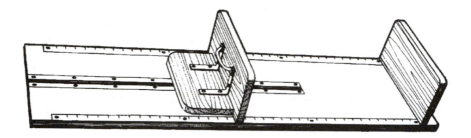

Figure 7–1 Measuring Board

up so that the child's line of sight is perpendicular to the measuring board. The assistant (clinic staff or parent) applies gentle traction to ensure that the child's head is firmly against the headboard until the measurement is completed.

The measurer then holds the child's knees together and pushes them down against the measuring board with one hand or forearm, thus *fully extending the child's legs*. With the other hand, the measurer slides the movable footboard to the child's feet until the *heels* of both feet touch the footboard (see Figure 7–2). The child's feet are then immediately removed from contact with the footboard with the measurer's one hand (to prevent the child from kicking and

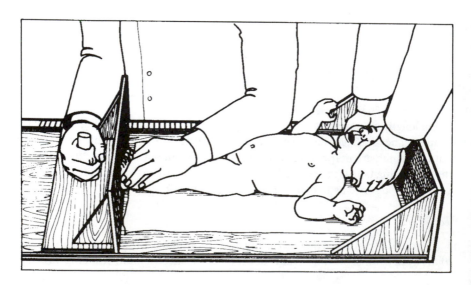

Figure 7–2 Technique for Measuring Child with Measuring Board

moving the footboard) while the footboard is held securely in place with the other hand.

The measurer reads the measurement to the nearest one-eighth of an inch. The measurement is repeated until two readings agree within one-fourth of an inch. The measurer reads aloud the second, confirming measurement and records it *immediately*.

Stature Measurement

Equipment

Platform scales with movable rods should *not* be used for measuring stature, since they tend to give inaccurate results. Rather, a vertical device (Figure 7–3) or a tape or measuring stick affixed to a true vertical surface, such as a wall, should be used. A movable headpiece, squared at right angles to the vertical surface, is essential. The "0" mark on the tape or measuring stick is at the foot level. The headboard must slide easily and not be loose or broken.

Technique

The patient should be told to stand "straight and tall" and to look straight ahead (Figure 7–4). The body is positioned so that the shoulder blades, buttocks, and heels are touching the wall or vertical surface of the measuring device. The feet must be flat on the floor, slightly apart, the legs and back should be straight, and the arms should be at the sides. The shoulders must be relaxed and in contact with the vertical measurement surface. The head is not necessarily in contact with the measurement surface.

The movable headboard is then lowered until it firmly touches the crown of the head, regardless of the patient's hairstyle. The stature is read to the nearest one-eighth of an inch. The assistant should ensure that the patient's knees are not flexed and the heels are not lifted from the floor. Adjustment of the headboard is repeated, and the child's stature is remeasured until two readings agree within one-fourth of an inch. The measurer then reads aloud the second, confirming measurement and records it *immediately*.

Weight Measurement

Equipment

For weight measurement, two types of beam-balance scales, with nondetachable weights, should be used. A pediatric scale with a pan (Figure 7–5) should be used

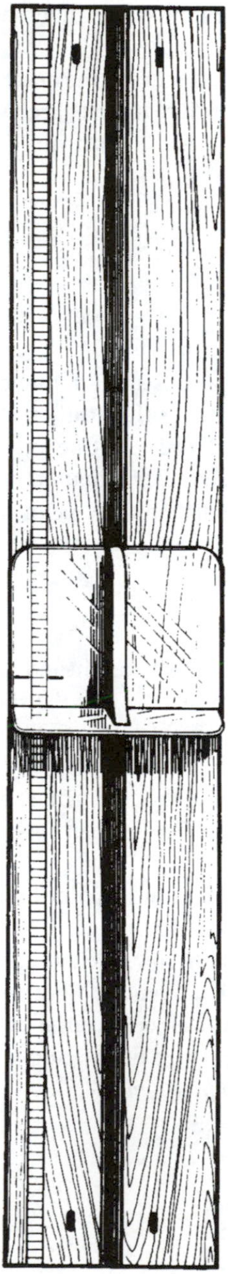

Figure 7–3 Vertical Measuring Device

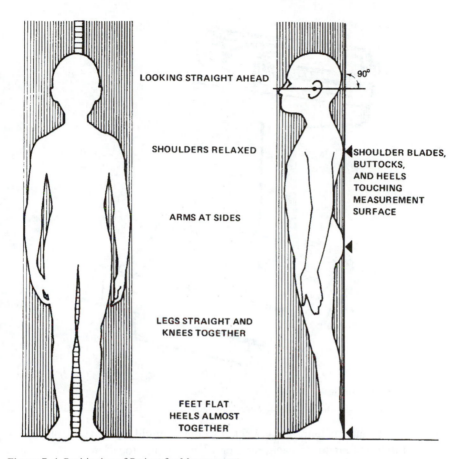

Figure 7–4 Positioning of Patient for Measurement

for infants and children who are too young to stand up or walk. They should be weighed lying down. This scale should be accurate to within one-half ounce (or ten grams). A standard platform-type, beam-balance scale (Figure 7–6) is suitable for older children. Bathroom or other spring-operated scales should *not* be used, as they are less reliable.

The horizontal beam needs to be checked for zero-balance several times a day. This requires removing any load, such as pads or clothing, from the scale. (If an infant is to be weighed on a pad or in a pan, the equipment must be zeroed with the pad or pan on the scale.) The weights on the main and fractional beams are placed directly over their respective zeros; then, by using the adjustment screw, the adjustable zeroing weight is moved until the indicator is centered and the

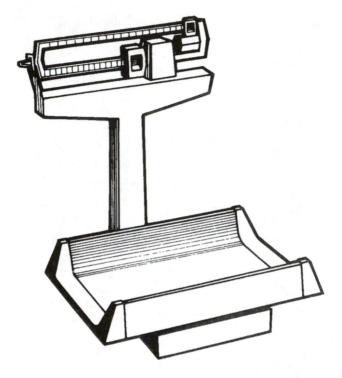

Figure 7–5 Pediatric Scale

scale is in balance (Figure 7–7). A set of weights should be used to calibrate the scale three or four times each year, or whenever the location of the scale is changed.

Technique

Infants may be weighed in a dry diaper if adjustment is made for diaper weight; all other patients should be weighed wearing *only* underwear or a clinic gown. Weighing passive infants is no problem, but there are difficulties with apprehensive infants and preschoolers. It is often best to use a standard beam-balance scale to weigh the mother alone and then weigh her carrying her child. However, though this method has a calming effect on the child, there is a disadvantage: two weights must be recorded, so the risk of recording error doubles.

Under some circumstances, patients must be weighed while they are dressed. In such situations, shoes *must* be removed, and the weight of the clothing worn must be determined and subtracted. Such details need to be recorded in the patient's record.

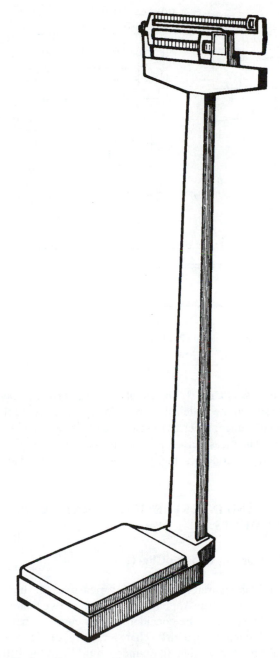

Figure 7–6 Standard Platform-Type, Beam-Balance Scale

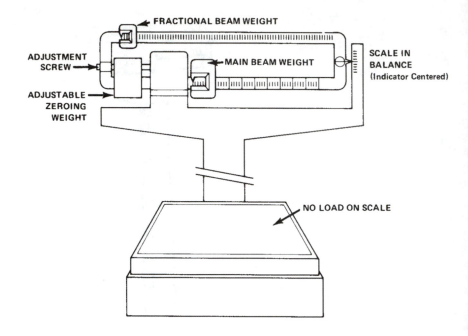

Figure 7–7 Checking the Scale for Zero Balance

In measuring weight, the sliding weights on the horizontal beam must be at the zero position so that the scale is in zero balance. Pediatric scales are read to the nearest one-half ounce; other beam-balance scales are read to the nearest one-quarter pound. The measurer weighs the child again until the first measurement is confirmed by a second; the measurer then reads it aloud and records it.

RECORDING AND INTERPRETING PEDIATRIC GROWTH MEASUREMENTS

Choosing the Correct Growth Chart

After the child is accurately weighed and measured, the next step is to choose the proper growth chart (see Appendix A). There are two factors to consider here. First, the child's sex must be considered. It is easy to arrive at an erroneous percentile level when using a girl's chart for a boy, or vice versa. For example, a five-year-old male weighing 34 pounds would be at the fifth percentile or at nutritional risk. However, if this value were plotted on a chart for girls, the child would appear to be above the tenth percentile (not at nutritional risk).

Second, the age of the child must be considered. For each sex there are three charts to choose from: (1) a chart for children birth to 36 months of age, (2) one for children 2 to 5 years old and (3) 2 to 18 years old. From birth to age two years, children must be supine when they are measured, and their measurements must be plotted on the birth to 36-month chart. When a child reaches two or three years of age, the child's infant chart should be attached to the new stature chart for that child (2 to 5 years). (Measurements for children aged 24 to 36 months can be recorded and plotted on any set of growth charts. If the child is supine when measured, measurements can be plotted on either set of growth charts. If the child is supine when measured, the length chart for ages birth to 36 months should be used. If the child is erect when measured, the stature chart for ages 2 to 5 or 2 to 18 years should be used.)

Inspection of charts aids in reviewing the child's growth pattern. The weights shown on the stature charts are for prepubertal children only—for girls from 2 to 10 years old and for boys 2 to 11½ years old. These charts should not be used for children who have begun to develop secondary sex characteristics.

Interpretation

Stature/length and weight data describe a child's size at a particular age. This information cannot be interpreted without making appropriate comparisons (1) with reference data, and/or (2) with earlier data obtained on the same child.

Reference Data Comparisons

Growth charts are based on the distribution of height and weight values for children in a reference population. The National Center for Health Statistics (NCHS) reference population is the one most widely used. This reference population is based on well-controlled body measurements data on children in the United States.[9] Growth curves based on these data have been developed in the form of both percentile curves and curves defined by standard deviations or z-scores.[10] Despite some technical limitations, these reference curves have proved to be highly useful for both clinical and public health use.[11] The World Health Organization has recommended these growth reference data for use internationally.[12] Updated growth charts based on the Third Health and Nutrition Examination Survey are planned, but data collection for this survey will not be completed until late 1994.[13]

Each growth chart contains a set of curved lines showing selected percentiles (5th, 10th, 25th, 50th, 75th, 90th, 95th). Plotting a height or weight measurement for a child on a growth chart permits evaluation of the child's size in relation to the reference population. For example, if the height measurement of a child falls on the 50th percentile curve of the growth chart, it means that the heights of half the children of the same age and sex in the reference population measured higher and half measured lower than that child's height. The child's growth pattern is thus average, compared with growth patterns for the reference population. The further away the plotted values are from the 50th percentile, the higher the probability that the child may have an abnormal growth pattern relative to the reference population (see Appendix A). However, most experts suggest that an abnormal growth pattern should be suspected only when a child's plotted values exceed the extreme percentiles (the 95th or the 5th).[14–20]

The growth chart is useful for detecting abnormalities of growth and thus for monitoring the nutritional status of children. It can give a continuous picture of major abnormalities or deviations from expected patterns of growth. Once such abnormalities have been detected, the chart provides a means of evaluating the impact of intervention measures (see Appendix A). Moreover, an explicit picture of the child's pattern of growth makes it easier to motivate parents during intervention efforts. The parents' support is imperative, for without it intervention efforts may be futile.

However, the growth chart is only as useful as the measurements are *precise* and *accurate*. To evaluate the growth status of an individual or of the population served, accurate measurements are essential. For example, a one-inch error in an infant's length can mean the difference between the child's growth being considered normal or needing follow-up.

Factors other than nutrition influence growth. Therefore growth data alone cannot be used to determine nutritional or health status. However, such data do allow the identification of children whose unusual growth patterns suggest nutritional or other health problems.

Common sense is the key to interpreting values for individual children. The NCHS growth curves provide a point of reference that is appropriate for most children. At the same time, familial and ethnic-group differences in growth patterns do exist and need to be considered. For example, the children of short parents are likely to be short themselves. Children who have a history of low birth weight or chronic illness, or who were subjected to economic deprivation early in life, such as those who are the children of refugee families, are likely to reflect this early experience in their growth status. Comparison of a child's growth with the reference population can help to identify the possibility of nutrition-related health problems and can also be used to monitor growth changes over time.

Generally, the following criteria indicate a potential problem and need follow-up:

- If a child's weight-for-height is at the 5th percentile or below, that child may be underweight (or "wasted") and should be referred for further assessment and counseling.
- If a child's height-for-age is at the 5th percentile or below, that child is at risk for linear growth retardation (or "stunting") and needs to be evaluated further.
- If a child has a weight-for-height at the 95th percentile or above, that child is overweight and possibly obese. A referral for further assessment and/or counseling is required.

Roche has described the growth assessment of handicapped children.[21] However, the nutrition problems for handicapped children who are severely disabled can be difficult to define.[22]

Comparison with Earlier Measurements

Although measurements at a single point in time provide insight into potential risk and the possible need for follow-up, data from several visits provide a more adequate basis for evaluating nutritional health. When plotted values obtained from a child during several visits are connected, the lines will follow or parallel the percentile lines if the child is growing normally. If the pattern of growth is irregular, it usually means either that the measurements are inaccurate *or* that one or more of the measurement values has been plotted incorrectly. "Flat" growth patterns or those that differ from the expected growth curve are cause for concern. Efforts should be made to identify the reason for such a growth pattern and, if necessary, to institute appropriate intervention.

For example, a girl aged 3½ years in a day care center was followed for one year (see Figure 7–8). Anthropometric measurements of height and weight were plotted on the growth chart, with her height within the normal range; however, her weight was consistently at or near the 5th percentile for her age. This consistent "slow growth" obtained over 12 months was of concern to the nurse for the day care program, who then initiated follow-up. The child was given a complete physical examination, laboratory analysis of a blood specimen, and a dietary evaluation. It was determined that she was anemic based on a comparison of her blood with accepted hemoglobin/hematocrit standards for her age and that she had a poor appetite along with an inadequate intake of nourishing foods. The nurse referred the parents to a dietitian, who provided nutrition counseling and further follow-up.

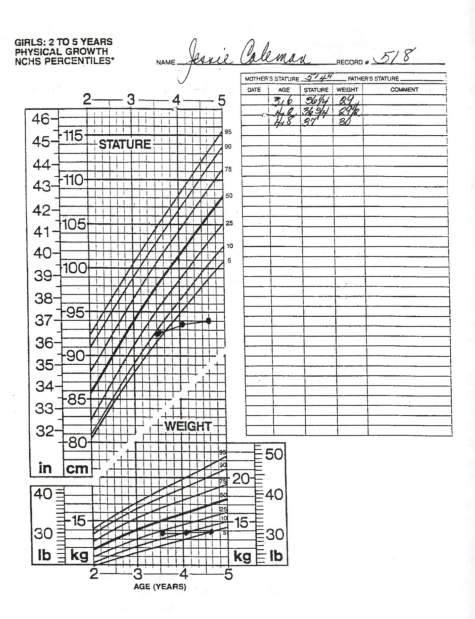

Figure 7–8 Weight Plotted on Growth Chart. *Source:* Used with permission from Moore WM and Roche AF. *Pediatric Anthropometry.* 2nd ed. Columbus, OH: Ross Laboratories, © 1983.

SELECTED BODY MEASUREMENTS

Mid-Upper-Arm Circumference

Equipment

A nonstretchable tape, 7 to 12 mm wide and made of fiberglass or laminated paper and plastic, is acceptable. Insertion tapes are preferred because they have a "window" for taking readings (Figure 7–9). A more flexible tape may be preferable for use with infants, since their soft arm fat is easily indented by a stiff tape, resulting in measurement errors.

Technique

The left upper arm* is measured midway between the top of the acromion process of the scapula and the olecranon process of the ulna, with the forearm flexed at 90° (Figure 7–10). A soft-tip pen is used to mark this location. While the arm is relaxed at the side, the insertion tape is drawn gently but firmly around the mid-upper arm (Figure 7–11). It should be pulled just tight enough to avoid

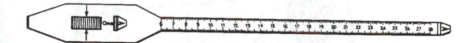

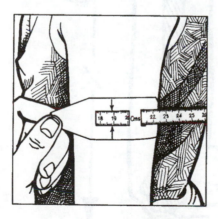

Figure 7–9 Insertion Tape

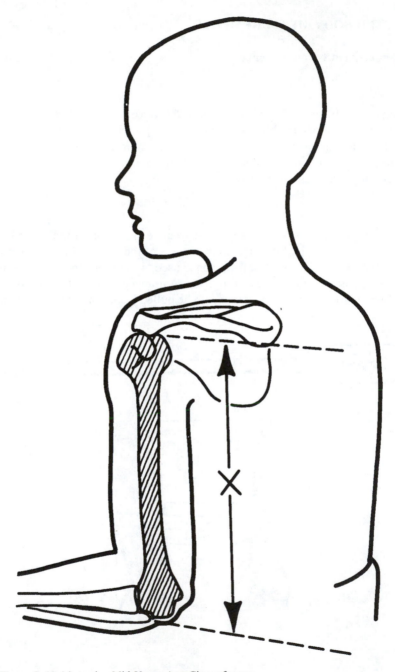

Figure 7–10 Measuring Mid-Upper-Arm Circumference

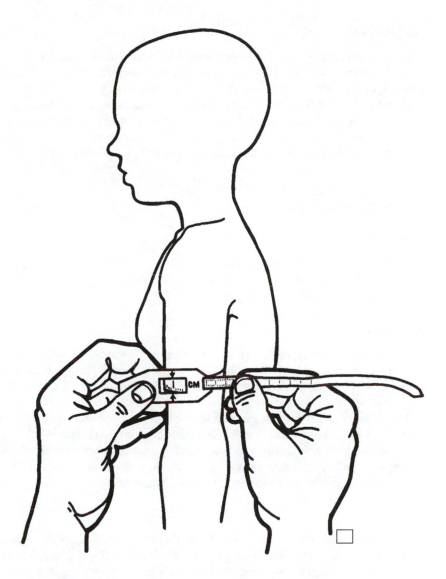

Figure 7–11 Use of Insertion Tape To Measure Mid-Upper-Arm Circumference

compression of the soft tissues. Readings are taken to the nearest millimeter; care should be taken not to crease the tape. When not in use, the tape should be hung on a hook or stored in some way that prevents folding or creasing the tape.

Interpretation

Reference standards for the interpretation of arm-circumference measurements have been developed from the same database used for developing height and weight standards—the National Health and Nutrition Examination Survey (NHANES–I) of 1971–1974.[23] Percentile distributions are presented for ages 1 to 74 years. As for height and weight, values that fall below the 5th percentile or above the 95th percentile, or that appear to be discrepant in relation to other anthropometric data for the individual, deserve follow-up evaluation.

Triceps Skinfold Thickness

Equipment

To measure triceps skinfold thickness, a flexible, nonstretchable tape measure and a skinfold caliper are required. A Lange, or Harpenden Holtain, or a reliable plastic caliper is suitable (see Appendix E).

Technique

While hanging freely, the left arm* is measured at its midpoint, as previously described. The skinfold parallel to the long axis of the arm is firmly grasped and slightly lifted between the finger and thumb of the left hand. Care should be taken not to include underlying muscle.

The calipers are applied at the midpoint of the arm about 1 cm below the measurer's fingers at the depth about equal to the skinfold (Figure 7–12). The skinfold should be held gently as it is measured. Excessive pressure should not be applied, and the reading should be made as quickly as possible. Three measurements should be made and the results averaged.

Interpretation

Norms for skinfold thickness based on the 1971–1974 HANES[23] permit evaluation of the percentile ranking of results by age and sex group. Triceps skinfold measurements may be combined with arm-circumference measurements to estimate arm muscle and arm fat areas. Such measurements may provide additional insight into the relative adequacy or excess of muscle and fat mass.

---

*Most current practice: The right arm is used for measurement in the US and the left arm is used for British measurement, regardless of favored side. (Telephone communication A. Roberto Frisancho, PhD, Professor of Anthropology, Research Scientist, Center for Human Growth & Development, University of Michigan, Ann Arbor, MI, August 18, 1994.)

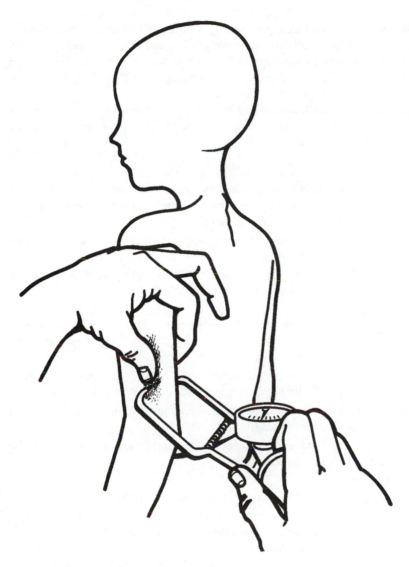

Figure 7–12 Measuring Triceps Skinfold Thickness

CAUSES OF INACCURACY

Measurement errors may not average out, either for individuals or for groups of children. Instead, certain errors may tend to occur in a consistent direction, resulting in biased results. For example, in clinics where many errors are made in measuring length, children, particularly infants, are commonly measured as being shorter than they really are. Since weight measurements generally are more accurate than length measurements in such situations, an artificially high proportion of children are reported as overweight for their length, and the prevalence of obesity may be exaggerated.

In general, the most frequent and most important causes of measurement inaccuracies are related to equipment, technique, and motivation. Some key factors that affect accuracy are as follows:

1. **Equipment**
   - The use of improper and inadequate equipment, such as bathroom and other spring-operated scales, and yardsticks or stretchable tapes not properly attached to a table or wall
   - Incorrect use of equipment (for example, failure to check periodically the zero balance on scales)
   - Inadequate maintenance of equipment, such as the use of worn, loose, or broken sliding headboards and footboards

2. **Technique**
   - Measuring the length of children when they are not properly positioned or extended; measuring infants without assistance; or trying to measure children who are unmanageable
   - The crown of the child's head should be firmly touching the headboard, and the head should not be tilting forward or backward
   - Failure to obtain a second, confirming measurement of the child's weight and stature or length
   - Failure to record measurements immediately and accurately on the child's record or growth chart

3. **Motivation**
   - Failure of measures to recognize the need for precision and accuracy
   - Lack of feedback to measurers, either on the accuracy of measurements they record or on the outcomes for patients who are referred for services because of measurements

---

REFERENCES

1. Waterlow JC. Classification and definition of protein-energy malnutrition. In Beaton GH, Bengoa HM, eds. *Nutrition in Prevention Medicine*. Geneva: World Health Organization; 1976: 530–555. World Health Organization micrograph series No. 62.

2. Waterlow JC, et al. The presentation and use of height and weight data for comparison of nutritional status of groups of children under the age of 10 years. *Bull World Health Org.* 1977;55:489–498.

3. *Expert Committee on Medical Assessment of Nutritional Status.* Geneva: World Health Organization; 1962.

4. Trowbridge FL, Hiney CD, Robertson AD. Arm muscle indicators and creatinine excretion in children. *Am J Clin Nutr.* 1982;36:691–696.

5. Chen LC, et al. Anthropometric assessment of energy-protein malnutrition and subsequent risk of mortality among preschool aged children. *Am J Clin Nutr.* 1980;33:1836–1845.

6. Moore WM, Roche AF. *Pediatric Anthropometry.* 2nd ed. Columbus, Ohio: Ross Laboratories; 1983.

7. United Nations National Household Survey Capability Program. *How to Weigh and Measure Children.* New York, NY: United Nations Dept of Technical Cooperation for Development; 1986. Statistical Office Publication DP/UN/INT-81-041/6E.

8. Cameron N. The methods of auxological anthropometry. In Faulkner F, Tanner JM, eds. *Human Growth: A Comprehensive Treatise.* 2nd ed. Vol 3. New York, NY: Plenum Press; 1986:3–46.

9. Hamell PV, et al. Physical growth: National Center for Health Statistics percentiles. *Am J Clin Nutr.* 1979;32:607–629.

10. Dibley MJ, et al. Development of normalized curves for the International Growth Reference: historical and technical considerations. *Am J Clin Nutr.* 1987;46:736–748.

11. Dibley MJ, et al. Interpretation of 2-score anthropometric indicators derived from the International Growth Reference. *Am J Clin Nutr.* 1987;46:749–762.

12. *A Growth Chart for International Use in Maternal and Child Health Care.* Geneva: World Health Organization; 1978.

13. Woteki CE, Briefel RR, Kuczmarski. Contributions of the National Center for Health Statistics. *Am J Clin Nutr.* 1988;47:320–328.

14. Fomon SJ. *Infant Nutrition.* St. Louis, Mo: Mosby-Year Book Inc.; 1993.

15. Shils ME, et al. *Modern Nutrition in Health and Disease.* Vol 2. Philadelphia, Pa: Lea & Febiger; 1994.

16. *Ross Growth Development Program.* Columbus, Ohio: Ross Laboratories; 1983.

17. Moore W, Roche AF. *Pediatric Anthropometry.* 3rd ed. Columbus, Ohio: Ross Laboratories; 1987.

18. *Measuring Change in Nutritional Status.* Geneva: World Health Organization; 1983.

19. Frisancho AR. *Anthropometric Standards for the Assessment of Growth and Nutritional Status.* Ann Arbor, Mich: University of Michigan Press; 1990.

20. Scott BJ, et al. Growth assessment in children: a review. *Top Clin Nutr.* 1992;8:5–26.

21. Roche AF. Growth assessment of handicapped children. *Diet Currents.* 1979;6:25–30.

22. Ekvall SW. *Pediatric Nutrition in Chronic Diseases and Developmental Disorders.* New York, NY: Oxford University Press; 1993:51–73.

23. Yetly E, Johnson C. Nutritional Applications of the Health and Nutrition Examination Surveys (HANES). *Ann Rev Nutr.* 1987;7:441–463.

Chapter 8

Adult Anthropometry

Barbara J. Scott, Sachiko T. St. Jeor, and Elaine B. Feldman

OVERVIEW

Anthropometry encompasses the physical, noninvasive measurements of the body's relative size and contours as well as the interpretation of these measurements including inferences of composition. Anthropometric measures at selected body sites vary depending on the intended use, practice setting, practicality, and intended applications, and utilize different available technologies. Measurements are interpreted in a variety of ways, including comparison with normative data and cutoff points or ranges indicating "normalcy" or risk. Various charts, nomograms, equations, and formulas are generally applied to help with the interpretation and utilization of anthropometric measures. These data are often used for public health and nutrition surveillance to monitor the health status of populations or at-risk subgroups. In clinical practice, individual reference values are used to monitor changes in nutrition status over time, assess the effectiveness of treatment or the course of disease, and evaluate overall health status or risk for development or exacerbation of disease.[1] As with any clinical tool or index, anthropometric measures have strengths and limitations. The strengths include ease of performance with relatively simple and inexpensive equipment, noninvasive techniques that can usually be performed in a clinic or field setting, and minimal training of personnel. The precision of measurements requires standardization of technique by trained individuals and the use of appropriate, accurate equipment. Examples of factors that can reduce precision include high staff turnover, poor equipment, and environmental conditions such as those encountered in a crowded clinic or temporary field site. The usefulness of anthropometric data for nutrition assessment for public health policy or for application to clinical practice may be limited by a lack of knowledge about certain population groups or by non-nutritional factors (such as genetics or disease) that impact the measurement results. These limitations can be minimized with good staff training and careful selection, use, and maintenance of equipment. Accurate interpretation of results must include an awareness of characteristics of the particular individual or group being studied and of the methods and populations used to derive assumptions and/or formulas being used.

Body weight is the most important single indicator of overall nutrition status in adults, and can be as important as the routinely assessed vital signs of body temperature, blood pressure, pulse rate, and respiration rate.[2] Height and weight should be measured routinely as part of the initial physical examination. Weight should be interpreted with reference to height, age, gender, and indicators of body fat distribution, and should be consistently monitored with each follow-up examination. The additional measures of body mass index, weight distribution, frame size, and body composition enhance the interpretation or usefulness of height and weight alone.

As a result of the current emphasis on fitness, the interest in and demand for personalized assessment of weight, weight distribution, and body composition have increased markedly. Consequently anthropometric measurements are now being done in nonclinical settings such as athletic departments of schools and universities, gyms, and health clubs. Body composition analyses are often accompanied by counseling regarding ideal weight and other diet and exercise recommendations. This increased interest in anthropometry necessitates a corresponding increase in the number of persons such as nutritionists, nurses, exercise physiologists, athletic trainers, and others who are *well trained* to both perform and interpret these measures with precision and accuracy. The *Anthropometric Standardization Reference Manual* reflects the consensus of experts in anthropometry for procedures for measurement of over 40 anthropometric dimensions and is an invaluable reference for such training.[3]

HEIGHT

Measurement

Most adults in developed countries can report their height with a reasonable degree of accuracy based either on previous measurements or on comparisons made with other adults. For this reason and because height is generally assumed to be static through the adult years, it is frequently assessed only by self-report. However, it is important to establish an accurate baseline height since this measure is integral to the evaluation of weight and the determination of body composition and is needed to assess shortening in later years caused by degeneration of intervertebral discs.

Staff members should receive initial training and periodic updates in performing careful measurement of height using a wall-mounted device (stadiometer) with a right-angle headboard that is wide enough to rest across the top of the head. The client should be measured in stocking feet and light clothing so that posture can be observed more clearly and positioning done correctly, with heels, buttocks, shoulders, and head against the wall and with the head positioned so the person is looking straight ahead, with the line of vision perpendicular to the body (Chapter 7, Figure 7–4). The measurer may need to stand on a step stool to be at eye level with the headboard and should record the height to the nearest 0.25 inch or 0.5 centimeter. Time of day (morning or afternoon) can also be recorded to allow for more accurate comparison with subsequent measures since height tends to be greater in the morning. When it is necessary to use the flexible rod on a balance beam scale, greater care is needed in positioning the patient and assuring that the rod is perpendicular to the upright section of the scale. Although frequency of height measurement is not as important in adults as in children, it should be done periodically (every three to five years) in younger adults and annually or biannually in persons over the age of 50.

Alternative Measures

Alternative measures may be needed to estimate stature in elderly individuals who have contractures or curvatures of the spine or who are unable to stand. Surrogate measures of long bone segments do not warrant repeated measurement in adults since they do not undergo significant reduction in length. The magnitude of reduction in height in the elderly varies widely (1.2 to 4.2 cm for every 20 years postmaturity) and can be attributed to postural changes (kyphosis or difficulty in standing fully erect due to muscular weakness) and to bone loss in the spine and/or legs.[4]

Special calipers are available[5] for measurement of knee height, which is highly correlated with stature.[6] This measurement is done with the person in a supine position, and can be used to estimate stature using a nomogram (not shown) or the equations developed by Chumlea et al[7]:

Women: Height (cm) = (1.83 × knee height [cm]) – (0.24 × age [yrs]) + 84.88

Men: Height (cm) = (2.02 × knee height [cm]) – (0.04 × age [yrs]) + 64.19

Similarly, it has been suggested that height can be estimated from arm span, measured as the distance between outstretched fingers of right and left hands, with arms extended laterally and maximally to the level of the shoulders.[3] The perception of equality between arm span and height dates back to the observations and drawings of Leonardo da Vinci and others, whose drawings of man in the square and circle were used as central themes of proportion in art and architecture. However, the earliest documented measures of span and height done in the 19th century demonstrated that span is more frequently greater than height.[8] More recently, investigation of the use of total arm length (TAL) (distance from the acromial process of the scapula to the end of the styloid process of the ulna) to estimate height in the elderly revealed a significant correlation (r = .63) between the TAL and height in 63 healthy subjects (mean age = 69.8 years).[9] This measure has greater ease of measurement than the arm span and may prove useful in the elderly for whom standing height is problematic. However, further studies are needed to completely validate this measure and provide useful conversion equations before it can be used clinically.

Interpretation of Measurement

Since height is used in conjunction with other parameters of weight and frame size, its independent interpretation is rarely necessary. However, any unexplained variations warrant remeasurement to verify accuracy, and decreasing measures over time should be noted. Height can be expected to decline with age at a rate of about 1.2 cm per 20 years postmaturity).[10] Height that decreases more rapidly than normal may be a sign of osteoporosis, which should be evaluated and treated.[11] Future studies that shed light on proportional distribution of height (sitting height, limb length, etc.) may be important in helping us to understand genetic differences and possible related risk for disease.

WEIGHT

Weight is the most widely used and misused anthropometric measurement. In addition to scientific and epidemiologic data that associate parameters of weight with health status, there are also very strong cultural and societal norms that associate weight, body size, and shape with beauty. Indeed, the obsession with weight supports a multimillion-dollar "diet" industry in the United States alone. Therefore, although the measurement of weight is simple, its interpretation can be problematic. Health professionals must be trained carefully to use accepted indices or standards and to avoid assumptions or conclusions influenced by their subjective judgment.

Measurement Methods

The platform balance scale is the preferred method for obtaining an accurate weight, and is available in most settings. Scales must be placed on a hard, level surface (never on carpet), and regular checking and calibration of scales is necessary to maintain accuracy. Scales should be set to zero, checked for balance after each weighing, and adjusted as necessary to achieve balance at the zero point. In addition, checking accuracy with standard weights should be done whenever a scale is moved and periodically depending on the frequency of use. This can usually be done annually by a representative of the state or county department of weights and measures. In a busy clinic or research setting, it is prudent to purchase a set of standard weights to use for monthly or quarterly checks.

In the hospital setting, it may be important to measure weight daily in some patients, and bed scales may be needed for patients who cannot stand. Detailed procedures and photographs of a commonly used bed scale are available.[12] Additional weights may be purchased to accommodate patients who exceed the upper limit of 350 pounds of most platform balance scales. Special platform scales are also available for weighing persons in wheelchairs. When body weight cannot be measured directly, it can be computed using the method described by Chumlea et al.[7] Weight of persons with amputations can be adjusted for comparison with tables of ideal weight if necessary by increasing their actual body weight by the percent "missing" as a result of their amputation. The contributions of weight by percent for individual body parts are: hand, 0.8 percent; foot, 1.8 percent; lower leg, 5.3 percent; upper leg, 11.6 percent; lower arm, 2.3 percent; and upper arm, 3.5 percent.[13]

Patients should be weighed under standard conditions to capture "true" weight, and measurements should be recorded to the nearest 0.25 pound or 0.1 kilogram. Ideally, clients should be weighed early in the morning, in underwear or paper gown, after having emptied the bladder and before eating or drinking. Practically, however, clinics should have clients remove shoes and outer clothing, empty their pockets, and remove heavy jewelry before weighing. When weight change is important for diagnosis or treatment, then time of day as well as food and fluid intake in the past two hours should be recorded to assist with interpretation of subsequent measures.

A comprehensive weight history can also provide valuable information that "fills in" the assessment picture of nutriture over time. Additionally, important psychological and behavioral factors regarding food intake and habits can be elicited and can contribute significant information to the interpretation of the resulting anthropometric measures. The history can include weight over the past 6 to 12 months, usual weight, preferred weight, highest and lowest adult weight, and patterns of normal weight fluctuation over time.[1]

Interpretation of Measurements

Although weight is readily available and simple to measure, it can be difficult to interpret. Because the components and distribution of weight (water, fat, lean tissue, and bone) can vary both within and among individuals, this deceptively simple measure must be interpreted with care when it is used to assess nutritional status.[14]

The most common use of the direct measure of weight is comparison with what is "ideal," "desirable," "recommended," or "healthy weight" for the person's height, age, and gender. Comparison with normative data is frequently done using tables developed in 1959 and 1983 by the Metropolitan Life Insurance Company[15,16] (see Appendix B). When the 1983 tables were first introduced, controversy and concern were expressed because the weight ranges had increased and because many believed that they overrepresented middle-class persons in good health and tended to exclude underweight (and possibly diseased) individuals and smokers. For these and other reasons, the 1959 tables were preferred over the more recent 1983 tables by many researchers[17–19] and were recommended for use especially in the presence of a family history or current indication of diseases or risk factors complicated by obesity.[20] Although the utility of these tables is limited by the purpose for which they were developed and the sample on which they were based, they continue to be used because of familiarity and ease of use. Recently, tables of "suggested weights for adults" have been published in conjunction with the 1990 dietary guidelines. These tables make no differentiation by gender but establish two categories of weight according to age (19–34 and 35 years and up) allowing for a little more weight (+10 to +16 pounds, depending on height) for older persons. The accompanying text indicates that the tables were developed using a combination of constructs associated with a long, healthy life, including weight-for-height standards and data indicating slight weight gain with age not associated with medical problems.[21] The scientific basis for these new suggested weights, which are higher than those previously recommended, is unclear, but there is concern that they may be based on analyses of life insurance data with inherent factors that bias the results toward optimal outcomes at higher relative body weights.[22]

Detailed reference data on mean weights of U.S. women and men aged 18 to 74 have been published by the National Center for Health Statistics. These detailed tables include percentile data (by gender, age, and height) derived from a relatively large and representative sample selected for the NHANES-I survey (1971–1974).[23] Although cumbersome, these tables allow for comparison by percentile of an individual's weight with that of an age-, gender-, and height-matched sample. Comparisons with population norms can provide some useful information, but they also raise additional questions such as how the population has changed since the survey was done, how closely the average weight represents the ideal, and how these data can be applied to persons over age 75. As the average life expectancy continues to increase, reference data for healthy persons in the 75- to 100-year range is increasingly necessary. A set of reference data for stature, weight, mid-arm circumference, triceps and subscapular skinfold thickness, weight over stature[2], and mid-arm muscle area has been developed based on a sample of 269 older persons aged 62 to 104 years.[7]

Several slightly different variations of a "rule of thumb" are frequently cited in nutrition texts to quickly and easily estimate ideal weight. For one commonly cited, an ideal weight for women of 100 pounds and for men of 106 pounds is assigned for 5'0", and an additional 5 pounds for women and 6 pounds for men is allowed for each inch above 5 feet.[24] For example, an ideal weight for a woman who is 5'6" would be 130 pounds (100 lbs + [6 in × 5 lbs]). Ideal weight for a man who is 6'2" would be 190 pounds (106 lbs + [14 in × 6 lbs]). In the above examples, the ideal weights estimated by the rule of thumb correspond to the 20th to 50th percentiles from the NHANES data for women and men (age 35–44 years) of these heights. Therefore, though rough, this method may yield reasonable results for healthy individuals whose usual weight is in the average range.

Significant controversy persists concerning whether the recommended weights should increase as the population gets heavier and what tables or guidelines to use for health screening or general health education. Reliance on normative data to establish healthy weight guidelines will continue to be fraught with difficulty until studies can establish the basis for identifying the weights associated with decreased morbidity and mortality.

Furthermore, the increasing prevalence of obesity and examination of the data on limited success of the myriad of weight loss programs have led some researchers to propose an additional type of more flexible weight guidelines to be used for overweight or obese persons. The concept of "achievable weight" or "reasonable weight" allows for individualization of treatment and modification of goals for persons in weight management programs whose weight has never been within the usual weight recommendations or for whom weight loss to recommended levels seems improbable.[25] Establishment of "reasonable weight" goals also allows for consideration of what is realistic given the patient's state of health, motivation, mobility, and metabolism. Thus recommended weight may be adjusted up or down as treatment of obesity progresses.

The phenomenon of weight loss followed by regain has received increased attention in recent years because of the association of weight gain with cardiovascular disease risk and overall mortality.[26] Studies have indicated significantly higher risk of cardiovascular disease in persons who both gained and lost large amounts of weight as compared with persons whose weight did not change or with persons who gained weight without a prior weight loss.[27] However, longitudinal epidemiologic studies are needed to distinguish systematic weight trends from normal or periodic weight fluctuations before clinicians can effectively counsel patients or provide intervention to prevent disease associated with weight fluctuation.

Self-Reporting of Weight and Height

The measurement of height and weight by researchers may not be feasible for large studies, and therefore collection of these data is often done by self-report from questionnaire or by in-person or telephone interview. Several studies of the difference between measured and self-reported height and weight have been done. The results vary depending on the type of self-reporting (in person or by telephone) and the population studied. A high degree of agreement for weight between measured and self-reported data has been reported in one study where 26 percent of the subjects reported their weight with no error, and 70 percent reported with a less than 2-kg difference.[28] On the other hand, results from another study where the height and weight data were collected in an in-home interview yielded different results.[29] In this study, all women tended to underreport their weight, while lower- and higher-weight men tended to respectively either overreport or underreport their weight. With regard to height, it was found that women (especially taller women) tended to underreport, and men (especially shorter men) tended to overreport. Based on these observations, regression equations were developed by gender for both height and weight that could potentially be used to adjust self-reported data for a large epidemiologic study. Another more recent study of the concordance between height and weight data collected by phone with measured data from previous participants in a weight loss program found a mean underreporting of weight in all subjects (female and male) of 2.3 kg, which did not seem to be influenced by gender, recency of weighing, or age.[30] However, degree of overweight did account for 10 percent of the variance observed between self-reported and measured weight, with greater discrepancies for the most obese persons. A mean overreporting of 1.8 cm of height was found with men, taller and older persons tending to overreport the most.

Some large studies will need to rely on self-reported weight and height data, and it appears that these data (especially those collected in person versus by mail questionnaire or telephone survey) may be used with some degree of confidence. Studies that use these data should attempt to identify the degree of accuracy or of under- or overreporting in different sample subgroups and include a discussion of the implications of these findings for the final results.

BODY MASS INDEX

Measures that represent relative weight for stature have been associated with mortality and morbidity.[31] The association of this measure of relative weight, or body mass index (BMI), with all-cause mortality exhibits a J-shaped curve. Lower values are associated with increased mortality from digestive and pulmonary diseases, and higher values are associated with increased risk for cardiovascular diseases, diabetes, and diseases of the gallbladder.[32] Different methods to express this relationship have been proposed that use some power of height in the ratio (wt/ht, wt/ht², wt/ht³, wt/htᵖ). The index developed by Quetelet many years ago [weight(kg)/height(meters)²] has become the most widely accepted index, and is the one that is most commonly referred to in discussions or applications of BMI. Whenever possible, attention should be given to the measurement of height and weight since reliance on self-reported weight and height can result in considerable underestimation of the BMI.[33]

This index may have advantages over height and weight used independently in that it is relatively easy to calculate and can be used readily for comparisons between women and men and persons of different heights. Nomograms have been developed to facilitate the determination of the BMI and can be used with measurements in pounds and inches or kilograms and centimeters.[6] Because the BMI does not distinguish weight from fat or lean tissue, its usefulness is enhanced by additional measures of body composition such as skinfold or circumference.

Interpretation

Several schemes or cutoff points have been developed for the interpretation of the BMI. In the United States, percentiles of weight for height were used to define ranges of BMI from the NCHS reference data (sample of 20- to 29-year-olds). Using these data, overweight was defined by the BMI at the 85th percentile for women (27.3) and men (27.8); severe overweight was defined by the BMI as greater than or equal to the 95th percentile (women = 32.3 and men = 31.1).[34] The cutoff points used in Canada also include the lower and middle ranges of BMI as follows: "BMI < 20 may be associated with health problems for some individuals, 20–25 is the 'Ideal' index range associated with the lowest risk of illness for most people, 25–27 may be associated with health problems for some people; and over 27 is associated with increased risk of health problems such as heart disease, high blood pressure, and diabetes."[35] Classification systems in Britain and Australia do not include the lowest BMI range, but extend the definitions on the higher ranges; normal range is 20–25; overweight is 25–30; severe overweight is 30–40; and massive overweight is over 40.[36] The interpretation of BMI using these cutoffs based on normative data must always include the following considerations: there is no assurance that the average weights of a population are healthy; by definition, these cutoffs will always define 15% of the adult population as overweight and 5% as obese; and as the average weight of the population increases, so do the cutoffs.[37] A nomogram to facilitate determining the BMI has been developed by Bray and is illustrated in Chapter 17.

FRAME SIZE

Measurement

Skeletal dimensions (bone length, density, and thickness) are important components of height and weight, and the measurement of stature is essentially equivalent to measurement of vertical bone length. Because measures of frame size are supplemental to height and estimate bone or body width, they are important contributors to the assessment and evaluation of body weight and can enhance the use of height-weight tables. Frame size can be conceptualized in different dimensions (general "body build," skeletal robustness, "big-boned," etc.). It cannot be measured directly; however, there is general agreement that measures used as surrogates for frame size should be distributed normally within a population, be highly correlated with lean or fat-free body mass, and not be correlated with fat. Many sites have been proposed for the estimate of frame size, including breadth measures (elbow, wrist, ankle, knee, shoulder, hip, and bony chest), ratio of height to wrist circumference, and biacromial and bitrochanteric diameters.[38] Comparison and evaluation of these methods are hindered by differences in the study samples of factors that are potentially related to frame size and may confound the data. These include age, gender, and ethnicity. There are no national reference standards for any of these measures except elbow breadth.

The ratio of the wrist circumference to height as proposed by Grant[39] to estimate frame size is widely cited, but has not been validated to meet the criterion of significant association with lean mass in a large sample of men and women and nonobese and obese individuals of varying ages. Measure of wrist breadth used alone has been validated as an indicator of frame size.[40]

In practice, the elbow breadth is currently the best measure of frame size for most applications because it has been validated, has reference standards, and is relatively simple and practical to measure.[41] In order to measure the elbow breadth, the subject raises the right arm perpendicular to the body, with the elbow flexed at 90 degrees and the back of the hand toward the investigator, who stands facing the subject. Calipers[42] are used to measure the distance between the bony protrusions of the elbow (epicondyles of the humerus). Slight pressure is applied to the calipers to compress soft tissue, and the measurement is done to the nearest 0.1 cm. Procedures for locating and measuring other sites using smaller sliding calipers or larger spreading calipers have been published.[43]

Interpretation

The elbow breadth is the indicator recommended for use with the 1983 Metropolitan Life Insurance Weight for Height Tables[16] (see Appendix B). Using NCHS data from both NHANES-I and -II, frame size has been defined at various ages for women and men by elbow breadth under the 15th percentile (small), in the 15th to 85th percentiles (medium), and over the 85th percentile (large).[44] Frisancho has also used the NCHS data to develop cutoff points that take into account the propensity to gain weight and lose height with age. An index (called Frame Index 2) was developed using the NCHS data to determine age- and sex-specific percentiles, where small, medium, and large frames correspond respectively to below the 25th, in the 25th to 75th, and above the 75th percentiles. Frame Index 2 is derived from the formula: [elbow breadth (mm)/stature (cm)] × 100. Tables are provided for gender and height by which the frame size can be determined from the Frame Index 2[14] (see Appendix B).

BODY COMPOSITION

Much work has been done over the past century to understand the composition of the human body and the progression and changes from childhood to old age. Many different methods have been devised to measure maturity and content of various structural tissues of fat, muscle, and bone.[45–47]

Measurements of the upper arm have been used traditionally in nutrition assessment as indicators of body stores of subcutaneous fat, and muscle mass has been measured as an indicator of tissue protein. Reference data are available for mid-arm triceps skinfold (TSF) (see Appendix C), arm circumference (AC) (see Appendix C), arm muscle circumference (AMC), and arm muscle area (AMA) (see Appendix C) for individuals from age 1 to 75 (NCHS) and for the elderly.[7] The AMA is generally thought to be a better index of muscle or lean tissue than the arm muscle circumference, and can be calculated from the fatfold and arm circumference using the formula $AMA(mm^2) = (ACmm - [3.14 \times TSFmm])^2/12.56$, or other formulas that help adjust for overestimation in overweight persons.[6] AMA can be determined readily from a nomogram[6] when a high degree of accuracy is not needed (see Appendix C). The measurements of arm circumference and triceps skinfold (Chapter 7, Figures 7–10, 7–11) are relatively easy to perform and are practical for most settings. Changes in these measures over time for an individual can be helpful to evaluate the efficacy of nutritional therapy or to diagnose protein-energy malnutrition.

Measures of percent body fat are used frequently as a component of fitness testing and in the evaluation of "ideal" weight. Underwater weighing has been the "gold standard" used to validate the more practical measures of circumference or skinfold. Newer methods that use simple physical measures to estimate body composition (primarily percent body fat) include bioelectrical impedance analysis (BIA)[48] and near-infrared interactance (NIR).[49]

Two types of medical calipers, the Lange and the Harpenden Holtain, are designed to measure the thickness of skin and subcutaneous fat, and provide constant tension between the jaws. The Harpenden Holtain calipers are preferred by some because the larger surface area at the jaws may reduce compressibility of skin and because the gauge can be read with a greater degree of precision. However, this requires the investigator to note the number of rotations on the inner dial for measures in multiples of 10 and to add incremental measures from the outer dial. Therefore the Lange calipers may be easier to interpret because the reading is taken directly from the gauge. Additionally, the jaws of the Lange caliper open wider and may be used with more obese subjects. The Harpenden Holtain calipers exert greater pressure/mm^2 and produce slightly lower values. Therefore investigators should use only one type of caliper to get reliable results.[50] Other types of less expensive, simpler calipers are available,[51] but little is known about the precision and accuracy of their measures.

Consistent and careful training and practice are required in order to achieve proficiency, reliability, and validity with skinfold measures. Personnel should be trained, certified, and recertified periodically by someone who is experienced in the use of skinfold calipers. The fatfold is grasped firmly between the fleshy end of the thumb and forefinger (fingernails cut short). Care must be taken to grasp only fat and not underlying muscle, and the subject can be asked to flex the underlying muscle if necessary to make this determination. The calipers are placed over the skinfold and in line with the contour of the body such that they neither push into the body nor pull the skinfold away. The "pinch" or grasp on the skinfold is maintained without undue compression as the calipers are placed and the reading is taken. The measurer's eyes should be directly above the gauge (using a step stool if necessary) in order to read it accurately. Three measures taken consecutively should agree within 0.5 mm before the average is recorded to the nearest 0.5 mm. Care should be taken to compress the handle of the calipers to completely open the jaws before removing them from the skinfold. Detailed procedures and photographs for measuring various skinfold sites[3,50] and for calibrating the Lange calipers[12] are available and should be utilized by all personnel who perform skinfold measurements.

Interpretation

Various prediction equations have been proposed for the estimation of body fat from different sites of skinfold measures and have been validated against underwater weighing. These vary depending on the sample used in the study (gender, degree of leanness or fatness, and age of the subjects). Sites commonly selected that reflect gender-appropriate upper and lower body adiposity include triceps, subscapular, chest, abdomen, suprailiac, and thigh.

Equations developed and validated by Jackson and Pollock for relatively diverse samples[52,53] contain skinfold measures for women and men that have been widely used:

> Women: % Body Fat = (495/Body Density) – 450
>
> Body Density = $1.0994921 - (0.0009929 \times a) +$
>
> $(0.0000023 \times a)^2 - (0.0001392 \times c)$

> Men: % Body Fat = (495/Body Density) – 450
>
> Body Density = $1.10938 - (0.0008267 \times b) +$
>
> $(0.0000016 \times b)^2 - (0.0002574 \times c)$

> a (women) = sum of triceps, thigh, and suprailium skinfolds
> b (men) = sum of chest, thigh, and abdomen skinfolds
> c (both) = age

Tables have been developed that use these equations to convert the sum of the skinfolds to percent body fat for adults 18 to $\geq$ 58 years (in five-year increments).[50] They also provide a method to establish a body composition profile for an individual by recording percent body fat and/or individual skinfold measurements on age-group- and gender-specific tables for comparison by percentile and descriptive categories (very lean to over fat).[50] Other widely cited equations to estimate body fat were developed by Durnin and Womersley.[54]

Additionally, Katch and McArdle have determined that combinations of circumference measures can be used to estimate body fat for moderately active younger (ages 17–26) and older (ages 27–50) adults of average weight (not very thin or very obese).[47] These include abdomen, right thigh, and right forearm (young women); abdomen, right thigh, and right calf (older women); right upper arm, abdomen, and right forearm (young men); and buttocks, abdomen, and right forearm (older men). The measurement methods and the five-step procedure to calculate percent body fat, fat weight, and lean weight from the circumferences are clearly described.

BODY FAT DISTRIBUTION AND WAIST TO HIPS RATIO

A recognition of the importance of adipose tissue distribution to disease risk has been growing. Much research remains to be done to clarify the exact mechanisms of this relationship and to develop adequate ways to measure this distribution.[55] Intra-abdominal adipose tissue is thought to be of particular significance to disease risk because of its high lipolytic activity and anatomic connection to the hepatic portal vein.[56] Several studies have demonstrated the importance of this pattern of fat distribution, upper versus lower body as characterized by the ratio of the waist to hip circumference (WHR), to risk for development of cardiovascular and other diseases. In this method of classifying obesity, the android (male, or "apple shape") type is characterized by predominance of obesity in neck, cheeks, shoulders, and upper half of the abdomen, in contrast to the gynoid (female, or "pear shape") type with obesity primarily in the lower abdomen, hips, buttocks, and thighs. Although both patterns of obesity occur in men and women, it is not clear whether the patterns of risk from upper body obesity differ by gender, and therefore whether the WHR is a more useful indicator of risk for men who may tend to deposit visceral fat at the waist than for women who may deposit subcutaneous fat.[57]

Although calculation of the WHR is simple, the measurement of waist and hips can be problematic, as evidenced by the varying definitions and methods used in studies of fat distribution in relation to disease risk. The anatomical landmarks for waist circumference have been defined in several ways: as the level of the umbilicus; as the midpoint between the lower rib margin and the iliac crest; or as the "natural waist" at the smallest waist circumference. Similarly, hip circumference has been measured at the iliac crest or at the maximum circumference of the buttocks. Depending on the definition used, these circumferences can be difficult to determine or pinpoint in very obese subjects and even in relatively normal weight persons with "beer bellies" or thighs that are larger than the buttocks. Therefore, for the purposes of standardization, the waist circumference should be represented by the "natural waist" (smallest waist circumference) and should be taken with a nonstretchable tape measure and recorded to the nearest 0.5 cm. The subject can breathe out gently as measurement is made and should stand erect with arms at the side and feet together. If there is no natural waist (as in the person with a "beer belly" or pendulous abdomen), the measure should be made at the level of the umbilicus, and this method should be noted.[57] Hip circumference should be represented by the maximum circumference of the buttocks and also be recorded to the nearest 0.5 cm.

Interpretation

A waist:hip ratio of over 0.8 for women and over 0.9 for men has been used as an indicator of risk for cardiovascular disease (CVD) and diabetes,[58] and a WHR of over 1.0 has been used for both genders to indicate a significant increase in CVD risk.[59] Abdominal obesity appears to be the important factor in disease risk. It is therefore necessary to use caution in the interpretation of the WHR in lean or normal weight individuals since it is possible that it is primarily the absolute abdominal size that contributes to the usefulness of the WHR.[60] It is clear that adipose tissue distribution is but one of the many factors contributing to the relationship of obesity and disease. An approach to estimating levels of risk (very low to very high) associated with overweight using a matrix of both BMI (five levels for both genders: 20–<25; 25–<30; 30–<35; 35–<40; and ≥40) and WHR (three levels: for women, <.70, .70–.85, and >.85; for men, <.85, .85–1.0, and >1.0) has been proposed.[37] In addition, top researchers at a recent workshop on obesity recommended that research initiatives aimed at building bridges between basic research and treatment and prevention practices be given high priority.[61] They particularly underscored the need for research aimed at better characterization and definition of obesity in various subgroups and the implications for etiology and treatment.

CONCLUSION

Overall, although the simplest anthropometric measurements of height and weight (vital signs) go a long way toward defining body size and composition, an array of other supplementary measures add to the sophistication and utility of anthropometry. All measures must be validated and performed with precision and accuracy. Personnel must be trained in the applications and interpretations of the results and be prepared to counsel and advise the subjects they examine.

Many researchers are currently pursuing a better understanding of the relationships of these anthropometric measures with other risk factors for disease. As practitioners, we will need to stay abreast of these rapidly emerging findings in order to provide the best services to our clients.

REFERENCES

1. St. Jeor ST, Scott BJ. "Weight" as a clinical indicator: adults. *Top Clin Nutr.* 1991;7:44–51.

2. Feldman EB. *Essentials of Clinical Nutrition.* Philadelphia, Pa: FA Davis Co; 1988:chap 3.

3. Lohman TG, Roche AF, Martorell R, eds. *Anthropometric Standardization Reference Manual.* Champaign, Ill: Human Kinetics Books; 1988.

4. Mitchell CO, Lipschitz DA. Detection of protein-calorie malnutrition in the elderly. *Am J Clin Nutr.* 1982;35:398–406.

5. Medical Express, 5150 S.W. Griffeth Dr., Beaverton, OR 97005. Phone: 503-643-1670.

6. Gibson RS. *Principles of Nutrition Assessment.* New York, NY: Oxford University Press; 1990.

7. Chumlea WC, Roche AF, Mukherjee D. *Nutritional Assessment of the Elderly Through Anthropometry.* Columbus, Ohio: Ross Laboratories; 1987.

8. Schott GD. The extent of man from Vitruvius to Marfan. *Lancet.* 1992;340:1518–1520.

9. Mitchell CO, Lipschitz DA. Arm length measurement as an alternative to height in nutritional assessment of the elderly. *J Paren Enter Nutr.* 1982;6:226–229.

10. Lipschitz DA, Mitchell CO. Nutritional assessment of the elderly—special considerations. In: Wright RA, Heymsfield S, eds. *Nutritional Assessment.* Boston, Mass: Blackwell Scientific Publications; 1984:131–139.

11. Remig VM, Shumaker NS, St. Jeor ST. Weight as a clinical indicator: elderly. *Top Clin Nutr.* 1993;8:16–25.

12. Jensen TG, Englert D, Dudrick SJ. *Nutritional Assessment: A Manual for Practitioners.* Norwalk, Conn: Appleton-Century-Crofts; 1983:53–64.

13. Brunnstrom MA. *Clinical Kinesiology.* 3rd ed. Philadelphia, Pa: FA Davis; 1981.

14. Frisancho AR. *Anthropometric Standards for the Assessment of Growth and Nutritional Status.* Ann Arbor, Mich: University of Michigan Press; 1990.

15. Metropolitan Life Insurance Company. New weight standards for men and women. *Stat Bull.* 1959;40:1–4.

16. Metropolitan Life Foundation. 1983 Metropolitan Height and Weight Tables. *Stat Bull.* 1983;64:2–9.

17. Schulz LO. Obese, overweight, desirable, ideal: where to draw the line in 1986. *J Am Diet Assoc.* 1986;86:1702–1704.

18. Weigley ES. Average? ideal? desirable? A brief overview of height-weight tables in the United States. *J Am Diet Assoc.* 1984;84:417–423.

19. Barn SM, Hawthorne VM. The "new" Metropolitan weight tables. *Am J Clin Nutr.* 1984;39:490–491.

20. Burton T, Foster WR, Hirsch J, VanItallie TB. Health implications of obesity: an NIH consensus development conference. *Int J Obes.* 1985;9:155.

21. US Dept of Agriculture, US Dept of Health and Human Services. *Nutrition and Your Health: Dietary Guidelines for Americans.* 3rd ed. Washington, DC: US Government Printing Office, 1990. Home and Garden Bulletin No. 232.

22. Willett WC, Stampfer M, Manson J, VanItallie T. New weight guidelines for Americans: justified or unjudicious? *Am J Clin Nutr.* 1991;53:1102–1103.

23. National Center for Health Statistics. *Weight by Height and Age for Adults 18–74 Years: United States, 1971–1974.* Hyattsville, Md: Dept of Health and Human Services; 1981. PHS publication no. 81-1669. Vital and health statistics: Series 11, Data from the National Health Survey; no. 219.

24. Dikovics A. *Nutritional Assessment: Case Study Methods.* Philadelphia, Pa: George F. Stickley Co; 1987.

25. Brownell KD, Wadden TA. Etiology and treatment of obesity: understanding a serious, prevalent, and refractory disorder. *J Consult and Clin Psychol.* 1992;60:505–517.

26. Ashley FW, Kannel WB. Relation of weight change to changes in atherogenic traits: the Framingham Study. *J Chronic Dis.* 1974;27:103–114.

27. Hamm P, Shekelle RB, Stamler J. Large fluctuations in body weight during young adulthood and twenty-five-year risk of coronary death in men. *Am J Epidemiol.* 1989;129:312–318.

28. Stunkard AJ, Albaum JM. The accuracy of self-reported weights. *Am J Clin Nutr.* 1981;34:1593–1599.

29. Pirie P, Jacobs D, Jeffery R, Hannan P. Distortion in self-reported height and weight data. *J Am Diet Assoc.* 1981;78:601–606.

30. DelPrete LR, Caldwell M, English C, Banspach SW, Lefebvre C. Self-reported and measured weights and heights of participants in community-based weight loss programs. *J Am Diet Assoc.* 1992;92:1483–1486.

31. Willett W. *Nutritional Epidemiology.* New York, NY: Oxford University Press; 1990.

32. Lew EA, Garfinkel L. Variations in mortality by weight among 750,000 men and women. *J Chronic Dis.* 1979;32:563–576.

33. Kuskowska-Wolk A, Bergstrom R, Bostrom G. Relationship between questionnaire data and medical records of height, weight and body mass index. *Int J Obesity.* 1992;16:1–9.

34. US Dept of Health and Human Services, Public Health Service. *The Surgeon General's Report on Nutrition and Health.* Washington, DC: US Government Printing Office; 1988. DHHS (PHS) Publication No. 88-50210.

35. *Canadian Guidelines for Healthy Weights. Report of an Expert Committee Convened by Health Promotion Directorate, Health Services and Promotion Branch, Health and Welfare, Ottawa.* Ottawa: Health and Welfare Canada; 1988.

36. National Academy of Sciences, National Research Council, Food and Nutrition Board. *Diet and Health: Implications for Reducing Chronic Disease Risk.* Washington, DC: National Academy Press; 1989.

37. Bray GA. Fat distribution and body weight. *Obes Res.* 1993;1:203–205.

38. Himes JH, Frisancho RA. Estimating frame size. In: Lohman TG, Roche AF, Martorell R, eds. *Anthropometric Standardization Reference Manual.* Champaign, Ill: Human Kinetics Books; 1988;121–124.

39. Grant JP. *Handbook of Total Parenteral Nutrition.* Philadelphia, Pa: WB Saunders Co; 1980.

40. Himes JF, Bouchard C. Do the new Metropolitan Life Insurance Weight-Height Tables correctly assess body frame and body fat relationships? *Am J Public Health.* 1985;75:1076–1079.

41. Frisancho AR, Flegel PN. Elbow breadth as a measure of frame size for US males and females. *Am J Clin Nutr.* 1983;37:311–314.

42. Inexpensive elbow breadth calipers are available from the Metropolitan Life Insurance Company, Health and Safety Education Division, One Madison Ave, New York, NY 10010.

43. Wilmore JH, et al. Body breadth equipment and measurement techniques. In: Lohman TG, Roche AF, Martorell R, eds. *Anthropometric Standardization Reference Manual.* Champaign, Ill: Human Kinetics Books; 1988:27–38.

44. Frisancho AR. New standards of weight and body composition by frame size and height for assessment of nutritional status of adults and the elderly. *Am J Clin Nutr.* 1984;40:808–819.

45. Forbes GB. Body composition in adolescence. In: Falkner F, Tanner JM, eds. *Human Growth: A Comprehensive Treatise.* Vol 2. New York, NY: Plenum Press; 1986:119–145.

46. Hill GL. Body composition research: implications for the practice of clinical nutrition. *J Paren Enter Nutr.* 1992;16:197–218.

47. Katch FI, McArdle WD. *Nutrition, Weight Control, and Exercise.* Philadelphia, Pa: Lea & Febiger; 1988.

48. Svendsen OL, Haarbo J, Heitmann BL, Gotfredsen A, Christiansen C. Measurement of body fat in elderly subjects by dual-energy x-ray absorptiometry, bioelectrical impedance, and anthropometry. *Am J Clin Nutr.* 1991;53:1117–1123.

49. McLean KP, Skinner JS. Validity of Futrex-5000 for body composition determination. *Med Sci Sports Exerc.* 1992;24:253–258.

50. Golding LA, Myers CR, Sinning WE, eds. *Y's Way to Physical Fitness.* 3rd ed. Champaign, Ill: YMCA of the USA; 1989.

51. Ross Laboratories, 625 Cleveland Avenue, Columbus, OH 43216.

52. Jackson AS, Pollock ML. Generalized equations for predicting body density of women. *Med Sci Sports.* 1980;32:563–576.

53. Jackson AS, Pollock ML. Generalized equations for predicting body density of men. *Br J Nutr.* 1978;40:497–504.

54. Durnin JV, Womersley J. Body fat assessed from total body density and its estimation from skinfold thickness: measurements on 481 men and women aged from 16 to 72 years. *Brit J Nutr.* 1974;32:77–97.

55. Seidel JC. Regional obesity and health. *Int J Obes.* 1992;16 (Suppl.2):S31–S34.

56. Terry RB, Stefanick ML, Haskell WL, Wood PD. Contributions of regional adipose tissue deposits to plasma lipoprotein concentrations in overweight men and women: possible protective effects of thigh fat. *Metab.* 1991;40:733–740.

57. VanItallie TB. Topography of body fat: relationship to risk of cardiovascular and other diseases. In: Lohman TG, Roche AF, Martorell R, eds. *Anthropometric Standardization Reference Manual.* Champaign, Ill: Human Kinetics Books; 1988;143–149.

58. Gray DS. Diagnosis and prevalence of obesity. *Med Clin North Am.* 1989;73:1–13.

59. US Dept of Agriculture. *Dietary Guidelines and Your Diet: Eat a Variety of Foods.* Washington, DC: US Government Printing Office; 1986. Home and Garden Bulletin No. 232-1.

60. Scott BJ, Brunner RL, St. Jeor ST. A closer inspection of the predictive value of waist to hips ratio for cardiovascular risk. Presented at the Annual Meeting of the North American Society of the Study of Obesity; October 1991; Sacramento.

61. St. Jeor ST, Brownell KD, Atkinson RL, et al. Obesity: workshop III. *Circ.* 1993;88:1391–1396.

Chapter 9

Interaction of Drugs with Foods and Nutrients

Mary J. Mycek

OVERVIEW

During the past two decades, the identification of a number of interactions between drugs (medications) and foods or nutrients led the Joint Commission on Accreditation of Healthcare Organizations to require dietitians to monitor such reactions. The importance of these interactions continues to command attention because many of them result in variability to the response to the medications or produce serious adverse effects compromising an individual's health.[1-7] For example, they may cause harm necessitating either a cessation of the drug's use, a decrease in dosage, or administration of an essential nutrient because the response to the drug has been altered or the nutrient availability affected. On the other hand, not all such interactions are untoward. Some are beneficial and indeed are the basis of the drug's action. This chapter will not be an exhaustive compilation of all such interactions. Those interactions that are most important or illustrate significant concepts will be considered, and the underlying mechanisms, that is, drug- or food-induced effects at the level of absorption, metabolism, utilization, and excretion will be examined.

Although all patients may experience drug–nutrient interactions, those receiving a relatively large number of drugs (five or more) over a long period of time are especially at risk. The chronically ill elderly fall into this category.[2] They frequently are treated with many medications, some of which have a potential for serious adverse effects if conditions alter their bioavailability (e.g., theophylline, digoxin). Thus it is no surprise that adverse drug reactions in the elderly have been reported to occur two to three times more frequently than in young adults. What fraction of these are due to drug–nutrient interactions has not been identified. This information is particularly difficult to acquire due to the lack of control of people's diets. With the number of elderly increasing, drug interactions will continue to be a significant problem with which to contend in this population. Optimal nutritional health and therapeutic benefit depend on the ability to anticipate and to recognize such interactions and on understanding the processes responsible for them.

BACKGROUND

The fact that foods or particular nutrients can have an influence on a response to a drug is not surprising since both are inextricably linked to the health of an individual. It is well established that the ingestion of diets deficient in nutrients can lead to disease states and that modification of diet can aid in preventing or reversing the problem. That foods or dietary constituents can produce "cures" or prevent certain conditions is an opinion widely held by the general public and even some scientists. Consider the use of chicken soup to alleviate flu symptoms and megadoses of vitamin C for the prevention of colds. Though controversial, data exist to support both viewpoints. Furthermore, some drugs may suppress appetite directly (anorectic agents such as phentermine [Fastin®]) or indirectly (the cancer chemotherapeutic agents, which often result in vomiting as a side effect), whereas other drugs can stimulate appetite directly (anabolic steroids) or indirectly (tranquilizers). The latter effects were expected since they were the basis for the drug's design or readily inferred from the drug's actions. Other interactions, though now readily understood, were not expected and have only become appreciated after being encountered in the clinical setting. No doubt, more will be identified in the future.

In developing new drugs, the measure of response to a drug is generally described by a dose–response curve, which relates the dose to a particular response, be it therapeutic or deleterious (toxic), in a population of subjects. On the basis of such information obtained in clinical trials, the pharmaceutical company markets the agent in particular dosage forms. A drug's safety depends on how close the toxic effect is to the therapeutic one. It is said to have a narrow therapeutic window if its effective therapeutic dose is very close to the dose that produces an untoward effect. Likewise, unwanted effects may be obtained if a drug has a steep dose–response relationship (that is, if a small increase or decrease in dose has a major effect on the response). Any situation that can alter the drug's level in the body (e.g., increasing the dose or availability of the drug) can favor an unwanted situation, for adverse effects are often seen at higher drug levels. Conversely, the availability of a drug can also be decreased (e.g., due to lowered absorption or rapid biotransformation) so that the desired beneficial effect is not achieved.

The manner in which the body handles a drug is no different from the way it handles dietary components; thus it is not surprising that interactions can occur. A review of processes that determine the fate of a drug in the body after oral administration may aid in comprehending the basis for the different types of interactions between foods or nutrients and drugs. The term applied to the processes describing the body's handling of drugs is *pharmacokinetics*.

Absorption of a drug after oral ingestion depends on many factors, such as the particle size of the medication (usually the smaller the drug particle after disintegration, the more soluble), the presence or absence of food in the stomach, the pH (either gastric or intestinal), and the presence of special transport systems. Unless transported, most drugs enter the circulation by passive diffusion down a concentration gradient, which relies on the drug's being soluble in the lipoprotein membranes of the gastrointestinal tract. This property is generally associated with the nonionized (undissociated) form of a drug. Depending on its structure (weak acid or base), the drug will undergo ionization in the stomach or farther along the gastrointestinal tract. For example, at the acidic pH of the stomach, the nonionized form of an acid will predominate ($R\text{-}COO^- + H^+ \rightleftharpoons R\text{-}COOH$), and the opposite will be true for a compound with an amine substituent ($R\text{-}NH_2 + H^+ \rightleftharpoons RNH^{3+}$). Thus the relatively nonpolar uncharged form of the acidic drug will be more readily absorbed in the stomach rather than in the intestine, where the more alkaline pH favors the ionized form of the acid, and vice versa for the basic drug. A special active transport system for a substance may exist (as in the case of some vitamins and sugars); drugs that are analogs of these may be absorbed through these pathways. Obviously, an individual's nutritional state may become impaired if the drug interferes in the absorption of the essential nutrient.

When taken with food, some drugs are partially destroyed or absorbed more slowly. The presence of food delays gastric emptying time, meaning that the time a medication resides in the acidic environment of the stomach contents is prolonged. This explains why effective plasma levels of a drug like benzylpenicillin are not attained if the drug is taken with food, since it is susceptible to acidic breakdown and destruction. To circumvent this problem, it is recommended that penicillin be taken on an empty stomach at least one hour prior to a meal, or that a more acid-stable antibiotic be employed. It is worthwhile remembering that elderly patients tend to have a longer gastric emptying time and so are more at risk when drugs are taken with meals. On the other hand, their gastric pH may be less acidic so that drugs usually destroyed by gastric acid may survive and be absorbed more readily. There are also clinical conditions, such as achlorhydria or the Zollinger-Ellinson syndrome, that affect gastric pH and influence drug absorption.

However, when taken with food, some solid drug preparations that are acid stable may undergo disintegration and slow dissolution in the gastric contents and eventually be absorbed (delayed absorption). Ingestion of some medications with food can reduce their irritant properties, as in the case of potassium supplements. In addition, the ingestion of a drug with food may result in higher blood levels of the drug compared with taking the drug in the fasting state. However, this is not common and is relatively undesirable because of the variability that might occur due to differences in the diets of patients.

In the systemic circulation, a drug usually exists in an equilibrium between being partially bound to a serum protein and being in the free state. The free drug distributes throughout most of the body and reaches the site(s) of action, whereas the bound drug acts as a reservoir from which the drug is slowly released. The major circulatory protein that binds many drug molecules electrostatically is serum albumin; other proteins, such as transcortin, bind specific drugs. The dose of a drug has been adjusted to reflect the fraction of drug bound to allow for desirable bioavailability. Although it is logical to expect that a patient with hypoalbuminemia may require a modification of drug dose, practically this does not appear to be an important problem since the drug may only be transiently elevated. Distribution and excretion of the drug readjust the levels.

After the drug arrives at its site of action and interacts with a specific macromolecule, termed a receptor, a sequence of biochemical processes is initiated that develop into a physiologic effect. Though there is a specific binding of the drug for the receptor, these macromolecules are not unique for drugs since they act as transducers for the action of endogenous substances. This underlines the fact that drugs act by modifying ongoing processes and use these pathways to accomplish their ends. No receptors have been found for gaseous anesthetics or alcohol.

Foods contain some compounds that are capable of exerting pharmacologic effects by interacting at receptors or altering endogenous enzymatic activity. For example, caffeine is consumed by many for its stimulating effects. As will be obvious below, certain biogenic amines, if not destroyed in the gastrointestinal tract or by the liver, may have very serious consequences.

Termination of a drug's effect ensues when the concentration of the drug at the active site falls. This results from a combination of processes: redistribution to other areas of the body, biotransformation to inactive metabolites, and excretion. The liver is the major site for drug metabolism, though biotransformation is not restricted to this organ. The enzymes responsible for most of these reactions are the mixed function oxidases that catalyze the oxidation and reduction of a wide array of drugs. This multienzyme system depends on the hemoprotein cytochrome P-450, which, when attached to a variety of apoproteins, gives rise to a family of isoenzymes, each with its own inherent specificity. The term *Phase 1 reaction* has been coined to cover the metabolism by oxidation, reduction, or hydrolysis to intermediate metabolites. Subsequently these products can undergo glucuronidation or sulfation (Phase 2 reactions) to yield more water-soluble compounds for ready urinary excretion from the body. The cytochrome P-450 enzymes can fluctuate in amount due to induction or inhibition by drugs and/or dietary components. This fluctuation contributes to the variability in drug response often observed clinically.

Excretion of the drug can be in either the feces or the urine. However, some drugs taken orally are not absorbed and exert their effects locally in the gastrointestinal tract—for example, cholestyramine (Questran®)—and thus will appear in the feces. In addition, drugs excreted into the bile and not reabsorbed are also found in the feces.

Most are excreted into the urine either as the parent drug or as a metabolite. The pH of the urine can influence whether a compound will be readily eliminated. If the agent is predominantly ionized, then it will be more readily excreted, whereas if it is largely uncharged it can be reabsorbed and thus result in a prolonged effect in the body. Diet influences the pH of the urine. The mean pH of a 24-hour sample is usually about 6 (range 4.5–8). Individuals consuming a diet high in animal protein have a urinary pH in the low range due to the presence of phosphoric and sulfuric acids. Conversely, people who ingest a vegetarian diet usually have higher urinary pH values.

It is self-evident that the body does not distinguish in the way it handles drug and food and thus that interactions can occur at all levels. These will be considered below.

SITES OF INTERACTIONS

Modification of Absorption

Many drug–nutrient interactions occur at the level of absorption. Table 9–1 lists a number of drugs that have a decreased or delayed absorption if taken with food. As discussed above, it is not surprising that absorption of antibiotics in the penicillin family is reduced by food since they are destroyed by the acidic environment of the stomach due to the longer gastric emptying time. To obviate this difficulty, the drugs are taken one hour before meals or two hours after. Labels with this information are affixed to drug containers. The importance of this caution should be made clear to the patient by health care personnel.

The drug captopril (Capoten®), an ACE (angiotensin-converting enzyme) inhibitor that is prescribed for many cardiac patients, must also be taken one hour

Table 9–1 Absorption of Drugs by Foods

Drug	Food/Food Component	Effect
Antibiotics		
Penicillins	Food—Decrease emptying;	Decrease
Tetracyclines	Dairy foods; chelates Ca++, Mg++, Fe++, etc.	Decrease
Ciprofloxacin	Dairy food; chelates Ca++, Mg++, Fe++, etc.	Decrease
Antiviral		
Zidovudine	Fat	Decrease
Cardiac Drugs		
Capoten (*Captopril*)	Food	Decrease
Digitalis (*Lanoxin*)	Bran fiber	Decrease
Propranolol (*Inderal*)	Food	Increase
Verapamil (*IsoptinSR*)	Food	Prolong
Hypocholesterolemic Drugs		
Lovastatin (*Mevacor*)	Bran fiber	Decrease
Pulmonary Drugs		
Theophylline (*Theo-24*)	High fat	Increase
Theophylline (*Theo-Dur*)	High fat	No effect
Antifungal Agent		
Griseofulvin (*Fulvicin*)	High fat	Increase
Antiparkinsonism Agent		
Levodopa (*Larodopa*)	Food; protein	Delays absorption; decreases peak levels

Note: Trade names of drugs are printed in italics.

prior to a meal. If taken with meals the absorption may be decreased 30 to 40 percent, thus leading to inadequate therapeutic levels. Interestingly, the absorption of the other ACE inhibitors such as enlapril (Vasotec®) and lisinopril (Prinivil®, Zestril®) is not affected by the presence of food in the gastrointestinal tract.

Absorption of other drugs may be retarded when food is present in the gastrointestinal tract and may minimize the peak-to-trough ratio of the drug levels in the plasma. This could be a desirable effect in some cases to preclude wide variations in the blood concentration of a drug that might be translated into adverse effects. For example, a sustained-release form of the antihypertensive agent and calcium channel blocker verapamil (Isoptin SR®) is intentionally taken with food to slow absorption. Ingestion of the short-acting form of the beta-blocker propranolol (Inderal®) with food may lead to increased blood levels in some patients.[8] This is a short-lasting phenomenon and has been attributed to a diminished "first-pass effect," that is, hepatic metabolism of the drug on its first pass through the liver. It is possible that some individuals taking this drug with food might experience a transient hypotensive episode. The exact mechanism remains to be determined. The slow-release (long-acting) form of this drug does not have the same problem; its absorption is not affected by food. It is important to stress to the patient that he or she observe the instructions of the physician and pharmacist as to whether to take a medication with meals.

Lipid Solubility

Solubility of a drug in the membrane lipoprotein is essential for its passive diffusion from the gastrointestinal tract into the circulation. However, when a drug has limited solubility in the gastrointestinal contents but adequate lipid solubility, its absorption may be facilitated by bile acids. Bile secretion is promoted by fats in the diet and thus the absorption of such drugs are favored by a fatty meal. This is illustrated by the antifungal agent griseofulvin (Fulvicin®), used in the treatment of dermatophytic infections of toenails or fingernails (Figure 9–1). Fungal growth is inhibited when the drug binds to the newly synthesized keratin; thus the drug must be taken until the nail grows out (6–12 months). Its poor absorption after oral administration was recognized early and led to studies showing that absorption could be enhanced by taking the drug with a high-fat meal. Patients were instructed to take griseofulvin with a fatty meal. This practice has been discontinued because of the availability of a micronized preparation that is more readily absorbed—fortunately sparing the cardiovasculature of possible lipid deposits.

Theophylline, a methylxanthine dilator of the bronchioles, is employed in the treatment of asthma, chronic obstructive pulmonary disease (COPD), and emphysema. This drug has a narrow therapeutic window; serum levels exceeding 20 micrograms/ml may precipitate serious harmful reactions, including hypotension and life-threatening cardiac arrhythmias. Long-acting preparations such as Theo-24® and Theo-Dur® have the advantage of maintaining therapeutic levels after the patient receives either one or two doses per day. Ingestion of a single daily dose of Theo-24® (greater than 900 mg) within an hour of a fatty meal, however, may result in potentially toxic serum levels.[9] Patients required to take this level of drug must be cautioned to take the drug in the fasting state, that is, more than an hour prior to a meal. Interestingly, Theo-Dur® does not appear to have this problem.

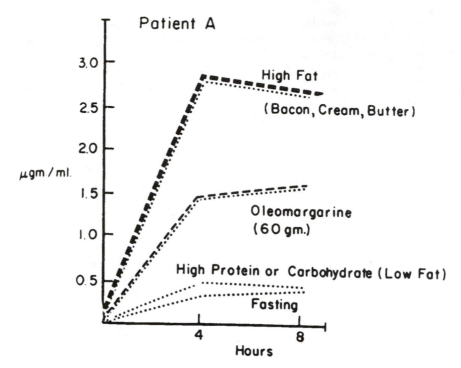

Figure 9–1 Absorption of Griseofulvin with Varying Dietary Fat Intake. *Source:* Reprinted from Crounse, R.G., Effective Use of Griseofulvin. *Archives of Dermatology*, Vol. 87, p. 177, with permission of the American Medical Association, © 1963.

It has been reported that the rate of absorption of the anti-AIDS drug zidovudine (AZT) is significantly slowed if it is taken with a high-fat meal.[10] Peak plasma levels are reached in about 1.9 hours as compared to 1 hour when taken in the fasting state. Furthermore, the peak serum level is reduced from about 5 μmol/L to 3 μmol/L (Figure 9–2). Because of the nausea associated with this medication, patients may take it with food. Consequently differences in diet may lead to variable absorption and response. The clinical significance of this study remains to be determined.

With the current interest directed to cholesterol's role in cardiovascular disease, there are several strategies to try to lower this compound when diet alone is not effective. One of these is the treatment with the basic anion exchange resin cholestyramine (Questran®) or colestipol (Colestid®).[11] After swallowing, these agents combine with bile acids in the intestine, and the complex is excreted into the feces. Since bile acids facilitate the absorption of lipid by emulsification, less cholesterol and other lipids are absorbed. The body compensates by oxidizing

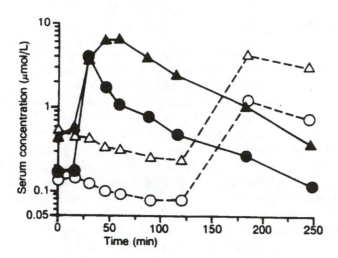

Figure 9–2 Oral administration of zidovudine (100 mg capsule) immediately after a high-fat meal considerably modulates both the peak and time to reach peak serum concentrations of zidovudine (○) and its 5'-glucuronidated metabolite (Δ) when compared with administration of the drug in the fasted state (● and ▲, respectively). (Unadkat et al., unpublished observations). *Source:* Reprinted from Collins, J.M., and Unadkat, J.D., Clinical pharmacokinetics of Zidovudine: An overview of current data. *Clinical Pharmacokinetics*, Vol. 17, No. 1, p. 2, with permission of Adis Press International, Ltd., © 1989.

---

endogenous cholesterol to bile acids and synthesizing more cholesterol, but more LDL receptors are also formed in the liver to take up the lipoprotein from the circulation, resulting in lowered serum cholesterol concentrations. However, the bile acids are also vital for the absorption of the fat-soluble vitamins A, D, E, and K. Because patients take the resins for years, deficiencies may develop. For example, hypoprothrombinemia has been reported due to inadequate levels of vitamin K. Other vitamins that are removed by binding to the resins are folate and Vitamin B_{12}. The resins also bind drugs, such as digoxin, and thus the scheduling of drug ingestion relative to intake of the resin is critical for proper therapy.

High-fiber diets are commonly used by individuals in the hope that they will lower serum cholesterol. Indeed, patients may try to supplement lipid-lowering drugs with such diets. That this practice may lead to therapy failure is supported by a report in which patients took the drug lovastatin (Mevacor®) along with pectin or oat bran.[12] In each case, LDL cholesterol rose, apparently due to postulated interference of the fiber in the absorption of the drug. Upon cessation of the bran diet, LDL fell to previous levels. Thus the suggestion has been made not to take the drug with brans. Furthermore, bran has been reported to decrease the absorption of digoxin.

Complex Formation

Ingestion of the tetracycline family of antibiotics irritates the stomach; hence patients tended to take them with milk. When it was appreciated that the effectiveness of the medication against an infection was reduced, a study revealed that an insoluble chelate had been formed with dietary calcium, thereby reducing the quantity of the drug absorbed. Not only dairy products but also mineral preparations (e.g., iron tablets) and antacids can interfere in absorption of these drugs if taken concomitantly with the medication due to the formation of inactive chelates with bivalent or trivalent cations, such as calcium, magnesium, zinc, iron, and aluminum. By affixing a label on the prescription vial indicating that the drug should not be taken with dairy products and antacids, the pharmacist calls the patient's attention to this problem. The medications may be taken with food to lessen the gastric irritation, but not with dairy products. The absorption of doxycycline (Vibramycin®) and minocycline (Minocin®) is not affected to the same extent as that of other tetracyclines. It should be noted that even the use of sodium bicarbonate to counteract the gastric upset can lower the absorption of tetracycline because it increases gastric pH and tetracycline absorption is favored by an acidic milieu.

Children under eight years old should not be treated with any of the tetracyclines, since calcification is affected. Tetracycline can not only deposit in newly forming dentition but also interfere in the formation of bone. This was documented in a study of premature infants whose skeletal development was arrested during a 30-day course of tetracycline therapy. Normal growth rate was resumed upon cessation of therapy (Figure 9–3). It is very likely that those individuals today have tetracycline deposited in their teeth and bones. The presence of the antibiotic does not affect the structure of those tissues, but the cosmetic disfigurement of the teeth (grey or yellowish lines) can have a psychological effect.

More recently, the effect of milk and yogurt on the absorption of the fluoroquinolone antibiotic ciprofloxacin (Cipro®) was examined.[13] This drug and other quinolone congeners were known to form insoluble chelates with ferrous sulfate, and bi- and trivalent cations of antacids with resulting significant decreases in absorption of the antibiotic. This study clearly showed that the dairy products also lowered the plasma concentrations of ciprofloxacin (Figure 9–4). The authors caution that therapeutic failures in combating infections may follow ingestion of large amounts of dairy foods with the antibiotic, especially if the microorganism is only moderately susceptible to the antimicrobial.

Effects on Transport Processes

A number of antiepileptic drugs are known to cause folate insufficiency ranging from a borderline problem to frank megaloblastic anemia.[14] These

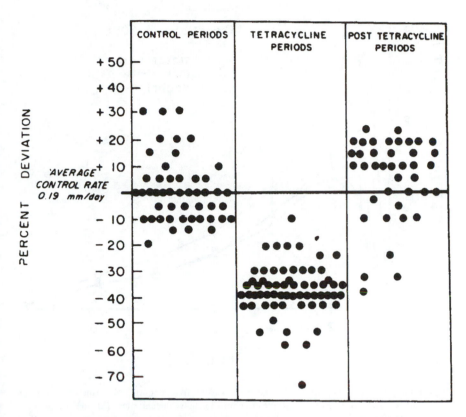

Figure 9–3 Rate of Skeletal Development in Premature Infants during a 30-Day Course of Tetracycline Therapy. *Source:* Reprinted from Cohlan, S.Q., Bevelander, G., and Tiamsic, T., Growth Inhibition of Prematures Receiving Tetracycline, *American Journal of Diseases in Children*, Vol. 105, p. 457, with permission of the American Medical Association, © 1963.

anticonvulsants must be given for the lifetime of the patient and include phenytoin (Dilatin®), phenobarbital, and primidone (Mysoline®). A number of mechanisms have been proposed to explain this observation, but not one of them has been accepted as definitive. One involves decreased absorption of folate by phenytoin as a result of direct inhibition of the intestinal conjugase α-glutamyl carboxypeptidase, the enzyme responsible for hydrolyzing the polyglutamate form of folate to the readily absorbable monoglutamate form. This postulate has been challenged and an alternate explanation offered. Phenytoin when dissolved has a pH of 12. It has been suggested that this high alkalinity in the microenvironment of the jejunum raises the pH above the optimum for the conjugase (pH 4.6). This explanation seems reasonable, but it has not been proved. Though

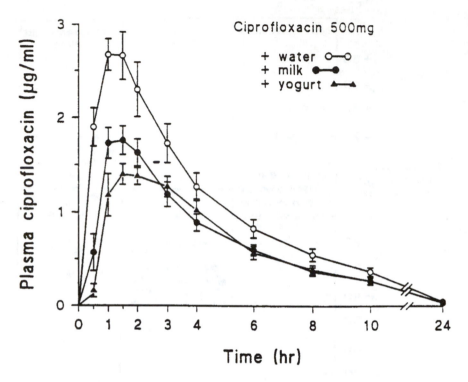

Figure 9–4 Effect of Concomitant Ingestion of Milk (300 ml) or Yogurt (300 ml) on the Absorption of Ciprofloxacin (500 mg), Reflected as Plasma Ciprofloxacin Concentrations (Mean ± SE) in Seven Subjects. The concentrations with milk and yogurt are significantly ($p < 0.05$) lower from ½ to 10 hours than with water, and with yogurt the concentrations are lower ($p < 0.05$) at 1 and 1½ hours than with milk. *Source:* Reprinted from Neuvonen, P.J., Kivistö, K.T., and Lehto, P., Interference of Dairy Products with the Absorption of Ciprofloxacin, *Clinical Pharmacology and Therapeutics*, Vol. 50, No. 5, p. 491, with permission of Mosby-Year Book, © 1991.

administration of folate can reverse the macrocytosis, supplementation may reduce the effectiveness of the phenytoin, and seizures have been known to occur; therefore the neurologist should be involved when supplementation with folate is contemplated. Indeed, doses of folic acid exceeding 5 mg can reduce the absorption of phenytoin if administered together.

A very important food-drug interaction at the level of transport explains the so-called "on-off" phenomenon seen in parkinsonian patients taking the drug levodopa (L-dihydroxyphenylalanine, Laradopa®). The parkinsonian syndrome has been traced to a deficit of the neurotransmitter dopamine in the nigrostriatal tracts of the brain. Because dopamine itself is rapidly metabolized by monoamine oxidase in the intestine and liver, it is ineffective therapeutically for this condition. More importantly, dopamine cannot penetrate the blood–brain barrier. Levodopa is effective in controlling the symptoms of parkinsonism because it can enter the central nervous system, where it undergoes decarboxylation to the neurotransmitter dopamine and relieves the symptoms.

Levodopa is a large neutral amino acid and, like other members of this group, is transported actively by a special transporter mechanism across the intestinal tract as well as into the central nervous system. Treatment failures were encountered initially due to the conversion of the levodopa to dopamine in the peripheral circulation by the pyridoxine-dependent enzyme L-amino acid decarboxylase. The dopamine was metabolized, and effective levels of levodopa could not be attained in the brain. This led to combining levodopa with carbidopa, an inhibitor of L-amino acid decarboxylase, which cannot penetrate the blood–brain barrier. Thus levodopa is not metabolized peripherally and is free to enter the brain. This combination is known as Sinemet®. Administration of vitamin B_6 to the levodopa regimen alone had resulted in therapeutic failures because it promoted the decarboxylation reaction. However, the vitamin has no effect on the Sinemet® formulation.

Some patients on this therapy exhibit symptoms of the disease intermittently, leading to the designation *on-off phenomenon*. Nurses were the first to associate the "off" reaction with meal consumption. Protein was shown to be the responsible agent. An elegant series of experiments has shown that the high-protein diet gives rise to large neutral amino acids, which compete with the levodopa for uptake into the brain.[15] Patients were monitored for tremor and dyskinesia while being maintained on an infusion of levodopa. (Tremor appears when there is insufficient dopamine in the striatum; dyskinesia is an indication of too much dopamine.) While infused, the patient received a high-protein meal. As can be seen in Figure 9–5, within a short time period, tremors returned. The same type of study was performed in which L-leucine or glycine was administered in place of the high-protein meal. Only when the large neutral amino acid leucine was given did the tremors appear, apparently due to the competition of the amino acid with levodopa for transport system; glycine had no effect. More meals with lower protein content spaced over the day have been recommended to help deal with this phenomenon.

Malabsorption

Neomycin, an aminoglycoside antibiotic, is used topically to treat skin infections or orally to eradicate intestinal bacteria either in cases of hepatic coma or prior to bowel surgery because it is not absorbed. When 4–6 g are administered per day, a malabsorption syndrome may develop due to intestinal

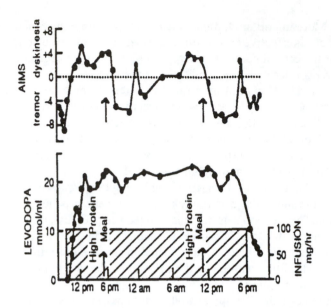

Figure 9–5 Effects of High-Protein Meals on the Plasma Levodopa Concentration and the Clinical Response during Intravenous Infusion of Levodopa in One Patient. The patient was also receiving carbidopa, 25 mg by mouth every two hours. AIMS denotes the algebraic sum of involuntary-movement scores (positive values indicate dyskinesia, and negative values indicate tremor). *Source:* Adapted from information appearing in Nutt, J.G., Woodward W.R., Hammerstad, J.P., et al., The On-Off Phenomenon in Parkinson's Disease: Relation to Levodopa Absorption and Transport, *New England Journal of Medicine*, Vol. 310, p. 486, with permission of the Massachusetts Medical Society, © 1984.

---

mucosal damage. It is classified as spruelike and characterized by diarrhea, steatorrhea, and azotorrhea. A variety of nutrients, including fat, protein, cholesterol, carotene, glucose, lactose, vitamin B_{12}, iron, Na^+, and Ca^{2+}, are poorly absorbed.

A drug-induced malabsorption-like condition may also develop with the chronic use of the antigout medications colchicine and indomethacin, or the laxative mineral oil. The latter solubilizes the fat-soluble vitamins and physically bars absorption.

Methotrexate, a folate antagonist used in cancer chemotherapy and in the treatment of psoriatic arthritis, has been reported to cause a dose-dependent malabsorption of calcium in children. Whether it has this effect at the doses used in arthritis in adults remains to be determined.

Aluminum-containing antacids may react with phosphates in the gut to form a compound that is excreted via the feces. Prolonged use of these antacids may cause hypophosphatemia.

INTERACTIONS AT THE DRUG RECEPTOR SITE

Perhaps no single food–drug interaction has made a greater impact on the medical profession than that of inhibitors of monoamine oxidase (MAO) and amines in the diet. A wide variety of compounds present in foods are capable of causing physiological effects either directly or indirectly. In most instances, the body is protected by enzymes that metabolize the potential offenders to innocuous products. Such is the case ordinarily with biogenic amines like tyramine (decarboxylated tyrosine), tryptamine (decarboxylated tryptophan), dopamine, and histamine (decarboxylated histidine). These agents ordinarily are oxidized by MAO in the gastrointestinal mucosa, liver, and other sites throughout the body. However, when that enzyme is inhibited the individual may be susceptible to very serious reactions.

In the early 1960s, a number of monoamine oxidase inhibitors (MAOI) were introduced as antihypertensive agents. These were pargyline (Eutonyl®), tranylcypromine (Parnate®), and phenelzine (Nardil®). Reports of hypertensive crises and fatalities due to cerebrovascular accidents in patients taking these medications led to the suggestion that food-associated amines might be involved. This was experimentally proven. Although no longer employed as antihypertensive agents, they are useful in the treatment of mental depression and may be beneficial in the treatment of narcolepsy and bulimia. It is imperative that patients taking these medications be cautioned to avoid foods containing amines.

The mechanism underlying the antidepressant effects of these three drugs and the nature of the interaction with food is incompletely understood. Normally, blood pressure is maintained by the constant release of norepinephrine (noradrenaline) from the nerve terminals of the sympathetic nervous system, which stimulates receptors on blood vessels to contract, thereby causing a pressor effect (this is sometimes referred to as "sympathetic tone"). MAO in the nerve terminals is responsible for regulating levels of norepinephrine and 5-hydroxytryptamine (serotonin). When the enzyme is inactivated, norepinephrine accumulates and inhibits its own synthesis to some extent; however, levels rise in the terminals and the adrenal. With the ingestion of foods containing tyramine, the dietary amine is free to enter the body and eventually is taken up by the nerve terminal and adrenal, where it displaces the accumulated norepinephrine. A barrage of norepinephrine exits the terminal and reacts with the receptor sites on the vasculature to cause vasoconstriction and hypertension. The patient complains of a throbbing headache, palpitations, profuse sweating, nausea, and vomiting. Patients in the supine position survive better. The effect usually occurs about 20–30 minutes after ingestion of the food and may last from 10 minutes to 6 hours or so unless there is an intervention.

A representative crisis in a patient on the MAOI pargyline is depicted in Figure 9–6. Upon ingesting 260 g of whole cooked broad beans (fava beans), his blood pressure climbed to life-threatening levels. Intravenous injection of phentolamine (Regitine®, a short-acting alpha blocker that interferes in the binding of norepinephrine to the receptor) terminated the crisis. Fava beans do not contain tyramine. Like other leguminous vegetables, they contain DOPA (dihydroxyphenylalanine) in the pods. This amino acid is converted to dopamine in the body, and this biogenic amine is taken up into the nerve terminals, where, like tyramine, it displaces the norepinephrine.

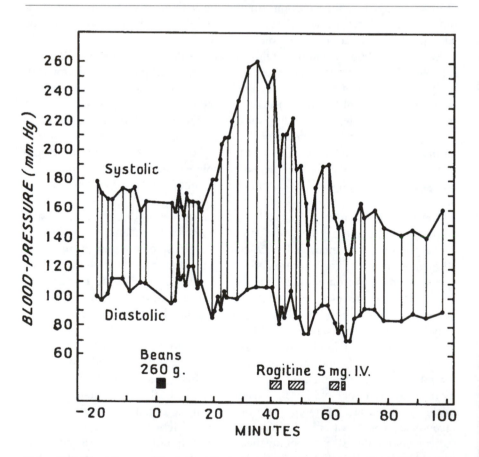

Figure 9–6 Blood Pressure Changes and Responses to Intravenous Phentoamine in Hypertensive Subjects after Ingestion of 260 g of Whole Cooked Broad Beans. *Source:* Reprinted from Hodge, J.V., Nye, E.R., and Emerson, G.W., Monoamine-Oxidase Inhibitors, Broad Beans, and Hypertension. *Lancet*, Vol. 1, p. 1108, with permission of *Lancet*, © 1964.

It is not surprising that patients with parkinsonism should generally not be treated with nonselective MAO inhibitors. A relatively selective MAO Type B inhibitor, selegyline [Eldepryl®] is sometimes used in combination with Sinemet® in patients whose parkinsonism has worsened. The dose of the selegyline is critical since cardiovascular difficulties may result. MAO exists in two forms, A and B; the former is intestinal, and the latter resides in the brain. Other MAO inhibitors are biotransformed to compounds that irreversibly and nonselectively inactivate both enzymes. It is fairly well established that inactivation of the B form (neuronal) is associated with the antidepressant action. Drugs specific for the neuronal enzyme are being developed. The rationale is to allow the A form to protect against exogenous amines, thus minimizing the capacity for hypertensive crisis.

Tyramine is formed during fermentation; therefore foods such as aged cheeses that are products of fermentative processes are rich sources of the amine and can provoke hypertensive crises. As little as 2 oz of a matured cheese has been known to cause such an attack. Levels of the amine in a particular food may vary, but it is generally accepted that 10 mg of tyramine can precipitate a crisis. Tables 9–2 and 9–3 list the tyramine content of a number of foods. It is note-

Table 9–2 Vasoactive Amines in Plant Food

Plant Substance		Amines in µg/gm or µg/ml*				
	Reference	Serotonin	Tryptamine	Tyramine	Dopamine	Norepinephrine
Banana peel	66	50–100	0	65	700	122
Banana pulp	66	28	0	7	8	2
Plantain pulp	66	45	—	—	—	—
Tomato	66	12	4	4	0	0
Red plum	66	10	0–2	6	0	+
Red blue plum	66	8	2	—	—	—
Blue plum	66	0	5	—	—	—
Avocado	66	10	0	23	4–5	0
Potato	66	0	0	1	0	0.1–0.2
Spinach	66	0	0	1	0	0
Grape	66	0	0	0	0	0
Orange	66	0	0.1	10	0	+
Eggplant	66	0	0	—	—	—
Pineapple juice	16,27	25–35	—	—	—	—
Pineapple, ripe	27	20	—	—	—	—
Passion fruit	26	1–4	—	—	—	—
Pawpaw	26	1–2	—	—	—	—

*A dash means that the food was not tested for this amine, 0 means that the level of the amine was below the detection threshold, and + indicates that the material contained a trace of the amine.

Source: Reproduced from *Toxicants Occurring Naturally in Foods.* National Academy Press, Washington, DC, 1973.

Table 9–3 Foods Reported To Contain Tyramine of Probable Microbial Origin

Food Substance	Tyramine (µg/gm)
Cheese	
Cheddar	120–1,500
Camembert	20–2,000
Emmenthaler	225–1,000
Brie	0–200
Stilton blue	466–2,170
Processed	26–50
Gruyere	516
Gouda	20
Brick, natural	524
Mozzarella	410
Blue	30–250
Roquefort	27–520
Boursault	1,116
Parmesan	4–290
Romano	238
Provolone	38
Beer and ale	1.8–11.2
Wines	0–25
Marmite yeast and yeast extract	0–2,250
Fish	
Salted dried fish	0–470
Pickled herring	3,000
Meat	
Meat extracts	95–304
Beef liver (stored)	274
Chicken liver (stored)	100
Miscellaneous	
Soya	1.76

Source: Reproduced from *Toxicants Occurring Naturally in Foods.* National Academy Press, Washington, DC, 1973.

---

worthy that avocado and oranges contain small amounts. This is unusual because they do not undergo fermentation. To the list can be added sour cream and chocolate, which also have high levels. There is a dilemma about providing depressed patients with a list of problem foods since the patient may use this route to suicide.

A patient taking MAO inhibitors may exhibit a variability in the hypertensive response to amine-containing foods. This may be partially explained by the variability in the levels of the amines in the food or by the presence of active MAO, presumably the intestinal/hepatic form.

Another drug that possesses some MAO-inhibitory activity is the anticancer agent procarbazine (Matulane®). Used in the treatment of lymphomas, procarbazine usually is administered for three to six days per cycle. The food interaction is generally seen if the patient has been taking the drug for five or more days.

Interactions with Alcohol

Alcohol is incompatible with many medications; Table 9–4 lists some of these. Many drugs have sedative properties either as a direct effect, such as barbiturates and tranquilizers, or as side effects, such as antihistamines used to treat allergies or cold symptoms, or drugs used to counteract motion sickness. A patient taking these medications should be cautioned not to drink alcohol since the sedative actions of alcohol and the medication will add to each other and the resultant CNS depression could be fatal. Interestingly, the antifungal drug griseofulvin also intensifies the effects of alcohol, though it has no sedative action of its own.

A number of drugs have what is termed an Antabuse® effect. Antabuse, the trade name for disulfiram, is used to treat alcoholism with the consent of the patient. Disulfiram inhibits aldehyde dehydrogenase, the enzyme responsible for metabolizing the acetaldehyde formed as a product of ethanol oxidation. The ingestion of alcohol by a patient taking disulfiram produces a very unpleasant array of reactions ranging from flushing and rapid heartbeat, to nausea and vomiting. Three antibiotics of the cephalosporin class, namely cefamandole, cefoperazone, and moxalactam, also produce an Antabuse-like reaction in patients who drink alcohol while being treated with them. Interestingly, these are the same three that act as vitamin K antagonists (see below). These antibiotics are administered intravenously so that the patient is usually in a health care facility and presumably can be monitored. Other agents that have the disulfiram-like property are the antimicrobial metronidazole (Flagyl®) and the oral antidiabetic agent chlorpropamide (Diabinese®). Since alcohol irritates the stomach lining, it may increase the bleeding that is a side effect of aspirin and other anti-inflammatory medications.

Alteration in Nutrient Demands

Drugs may increase the demand for certain nutrients or minerals. A number of medications owe their action to their ability to interfere in the function of vitamins, for example, methotrexate's interference with folate and warfarin (Coumadin®)'s interference with vitamin K. Other drugs may react with a vitamin to render it inactive, such as hydralazine (Apresoline®) with vitamin B_6,

Table 9–4 Interactions of Drugs with Alcohol

Drugs	Effect
Those That Lead to Increased CNS-Related Effects	
Antihistamines (*Benadryl, ChlorTrimeton, Contact, Dristan*)	Drowsiness, confusion, increased intoxication, loss of consciousness, may be fatal
Muscle relaxants (*Soma, Robaxin*)	
Motion-sickness medications (*Dramamine*)	
Tranquilizers (*Valium, Xanax, Ativan*)	
Sleep medications (*Dalmane, Halcion*)	
Antidepressants (*Tofranil, Prozac, Elavil*)	
Narcotic pain relievers (Codeine, *Percodan,* etc.)	
Antianginal drugs (Nitroglycerin, *Isordil*)	Lightheadedness, dizziness, may cause ataxia, fainting
Griseofulvin (*Fulvicin*)	Intensifies intoxication
Those That Lead to Systemic Effects	
Metronidazole (*Flagyl*)	Disulfiram (*Antabuse*)-like reaction, i.e., headache, flushing, tachycardia, nausea and vomiting
Specific antibiotics (*Mandol, Cefobid*)	
Specific oral antidiabetic agents (*Diabinease,* rarely *Micronase*)	
NSAIDS (Aspirin, ibuprofen, *Naprosyn, Feldene*)	Stomach irritation may cause bleeding
Potassium tablets	

Note: Trade names of drugs are printed in italics.

---

or increase the demand by stimulating metabolism of the vitamin, such as phenytoin with vitamin D. The consequences of these drug/nutrient interactions can be deleterious but are usually corrected by supplementation with the vitamin.

Folic Acid

Folic acid plays a key role in cellular metabolism. It is the precursor of a family of coenzymes that are required for one-carbon metabolism. Methotrexate is an analog of folic acid and was specifically designed to antagonize that vitamin in cancer chemotherapy after it was realized that many neoplastic cells had a higher demand for the folate than normal cells. Clinically, it is used in the treatment of a number of neoplastic states as well as psoriatic arthritis. The drug specifically binds to and inhibits the enzyme dihydrofolate reductase, which catalyzes the reduction of dihydrofolate to the active tetrahydro form. The affinity of methotrexate for the enzyme is several orders of magnitude greater than that of the natural vitamin, and thus cells become "starved" for tetrahydrofolate. This in turn decreases the availability of the metabolically active folate coenzymes essential in the biosynthesis of purines and the pyrimidine thymine. Neoplastic cells become deprived of important growth factors, thus resulting in cell death.

However, normal cells are also depleted of the active form of the vitamin. Cells undergoing rapid turnover, such as those in the bone marrow and oral intestinal mucosa, are particularly susceptible, leading to megaloblastic anemia and ulcerative stomatitis. By administering Leucovorin® (folinic acid, 5-formyl tetrahydrofolate), some of the normal cells may be rescued and the toxicity reversed. Leucovorin bypasses the blocked dihydrofolate reductase and enters cell metabolism. A knowledge of the pharmacokinetics of these agents is required so as to schedule the rescue properly in order not to jeopardize the antineoplastic effects of methotrexate.

Low serum levels of folate have been reported in epileptic patients receiving phenytoin, and this can sometimes express itself as macrocytosis or even megaloblastic anemia, which can be reversed by folate administration. As mentioned above, phenytoin may decrease the absorption of the vitamin. However, there is also evidence that phenytoin interferes in the function of the folate coenzymes. The hydantoin structure of phenytoin closely resembles that of two coenzyme forms of folate, namely N^{5-10}-methenyl- and N^{5-10}methylene tetrahydrofolate. At the present time the underlying mechanism of the interaction remains undefined.

Vitamin B$_6$ (Pyridoxine)

Like folate, vitamin B$_6$ is a cofactor for many enzymes. Principal among these are the amino acid transaminases and decarboxylases. For example, it plays a central role in the nervous system, where it is the cofactor for the decarboxylation of both L-dihydroxyphenylalanine (DOPA) to dopamine in the biosynthetic pathway forming norepinephrine and 5-hydroxytryptophan to 5-hydroxytryptamine (serotonin). Vitamin B$_6$ exists in three forms in nature: pyridoxine, pyridoxal, and pyridoxamine. They are interconvertible enzymatically; pyridoxal phosphate has been shown to be the most important as a cofactor.

Chronic treatment with the anti-TB drug isoniazid (INH), the antihypertensive drug hydralazine (Apresoline®), or the antiarthritic drug penicillamine

(Cuprimine®) results in lowered serum levels of the vitamin. In about 2 percent of those on isoniazid and 10 percent of those taking hydralazine, paresthesias (tingling in the extremities), a sign of B_6 deficiency-induced peripheral neuropathy, have been reported to develop.[16] Administration of the vitamin reverses the symptoms. It has been reported that INH can achieve levels in breast milk that are high enough to cause a B_6 deficiency in the nursing infant unless the mother is supplemented with the vitamin. The decrease in the vitamin has been attributed to a chemical reaction of the drug with pyridoxal to yield the inactive hydrazone through a condensation of the aldehyde group of pyridoxal and the amino group of the drug. The product does not retain the activity of either the drug or the vitamin and is excreted from the body.

The use of oral contraceptive agents containing ethinyl estradiol may increase the demand for pyridoxine, especially in those who are not adequately nourished.[17,18] Early studies were carried out in the traditional manner of evaluating pyridoxine deficiency, that is, by examining urinary products of tryptophan metabolism after a loading dose of tryptophan. Pyridoxal serves as a cofactor for a number of the enzymes in this pathway, and deficiency is manifested by increased excretion of xanthurenic and/or kynurenic acid. This was found and could be reversed by administration of the vitamin. One explanation offered for the hormone induced B_6 "deficiency" was that the estrogen led to increased levels of transcortin, the serum protein that transports cortisone. The diminution of free cortisone would then be perceived by the adrenal cortex, which would compensate by stimulating the synthesis of cortisol. The hormone in turn would trigger the synthesis of hepatic tryptophan oxygenase and accelerate tryptophan metabolism, leading to a greater demand by the body for the vitamin. Thus the demand for B_6 would increase because estrogen accelerates tryptophan oxidation indirectly. Though an attractive hypothesis, its validity and the use of the tryptophan load experiments have been questioned by a study in rats that showed that estrone sulfate inhibits kynureninase, an enzyme in the tryptophan metabolic pathway.[19] Hepatic kynurenine levels rise, leading to enhanced excretion of xanthurenic and kynurenic acids. The reversal by supplementation with the vitamin in this study was shown to be due to an increase in kynureninase. These results seemingly challenge whether estrogen decreases B_6.

However, direct measurement of plasma pyridoxal phosphate found that about 20 percent of women on these drugs for at least six months had depressed levels. Thus at the present time it is not clear how oral contraceptives cause the B_6 "deficiency." Most of the studies were performed with oral contraceptives containing 0.05 mg of ethinyl estradiol, which is roughly double the amount present in today's oral contraceptive preparations. It remains to be determined whether levels of the vitamin are lower in these patients.

Furthermore, many postmenopausal women are being treated with conjugated estrogens for the treatment of symptoms associated with the menopause as well as to deter osteoporosis. It would be interesting to evaluate them for their B_6 status. Some reports indicate that 75 percent or more receiving conjugated estrogen (Premarin®) may have low levels, but overt peripheral neurological symptoms have not been reported.

Vitamin D

Treatment of epilepsy with phenytoin and/or phenobarbital has been shown to produce vitamin D deficiency, manifesting itself sometimes as osteomalacia or even frank rickets. The latter is relatively uncommon since vitamin D is consumed in milk and exposure to sunlight increases synthesis of the vitamin in the skin. Institutionalized patients who receive insufficient sunlight are particularly at risk.

Figure 9–7 illustrates a case of a young patient institutionalized in Great Britain, where milk was not supplemented with vitamin D and the patient was confined to the institution.[20] He was receiving three anticonvulsant agents,

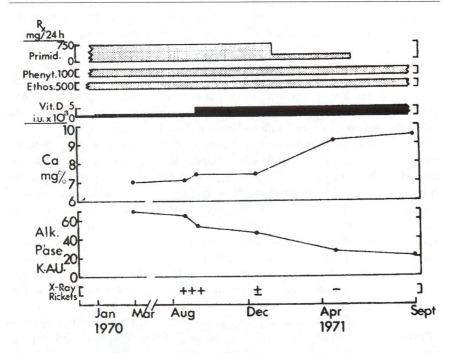

Figure 9–7 Progress in Anticonvulsant Therapy on Rickets. *Source:* Reprinted from Stamp, T.C.B., Effects of Long-Term Anticonvulsant Therapy on Calcium and Vitamin D Metabolism, *Proceedings of the Royal Society of Medicine*, Vol. 67, p. 64, with permission of the *Royal Society of Medicine*, © 1974.

phenytoin, phenobarbital,and primidone. It can be seen that the rickets were corrected and serum calcium rose only after the dose of primidone was reduced and the patient was being treated with 0.25 mg of vitamin D_2 on alternate days. In another study, doses of 6,000 IU to 15,000 IU of vitamin D_2 were required to correct the rickets that had developed in children being treated with the antiepileptic drugs plus conventional doses of vitamin D_2.[21] Administration of 50 IU of the 25-hydroxycholecalciferol (25-(OH)D) was also effective in reversing the rickets. The explanation for these observations was that the vitamin had been metabolized to inactive products.

Vitamin D is hydroxylated by the hepatic cytochrome P-450 enzymes to 25-(OH)D, which is converted subsequently by the kidney to what is believed to be the active hormonal form, 1,25-dihydroxycholecalciferol (1,25-(OH)$_2$-D). Phenytoin and phenobarbital are excellent inducers of the hepatic cytochrome P-450 enzymes and thus enhance the metabolic capacity of these oxidative enzymes. Located in the endoplasmic reticulum of the liver, the enzyme levels may vary depending on diet (see below) and various drugs. These enzymes not only are able to metabolize vitamin D to 25-(OH)D but can form inactive metabolites by extended biotransformation of the vitamin. Thus it has been postulated that with chronic use of the antiepileptic drugs, vitamin D requirements are increased due to increased metabolism.

Low serum levels of calcium can provoke seizures and therefore exacerbate epilepsy. If the condition is not recognized, the dose of anticonvulsant may be increased, which can result in further elevation of the cytochrome P-450 enzymes. This may explain the case in Figure 9–6, where the serum calcium rose only after the dose of primidone had been lowered.

However, the above hypothesis has been challenged by the discovery that even though serum concentrations of 25-(OH)D tended to be depressed in anticonvulsant treated patients, the levels of 1,25-(OH)$_2$D were elevated.[22] The latter response is to be expected in hypocalcemia and secondary hyperparathyroidism. Consequently even though 25-(OH)D may have been decreased due to enhanced metabolism, enough of the sterol was available to form adequate quantities of the 1,25-(OH)$_2$D. Thus either 25-(OH)D plays a more important role in calcium homeostasis than hitherto believed, or the drugs may additionally reduce the responsiveness of the receptors in the gut and bone for the 1,25 dihydroxy vitamin. The exact mechanism underlying the anticonvulsant-induced osteomalacia and its relationship to vitamin D metabolism remain to be elucidated.

Treatment with prednisone and other glucocorticoids is accompanied by a loss of calcium secondary to the effects on vitamin D. Serum levels of 1,25-(OH)$_2$D are depressed. The glucocorticoids are known to be inducers of the hepatic cytochrome P-450 system in experimental animals. This would suggest that 25-(OH)D is metabolized to inactive products and that not enough of the 1,25-dihydroxy form is synthesized.

Vitamin K

The vitamin K antagonist anticoagulants do what the name implies: they antagonize the effects of the vitamin and lead to hypoprothrombinemia, that is, decreased prothrombin and clot formation. Clinically, they are employed in cases of acute myocardial infarction and in other vascular problems. These drugs, warfarin (Coumadin®) and dicumarol, interfere in the carboxylation of the glutamyl residues in the various clotting factor proteins. The adverse effects of these agents (bleeding or hemorrhage) may be reversed by the administration of vitamin K_1, but it takes 24 hours to reverse the hypoprothrombinemic state; thus whole blood is sometimes employed, depending on the severity of the problems.

Patients can inadvertently influence their prothrombin times by eating vegetables high in vitamin K. For example, a patient with atrial fibrillation was admitted for cardioversion and anticoagulated with heparin followed by warfarin. After discharge from the hospital on warfarin, her prothrombin time was never within the therapeutic range.[23] Careful questioning revealed that she ate a pound of broccoli a day—a vegetable high in vitamin K. Thus what might have been interpreted as resistance to the anticoagulant was readily explained by the patient's dietary habits. Similarly, patients who appear to be resistant to these anticoagulants may be supplementing their nutrition with liquid nutritional preparations, some of which contain significant levels of vitamin K. It is important to advise them to use preparations without vitamin K.

Antimicrobials may also decrease intestinal bacterial flora that are normally a source of vitamin K for the host, thereby leading to bleeding problems. This is of concern in malnourished patients receiving the antibiotics and especially if they are also being treated with an anticoagulant like warfarin. It is less of a concern in the well-nourished patient. Supplementation with vitamin K is required for patients receiving either cefoperazone (Cefobid®), cefamandole (Mandol®), or moxalactam (Moxam®) because these act as vitamin K antagonists.

ROLE OF FOOD IN STIMULATING AND INHIBITING METABOLISM OF DRUGS

It is well recognized that individuals may respond to a drug differently or to varying degrees. This may be ascribed partly to substances in the diet that affect levels of the oxidative enzymes that metabolize these medications. The cytochrome P-450 system mentioned above and found throughout the body but especially in the liver is responsible for metabolizing a wide variety of drugs. Indole compounds found in the *Brassecea* vegetables—that is, broccoli, cabbage, cauliflower, and brussels sprouts—are capable of increasing the hepatic levels of this enzyme system and can result in an elevated metabolism of a drug, leading to decreased levels of the free drug and/or a shorter duration of action.[24] This reminds us of the cardiac patient who ate a pound of broccoli per day. She was not only replacing the vitamin but possibly also accelerating the metabolism of the anticoagulant.

It has also been shown that a high-protein diet will accelerate the metabolism of theophylline over that of an isocaloric high-carbohydrate diet.[25] This is particularly important for asthmatics. The therapeutic range of theophylline is very narrow, and if the drug is more rapidly metabolized, then effective levels may not be available to protect the asthmatic patient (Figure 9–8). Unfortunately, the pharmacological effects were not evaluated in the patients in this study.

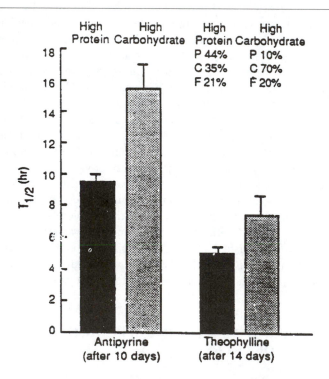

Figure 9–8 Effects of Exchanging Protein and Carbohydrate in the Diet on Drug Metabolism in Six Normal Subjects. A high-protein diet (44% of total calories as protein) was fed for two weeks, followed by a high (70%) carbohydrate diet also for two weeks. As indicated by the values shown for dietary compositions, the study entailed an isocaloric substitution of carbohydrate for protein while dietary fat content remained the same. Antipyrine and theophylline metabolism were studied on days 10 and 14, respectively, of each dietary period. Half-lives (mean ± SE) for these drugs are shown. *Source:* Reprinted from Anderson, K.E., Conney A.H., and Kappas, A. Nutrition and Oxidative Drug Metabolism in Man: Relative Influence of Dietary Lipids, Carbohydrate, and Protein, *Nutrition Review*, Vol. 40, No. 6, p. 161, with permission of Springer-Verlag, © 1982.

Preparation of food may also alter drug levels, as shown by a study in which subjects were kept on a diet of hamburger that was broiled either directly over a charcoal fire or with aluminum foil interface blocking direct exposure of the meat to the fire.[26] The peak serum levels of the drug phenacetin were much lower if the subject had ingested the former diet previously. Studies in rodents where a similar effect was obtained showed that the drug had undergone metabolism in the intestinal mucosa, where the cytochrome P-450 enzymes had been increased by the aromatic hydrocarbons formed during the preparation of the meat.

Alternatively, the metabolism of a drug may be inhibited by diet components. For example, grapefruit juice has been shown to hinder the metabolism of the calcium channel blocker felodipine (Plendil®).[27] A study compared the absorption of the drug in men taking it either with water or orange or grapefruit juice. The bioavailability of the drug was increased more than twofold in all of the men who had taken it with grapefruit juice. What is present in the grapefruit juice that can cause this? It is known to contain certain bioflavonoids (quercetin, kaempferol, and naringenin) that are absent in orange juice and that are known to inhibit the cytochrome P-450 system, particularly the isozyme CYP3A4. Furthermore, the effects of the drug on diastolic blood pressure and heart rate were also increased. Interestingly, the effect of juice is not seen with the slow-release preparation of felodipine. Though grapefruit juice has a similar effect on the other dihydropyridine calcium channel blockers (e.g., nitrendipine), it is not as dramatic as with felodipine.[28] It is clear that patients should be advised not to take felodipine with grapefruit juice.

DRUG-INDUCED LOSS OF MINERALS

Table 9–5 summarizes some of the drugs that affect minerals in the body. Many patients take diuretics for hypertension. Both the thiazides (Diuril® and others) and furosemide (Lasix®) cause a loss of potassium, which must be replenished by potassium supplementation either by foods such as bananas, oranges, and potatoes or by potassium preparations. The usual loss of K^+ is 25 to 40 meq per day. If it is not corrected, the patient will feel weak and his or her cardiac function may be threatened, particularly if the patient is being treated with digoxin. The loss of potassium sensitizes the heart to the digoxin toxicity. Furosemide also causes a loss of calcium and magnesium; indeed, furosemide can be used to treat hypercalcemia. The newest so-called high-ceiling diuretic, bumetanide (Bumex®), also leads to hypocalcemia. The thiazide diuretics, on the other hand, cause calcium retention.

It was already mentioned above that a loss of calcium occurs with phenytoin or glucocorticoid therapy secondary to their effect on vitamin D.

Table 9–5 Drugs That Affect Mineral Levels

Mineral	Drug	Effect	Mechanism
Calcium	Methotrexate	decrease	decreased absorption
	Furosemide	decrease	increased excretion
	Bumetanide	decrease	increased excretion
	Thiazides	increase	renal reabsorption
	Phenytoin	decrease	secondary to decreased vitamin D
	Glucocorticoids	decrease	secondary to decreased vitamin D
Potassium	Diuretics	decrease	increased excretion
Magnesium	Diuretics	decrease	increased excretion
Iron	Nonsteroidal anti-inflammatory agents (NSAIDS)	decrease	secondary to blood loss

Nonsteroidal anti-inflammatory drugs such as aspirin and ibuprofen may lead to a secondary loss of iron due to irritation and bleeding from the gastrointestinal tract.

EFFECT OF URINARY pH ON DRUG EXCRETION

The ionized form of a drug is usually more water soluble and more readily excreted in individuals who eat a normal diet. However, if the pH of the urine is raised, as may happen in vegetarians or individuals abusing antacids, it may affect the excretion of a drug, which may become nonionized at that pH. Consequently the drug would be reabsorbed in the kidney and would eventually lead to higher drug levels. A case has been reported in which a patient was being treated with the antiarrhythmic drug quinidine for two years without any problems when he entered the emergency room with arrhythmias.[29] His quinidine level was in the toxic range. When questioned about self-medication and diet, he admitted to ingesting eight Mylanta® tablets daily and drinking about one quart of orange-grapefruit juice per day. Urinary pH was not measured, but the reporting physician pointed out that the magnesium hydroxide and aluminum hydroxide in the antacid could alkaline the urine, as could the ingestion of about 50 meq of bicarbonate daily in the fruit juice. He verified his hypothesis by giving normal subjects Mylanta or fruit juice or both. The combination persistently alkalinized the urine, although the specific data were not reported. In view of the observed effect of grapefruit juice on felodipine, it would be of interest to determine whether quinidine metabolism may have also been compromised by the juice.

CONCLUSION

Many food–drug or drug–nutrient interactions were considered and many were not. It is the responsibility of the dietitian/nutritionist to be aware of potential interactions and to educate the patient and other health personnel to them as mandated by the Joint Commission on Accreditation of Healthcare Organizations.

The implementation of an effective program to identify interactions and educate may take many forms.[30] In most instances cooperation among the health professionals, such as the pharmacists, nurses, and physicians along with the clinical nutritionists or dietitians, can lead to development of counseling programs and instructional materials. The informed patient who understands the potential problems is in a position to avoid or identify them and thus preclude more serious clinical predicaments. The welfare of the patient can thus be safeguarded and the quality of medicine improved.

REFERENCES

1. Roe DA. *Diet and Drug Interactions.* New York, NY: Van Nostrand Reinhold; 1988.

2. Roberts J, Rumer N. Age and diet effects on drug action. *Pharmacol Ther.* 1988;37:111–149.

3. Pinto J. Pharmacokinetics and pharmacodynamics of interactions of food and drugs. *Top Clin Nutr.* 1991;6:14–33.

4. Theuer RC, Vitale JJ. Drug and nutrient interactions. In: Schneider HA, Anderson CE, Coursin DB, eds. *Nutritional Support of Medical Practice.* New York, NY: Harper & Row; 1977:297–305.

5. Roe DA. Interactions between drugs and nutrients. *Med Clin North Am.* 1979;63:985–1007.

6. Toothaker RD, Welling P. The effect of food on drug bioavailability. *Annu Rev Pharmacol Toxicol.* 1980;20:173–199.

7. Trovato A, Nuhlicek DN, Midtling JE. Drug-nutrient interactions. *Am Fam Physician.* 1991;44:1651–1658.

8. Liedholm H, Melander A. Concomitant food intake can increase the bioavailability of propranolol by transient inhibition of its presystemic conjugation. *Clin Pharmacol Ther.* 1986;40:29–36.

9. *FDA Drug Bull.* Theo-absorption with meals. 1984;14:3.

10. Collins JM, Unadkat JD. Clinical pharmacokinetics of zidovudine: an overview of current data. *Clin Pharmacokinet.* 1989;17:1–9.

11. Levy RI, et al. Dietary and drug treatment of primary hyperlipoproteinemia. *Ann Intern Med.* 1972;77:267–294.

12. Richter WO, Jacob BG, Schwandt P. Interaction between fibre and lovastatin. *Lancet.* 1991;338:706. Letter.

13. Neuvonen PJ, Kivistö KT, Lehto P. Interference of dairy products with the absorption of ciprofloxacin. *Clin Pharmacol Ther.* 1991;50:498–502.

14. Stebbins R, Scott J, Herbert V. Drug-induced megaloblastic anemias. *Sem Hematol.* 1973;10:235–251.

15. Nutt JG, Woodward WR, Hammerstad JP, et al. The on-off phenomenon in Parkinson's disease—relation to levodopa absorption and transport. *N Engl J Med.* 1984;310:483–488.

16. Raskin NH, Fishman RA. Pyridoxine-deficiency neuropathy due to hydralazine. *N Engl J Med.* 1965;273:1182–1185.

17. Bosse TR, Donald EA. The vitamin B$_6$ requirement in oral contraceptive users. 1. Assessment by pyridoxal level and transferase activity in erythrocytes. *Am J Clin Nutr.* 1979;32:1015–1023.

18. Rose DP. The interactions between vitamin B$_6$ and hormones. In Harris RS, Munson PL, eds. *Vitamins and Hormones.* Vol. 35. New York, NY: Academic Press, Inc; 1978:53–99.

19. Bender DA, Wynick D. Inhibition of kynureninase (L-kynurenine hydrolase, EC 3.7.1.3) by oestrone sulfate: an alternative explanation for abnormal results of tryptophan load test in women receiving oestrogenic steroids. *Brit J Nutr.* 1981;45:269–275.

20. Stamp TCB. Effects of long-term anticonvulsant therapy on calcium and vitamin D metabolism. *Proc Roy Soc Med.* 1974;67:64–68.

21. Maclaren N. Lifshitz F. Vitamin D-deficiency and rickets in institutionalized mentally retarded children on long term anticonvulsant therapy. II. The response to 25-hydroxycholecalciferol and to vitamin D$_2$. *Pediatr Res.* 1973;7:914–922.

22. Bell RD, Pak CYC, Zerwkh J, et al. Effect of phenytoin on bone and vitamin D metabolism. *Ann Neurol.* 1978;5:374–378.

23. Kempin SJ. Warfarin resistance caused by broccoli. *N Engl J Med.* 1983;308:1229. Letter.

24. Pantuck EJ, Pantuck CB, Garland WA, et al. Stimulatory effect of brussels sprouts and cabbage on human drug metabolism. *Clin Pharmacol Ther.* 1979;25:88–95.

25. Anderson KE, Conney AH, Kappas A. Nutritional influences on biotransformations in humans. *Nutr Rev.* 1982;40:161–171.

26. Conney AH, Pantuck EJ. Hsia K-C, et al. Enhanced phenacetin metabolism in human subjects fed charcoal-broiled beef. *Clin Pharmacol Ther.* 1976;20:633–642.

27. Bailey DG, Spence JD, Munoz C, et al. Interaction of citrus juices with felodipine and nifedipine. *Lancet.* 1991;337:268–269.

28. Soon PA, Vogels BAPM, Roosemalen MCM, et al. Grapefruit juice and cimetidine inhibit stereoselective metabolism of nitrendipine in humans. *Clin Pharmacol Ther.* 1991;50:394–503.

29. Zinn MB. Quinidine intoxication from alkali ingestion. *Tex Med.* 1970;66:64–66.

30. Huyck NI. Patient education: implementing a food and drug interaction program. *Top Clin Nutr.* 1991;6:34–41.

Chapter 10

Dietary Intake Methods

Helen Smiciklas-Wright and Helen A. Guthrie

OVERVIEW

In this chapter, we consider methods for assessing dietary intakes of individuals and groups of individuals. Assessment of dietary intake involves the collection of information on foods and beverages consumed. The consumption data can be used to compute intake of energy, nutrients, and other food components as well as the consumption patterns for specified food groups. The basic methods for assessing dietary intake have been used for a long time,[1] but there has been a significant expansion in the attention paid to dietary intake methodology with the national focus on nutrition monitoring and with the epidemiological and clinical interests in the relationships between diet, health, and disease.[2,3]

PURPOSE OF DIETARY ASSESSMENT

Dietary data are collected for many different purposes. They may be used to estimate population prevalence of particular foods or food components, to study time trends in consumption patterns, to compare intakes of groups, and to study the relationships between intake and health outcomes.[4] They are also used by nutritionists and other health professionals to design nutritional care plans and to evaluate the effectiveness of therapeutic and educational interventions. Dietary assessment can be a challenging undertaking. Success depends on the commitment and ability of respondents to provide information on both quantity and type of foods consumed as well as on the training and supervision of staff responsible for assessment.

A number of methods are available for dietary assessment, but no single method is considered to be generally accepted for all of the purposes. There have been several recent reviews of methods.[3-9] The selection of a method depends upon the proposed use of the data, the abilities and commitment of subjects, and the resources available for data collection and analyses.

The most commonly used dietary data collection methods are 24-hour food recalls, food records (i.e., diaries), the diet history, and food frequencies. These methods have been categorized in a number of ways. Some researchers categorize the methods as retrospective and prospective, with retrospective methods (e.g., the 24-hour food recall, food frequencies) requiring memory for foods eaten and prospective methods involving record keeping concurrent with intake.[5] Other investigators categorize methods as quantitative daily consumption methods (i.e., food recalls, food record), which attempt to capture the actual food consumption in a day, and food frequency methods, which attempt to collect data about food use patterns across longer, less precisely defined time periods.[4] Before reviewing the methods, it is well to remind ourselves that the goal of any dietary study is to discover what people are accustomed to eating and what and how much they freely choose to eat.

METHODS OF COLLECTING DIETARY DATA

Twenty-Four-Hour Food Recall

Recall of food intake may be for any period of time. Since it is almost always administered for a 24-hour period, the method is generally termed the 24-hour recall. The recall may be obtained by interview or by a self-administered questionnaire. The choice depends on cost and the ultimate use of the recall information. If the purpose of the study is to obtain a more qualitative dietary assessment and subjects can be instructed to provide good information, self-administered recalls may be acceptable. Interviewer-administered recalls may be conducted in person or by telephone.[10,11] There has been increasing use of computers for collection and computation of 24-hour recall data.[12]

The typical 24-hour recall asks the client to recall all food eaten and to estimate the quantities in ordinary household measures or by shape and dimensions. The 24-hour recall has become a favored way of obtaining dietary data. It requires only about 15 to 20 minutes of interview time. It is often taken at an unannounced time or with no prior indication of the nature of the data to be requested. This approach minimizes the likelihood that the subjects will modify their food habits in recall. It can provide detailed information about specific foods.

Well-conducted recalls can provide estimates of group average intakes for large groups of subjects.[13] They can also be a helpful screening tool for examining intakes of individuals, especially if information relating to the typical nature of the recall and the ways in which it deviates is integrated with the 24-hour recall data.

An example of a form for recording 24-hour recall data is shown in Exhibit 10–1. The form is modified slightly from that used to collect data in the National Health and Nutrition Examination Survey III.[14] The 24-hour recall form shown in Exhibit 10–1 provides an opportunity for clients to describe not only what foods and what amounts of foods are eaten but also when and where foods are eaten. Time and place of food consumption may be important factors to consider when developing nutrition care plans and designing therapeutic and educational interventions. When using a form such as the one shown, be sure to provide enough space to allow people to list and adequately describe all items eaten.

Several questions are included in Exhibit 10–2 to suggest additional information that may be collected along with the actual food recall. Questions about vitamin and mineral supplement use are sometimes included in surveys but are seldom included in the computed data on vitamin and mineral intake. Yet from one-third to one-half of Americans consume vitamin and/or mineral supplements regularly.[15] About 70 percent take multivitamin and mineral supplements. It is often difficult to quantify supplement intake data because clients may not remember what they use or may use supplements irregularly and because the actual nutrient content of supplements may be uncertain. However, information about supplement use may be helpful in reviewing dietary adequacy.

Another category of questions that can be added to a recall is questions about overall food availability and the resources to obtain food. These are referred to as food security questions and might include such items as "How often are you hungry but you don't eat because you can't afford enough food?"[16] or "Did you skip any meals yesterday because there wasn't enough money to buy food?"[14]

The 24-hour recall method is subject to criticism about accuracy. People may not be able to remember what they ate or know how much they ate. To recall intake, a respondent must have acquired specific memories about food and be able to retrieve the information. Some people may lack the cognitive ability to recall foods eaten, some may have little awareness of what they eat, and others may recall a "good" diet rather than what was actually eaten. Foods that are viewed as unacceptable (e.g., alcohol, fats) may be selectively forgotten.[17]

Several strategies are recommended for helping a client recall food intake. It is important that a nutritionist be well trained in conducting interviews and avoiding leading questions and verbal and nonverbal cues that appear to be judgmental about the recalled diets. The American Dietetic Association has

Exhibit 10–1 A 24-Hour Recall Form

Name or I.D.: _____   Date of Recall: _____
                                            Day of Week of Recall: _____

Time of Day   Foods and Beverages Consumed

Hour	A P M N	Meal	Place	Food Item	Description	Amount

Codes: *Time of Day*   *Meal*
          A—morning   BRE—breakfast
          P—afternoon/evening   BRU—brunch
          M—midnight   LUN—lunch
          N—noon   DIN—dinner/supper
                                                     SNA—snack

          Place   *Amount*
          COM—community feeding program   t—teaspoons
          DAY—day care   T—tablespoons
          FRI—friend's/someone's house   C—cups
          HOM—home   Oz—ounces
          OTH—other   Sm—small serving (unit)
          RES—restaurant   L—large serving (unit)
          SCH—school
          STO—store
          WOR—work

Exhibit 10–2 24-Hour Recall Supplementary Questions

1. How does the amount of food you consumed yesterday compare with the amount that you usually consume for that day of the week?
   _____ much more than usual
   _____ usual
   _____ much less than usual
   _____ don't know

2. Do you take nutrient supplements?
   _____ Yes For how long have you taken them? _____ months
   _____ No   _____ years

   If yes,

Type	Yes	No	How many? Per day/ wk, etc.	Brand	Strength (mg, I.U., etc.)
Multivitamins	_____	_____	_____	_____	
Multivitamins & Minerals	_____	_____	_____	_____	
Vitamins					
Vitamin C	_____	_____	_____	_____	_____
Vitamin E	_____	_____	_____	_____	_____
Others	_____	_____	_____	_____	_____
Minerals					
Calcium	_____	_____	_____	_____	_____
Iron	_____	_____	_____	_____	_____
Others	_____	_____	_____	_____	_____
	_____	_____	_____	_____	_____
	_____	_____	_____	_____	_____

made available an audiocassette guide describing appropriate interviewing skills for the diet interview.[18]

A multiple-pass method may increase retrieval of food memory. The client is first asked to recall all foods eaten in the previous 24 hours but not necessarily to describe them or to give amounts. The client may use memory guides such as time and place of eating. In the next pass, the interviewer begins to ask more probing questions about type of food and amount. In a final pass, the nutritionist may say, "Now I will read to you what I have written (recorded) about the foods you ate and the amounts. Let me know if I have done so correctly."

Computer programs have been developed to provide standardized and consistent probes.[12]

Twenty-four-hour food recalls rely on a respondent's ability to remember the amounts (i.e., portions) of foods and beverages consumed. There is considerable evidence that people cannot accurately describe the amounts of foods they eat.[19–21] Various aids are used to help with portion size estimation. These include measuring utensils, food models and pictures of foods or utensils. Using aids or training people to estimate portion sizes increases portion size estimates, but not for all foods.[22,23]

The 24-hour food recall is subject to further criticism that an individual's usual intake is not likely to be well described in a single 24-hour recall. There has been an extensive literature on the day-to-day variability in intake.[24–27] Several investigators have published data on the number of days of dietary data needed to estimate typical intakes for individuals and for groups of people. For some nutrients such as vitamin A, more than 100 days may be needed to estimate an individual's true average intake.[27] Obviously this is not practical in many situations. Generally a good estimate of a group's mean intake may be estimated from one 24-hour recall, but several recalls, preferably on random rather than consecutive days, should be administered to get a better estimate of an individual's typical intake.[28,29]

In summary, the 24-hour recall is commonly used because it minimizes respondent burden and is reasonably quick to administer. A number of strategies can be used to reduce errors in accuracy. Multiple days of recall can improve estimates of an individual's usual intake.

Food Records

Food records or diaries, like 24-hour recalls, allow for estimates of foods actually consumed during a specified time period, and are preferably done throughout the day to minimize memory errors.[3] Records may be kept by staff, subjects themselves, or surrogates. Records are usually kept for one to seven days, although satisfactory record keeping has been reported for periods of a month to a year with highly motivated persons.[29,30] The shorter the period, the less likely the record will reveal usual eating patterns. On the other hand, the longer the period, the more tedious it may become to keep the record. Gersovitz et al. found that 85 percent of subjects 60 years of age and older who kept seven-day records returned at least two usable records, but only 60 percent returned seven good records.[13] People who returned complete records for seven days were more likely to be the more highly educated of the sample. The results or nature of findings of a study could obviously be influenced by those who dropped out of the study or returned poor records. Generally, multiple days are needed to be representative of usual intake and should preferably be nonconsecutive days.

The perceived strengths of food records are that people can be instructed in advance so that recording errors are minimized and errors of recall are reduced. Multiple days of records may be obtained with less staff time committed to the data collection.[5] Potential limitations are that literacy is required, the act of recording may alter the typical intake, and the costs of coding and analysis are high.[5] Questions are also raised about subjects' abilities to estimate portion sizes and the relevance of a one-day record for describing typical intake.

The level of detail recorded and units of measurement (i.e., estimations by household measure versus weighed measurements) will reflect the purpose(s) of the record keeping. For example, clients may be asked to keep records as self-management tools in weight management and dietary management programs. Such records may not need a high level of detail and yet may be valuable in predicting success of dietary management programs.[31] Clients may be asked to include information not only about the foods and amounts eaten, but also about locations, times, and events associated with eating. This information may help to identify the best targets for change.

Another setting in which a high level of detail may not be necessary but a procedure for routine recording of intake is essential is in long-term care institutions. Many institutions monitor intake regularly on food intake record forms that list menu items served. These serve as checklists and enable a staff person to note how much of each item was eaten by a resident (e.g., all of it, one-half of it, one-quarter of it, none).

When more detailed food records are necessary, subjects must be given good instructions about record keeping, and completed records must be reviewed thoroughly by staff. The U.S. Department of Agriculture is responsible for nationwide food consumption surveys in which participants are asked to keep records. The department prepares booklets for subjects telling them how to describe foods and beverages and report as accurately as possible how much was eaten.[32] The instructions can be a useful guide for anyone working with food records. The level of detail may be modified for specific study purposes.

The Diet History

The dietary history is designed to determine a client's usual intake over a specified time period. The diet history as described by Burke includes several techniques to estimate usual dietary intake.[33] Burke's dietary history combined questions about subject's health habits with a 24-hour recall and questions about the usual eating pattern by asking, "What do you usually have for breakfast?" The history included a cross-check in the form of a detailed list of foods, with questions about use, likes, and dislikes. An added cross-check was available in the form of a three-day food record.

Jean Hankin, who has made significant contributions to the field of dietary assessment, described the diet history as a method designed to cover the total intake and one that requires highly trained dietitians and nutritionists to administer.[34] This requires considerable interviewer time and requires clients to be quite observant of food intakes.[35] The history may be difficult to complete if a client has no well-defined eating pattern.

The term *diet history* is often used synonymously with food frequency methods. In general, the diet history is intended to focus on foods in the total diet, whereas food frequencies may be designed for total diet assessment or be directed on selected foods reflecting specific dietary concerns (e.g., lipids, use of fruits and vegetables).[34]

Food Frequency Questionnaires

Food frequency questionnaires (FFQs) have become widely used, particularly in epidemiologic studies. There are numerous FFQs essentially consisting of two parts: a list of foods or food groups and a set of response options indicating how often foods or food groups are consumed during a specific time period.[36–41] The list of foods may vary considerably, from a brief list focusing on a specific nutrient to a list of several hundred foods designed to assess the total diet. The frequency of response options may be general (e.g., "often," "sometimes," "never") or more elaborate and specific (e.g., number of servings per day, per week, per month). Finally, the period of recall may vary, normally from one month to one year, and may be the period preceding the completion of the questionnaire or at some distant time.

FFQs with food lists and response options are generally referred to as qualitative FFQs; such FFQs ask about numbers of servings or units of foods consumed, but not amounts. An example of a qualitative FFQ is shown in Exhibit 10–3, which shows a portion of the questionnaire that is being used for NHANES-III.[14]

Various food questionnaires are termed *semiquantitative* in that they ask respondents questions about portion size. Some questionnaires ask respondents to describe a "typical" portion size, some state the amount of a "medium" serving and ask a client to indicate whether his or her intake of a food is "small," "medium," or "large,"[36] and still others use pictures to illustrate different portion sizes.[34]

FFQs are considered to be cost-effective tools for dietary data collection. They can be self-administered, interviewer administered in person or by telephone, or administered using computerized precoded questionnaires.[42]

Exhibit 10–3 A Portion of the NHANES-III Food Frequency Questionnaire

Now I'm going to ask you how often you usually eat certain foods. When answering think about your *usual* diet over the *past month*. Tell me how often you usually ate or drank these foods per day, per week, per month, or not at all.

Times	Day	Week	Month
___ ___	per 1☐ D	2☐W	3☐M
	Never	Don't Know	
	or 4☐N	9☐DK	

1. *MILK AND MILK PRODUCTS*

First are milk and milk products. Do not include their use in cooking.

a. How often did you have chocolate milk and hot cocoa?   ___ ___ per 1☐D 2☐W 3☐M or 4☐N 9☐DK

b. How often did you have milk to drink or on cereal? Do not count *small* amounts of milk added to coffee or tea.   ___ ___ per 1☐D 2☐W 3☐M or 4☐N 9☐DK

c. CHECK ITEM. REFER TO RESPONSES IN 1a AND 1b.
   ☐ "Never" in both 1a and 1b (1e)
   ☐ Other

d. What type of milk was it? Was it *usually* whole, 2%, 1%, skim, nonfat, or some other type?
   ☐ whole/regular
   ☐ 2%/low fat
   ☐ 1%
   ☐ skim/nonfat
   ☐ buttermilk
   ☐ evaporated
   ☐ other _____
               specify
   ☐ DK

e. Yogurt and frozen yogurt   ___ ___ per 1☐D 2☐W 3☐M or 4☐N 9☐DK

f. Ice cream, ice milk, and milkshakes   ___ ___ per 1☐D 2☐W 3☐M or 4☐N 9☐DK

g. Cheese, all types including American, Swiss, cheddar, and cottage cheese   ___ ___ per 1☐D 2☐W 3☐M or 4☐N 9☐DK

continues

Exhibit 10–3 continued

h. Pizza, calzone, and lasagna	___ ___ per 1 ☐ D 2 ☐ W 3 ☐ M or 4 ☐ N 9 ☐ DK
i. Cheese dishes such as macaroni and cheese, cheese nachos, cheese enchiladas, and quesadillas	___ ___ per 1 ☐ D 2 ☐ W 3 ☐ M or 4 ☐ N 9 ☐ DK

Source: National Health and Nutrition Examination Survey III Data Collection Forms, US Dept of Health and Human Services, Public Health Service, Centers for Disease Control, National Center for Health Statistics, Hyattsville, MD, March 1990.

There are concerns about the cognitive demands of FFQs, both memory and mathematical computations. FFQs make demands on long-term memory. They assume the existence of a pattern that may or may not exist. Food lists that are very limited will not reflect total food intake. Those that are too extensive, on the other hand, may be tedious to complete, and clients may mark items indiscriminately, with the quality of the data deteriorating throughout the checklist. Questionnaires that ask about portion sizes require more judgments on the part of respondents.

In summary, FFQs are valuable as descriptors of dietary patterns. They are particularly useful in describing intake of foods that may be consumed periodically (e.g., alcohol) but less able than recalls or records to elicit information about intake of specific foods and amounts.[43]

Data Collection Completion

There are several ways of completing food intake data collection, primarily by interview or self-completion by clients. Interviewers may complete data collection for 24-hour recalls and food frequency questionnaires with face-to-face or phone interviews. Clients may complete their own records or questionnaires during a clinic visit or may be contacted and return data by mail. Validity of the data, response rates, and cost of obtaining and preparing data for analysis are all considerations in selecting a method.

Interviewer-completed data allow for standardized data collection procedures, for clarification, and for guiding clients in use of portion-size aids. Home-based interviews can provide opportunities for probing for food brands and for nutrient supplements. However, the staff time and associated costs of interviews may limit interviewer-completed recalls, particularly multiple recalls.

Telephone interviews are an alternative to face-to-face interviews. The advantages include the relative speed of data collection, good response rates, and relatively low costs.[6,10] Telephone interviews for 24-hour recalls can provide food energy intake data comparable to that of face-to-face interviews. A disadvantage of phone interviews is that contact times convenient for clients may not be convenient for clinical staff.

There are also advantages and disadvantages to self-completed data. Less time is required for training of interviewers and data collection. It may be possible to obtain data from more people and from people who could not or would not be available for an interview. Respondents have a greater sense of privacy and less time pressure, and may feel freer to provide information that they believe to be personal. A problem with self-completed data is possible misinterpretation of the task. The nutritionist needs to provide instructions that are clear and sufficiently detailed and yet not overwhelming to clients. Another problem may be response rate, particularly for mailed data. Finally, considerable staff time may be given to the cleanup of data in preparation for data analysis.

Guidelines in Selecting an Appropriate Method

It is difficult to give clear-cut advice about the best method for dietary assessment. The single, most useful piece of advice is probably that of Christakis, who suggested that the method selected should be no more detailed, no more cumbersome, and no more expensive than necessary.[44] With these words in mind, the following may serve as guidelines in the dietary assessment of groups and individuals and as a means of developing a database for counseling.

Groups

The 24-hour recall, diet records, and food frequencies have been the methods used in recent nationwide surveys. A 24-hour recall or one-day record can provide estimates of population group average intakes on the assumption that if enough subjects are chosen, the range of usual intake of the population from which they are selected will be represented. However, this method does not provide reliable estimates either of usual intake of an individual or of the distribution of usual intakes for a population. Some years ago Beaton and coworkers[45] recommended that in order to get more data about usual intake distributions, study designs of large groups should provide for a replicate examination of a subsample of the group. This idea is receiving consideration in the most recent nationwide surveys.[42]

Individuals

The method for assessing the dietary intake of individuals should be compatible with the purpose of the assessment. If the goal of the study is to relate dietary intake data to biochemical determinations, the dietary information should be collected for a long enough period to permit meaningful analysis to relate it to the laboratory data. Multiple days of data are advisable and likely to be more feasible than records kept for a longer time period.

Data for Dietary Counseling

If the purpose of the assessment is to develop a database for counseling, food frequencies, recalls, or records may all provide the nutritionist with some insight about a person's diet and help to establish a base for further inquiry and probing. How extensive that probing will be is likely to be limited by time or the person's ability to provide more information. In this situation, if time is very limited, a simple food frequency may be more valuable than a 24-hour recall, especially for foods such as salad dressings, gravies, snacks, and alcoholic beverages that are frequently overlooked by respondents.

THE USE OF DIETARY INTAKE DATA

Analysis

An evaluation of dietary adequacy has two major components: (1) the collection of information about the kinds and amounts of foods consumed, and (2) the translation of that information into nutritional terms. The translation or analysis of dietary intakes ranges from describing intake of foods and food group methods to computations for energy, nutrients, and other food components.

Food-scoring systems, the fastest way of analyzing data, can provide considerable information on which to base counseling. The scores are usually based on food groups. The scoring system shown in Table 10–1 is based on the Food Guide Pyramid.[46] Guthrie and Scheer studied the relationship between a food group dietary score and computed nutrient values. They found the score to be an appreciably sensitive tool for assessing dietary adequacy, and concluded that it could be used to evaluate nutrition intervention programs and monitor changes in dietary intakes over time.[47] Food scores may also be designed to rate specific foods. For example, the multiple risk factor intervention trial (MRFIT) used a food-scoring system as an assessment and teaching device for men who were identified as being at risk of developing coronary heart disease. The scoring system was based on a scaling of the foods that are main contributors to serum cholesterol elevation.[48]

Table 10-1 Dietary Score Based on a Guide to Daily Food Choices

Food Choice Examples	Many Women, Older Adults (~1600 Kcals)	Children, Teen Girls, Active Women (~2200 Kcals)	Teen Boys, Active Men (~2800 Kcals)
	*Maximum Points/Food Group**		
Bread Group			
1 slice bread			
1 oz RTE cereal			
½ C cooked cereal, rice, pasta	6	9	11
Vegetable Group			
1 C raw leafy			
½ C other—cooked or			
chopped raw			
¾ C juice	3	4	5
Fruit Group			
1 medium apple, banana, etc.			
½ C chopped, cooked, canned			
¾ C juice	2	3	4
Milk Group			
1 C milk or yogurt			
1 ½ oz cheese			
2 oz processed cheese	2 (3)**	2 (3)**	2 (3)**
Meat Group			
2-3 oz meat			
½ C beans, 1 egg			
2 T peanut butter =			
1 oz meat	2 (total 5 oz)	2 (total 6 oz)	3 (total 7 oz)
Total points	15 (16)**	20 (21)**	25 (26)**

*1 point/serving in each food group.
**For women who are pregnant or breastfeeding, teenagers, and young adults to age 24, who need three servings from milk group, total points are increased by 1.

Scoring systems based on the major food groups are likely to be inadequate for some purposes. They may not be applicable to hospital diets based on unconventional foods, such as liquid or semisolid regimens or supplemental formula foods. The systems may not account for many foods that are not in the target food group yet add significantly to the nutrient and caloric intake of the diet. Nevertheless, if the data that have been gathered are primarily qualitative, scores may serve as a useful proxy for actual nutrient values.

More detailed nutrient computations may be made on the basis of food composition tables. The standard reference tables are contained in the U.S. Department of Agriculture's *Composition of Foods, Raw, Processed and Prepared* (Handbook No. 8).[49] The 1963 edition has been updated into a 21-volume loose-leaf form publication. Each volume covers nutrient values for a major food group. Other food composition and computer software databases draw extensively on the Agricultural Department's Handbook-8 data, adding additional foods depending on the focus of the table. Additional data may be needed for mixed dishes calculated from recipe information or processed foods provided by food companies. Reference tables are now being expanded to provide data on more nutrients. The professional should be aware of how complete the database is for each nutrient before making conclusions about dietary adequacy.

Nutrient calculations may be made manually from food records. However, the computation can be laborious and tedious; thus computer calculations have become increasingly common. The foods listed in the Agriculture Department's Handbook-8 are provided with code numbers for computer calculations.

Computers are playing an increasingly important role in dietary analysis, facilitating the development and organization of large nutrient composition data banks. However, computers have not solved all dietary intake calculation problems. The variety of foods available and consumed by clients often require that dietitians interpret and select a best-fit food before coding for analysis. Considerable variability in estimated nutrient intake can be the result of variability in coding intake.[50]

Interpretation

Standards

Once dietary nutrients have been determined, they are generally compared to some standard. The dietary standard in the United States is the recommended dietary allowances (RDAs).[51] Except for calories (energy), RDAs are set at levels that exceed the requirements of the vast majority of healthy people for most nutrients. The allowances state very clearly that intakes below the recommended allowances for a nutrient are not necessarily inadequate. Failure to consume the recommended amounts cannot necessarily be interpreted as a dietary deficiency. This warning against misinterpretation is particularly critical with analysis of one-day intakes.

There are several approaches for determining adequacy of diets.[52] The most widely used method is the cutoff method, which estimates the intake of a nutrient below a given value of the RDAs. Many different cutoff points have been used (80 percent, 66 percent, 50 percent). A value of 77 percent of the RDA is a value that represents the "average" requirement for a given age and sex group. If the RDAs are considered to represent the mean requirement +2 S.D., and the S.D. is 15 percent of the mean, as in most biological measures, then RDA equals 130 percent of the mean. The average requirement is represented by 77 percent of the RDAs (e.g., 100/130). The requirement of half the population is below 77 percent of the RDAs.

It is not appropriate to consider that levels falling below the RDAs or any value of the RDAs indicate dietary deficiencies, although it is appropriate to consider levels well below the RDAs to indicate risks to dietary adequacy. The existence of deficiencies must be confirmed or rejected on the basis of biochemical and/ or anthropometric data.

An alternative to the cutoff approach is the probability approach, which assesses the percentages of a population whose usual intakes are below their individual requirements. This method requires that the distribution of requirements as well as the distribution of intakes be known. An excellent review of these approaches has appeared recently.[52]

Criteria for Assessing Nutrient Quality of Food

The nutrient quality of a food or a diet in regard to any one nutrient is often expressed as an Index of Nutrient Quality (INQ) representing the nutrient density of the food or diet. This is the ratio of the percentage contribution of a food to the requirement for a specific nutrient to its percentage contribution to the need for calories; that is,

$$INQ = \frac{\% \text{ RDA for a nutrient}}{\% \text{ energy requirement}}$$

Because both the RDA for a nutrient and the need for calories will vary with the age and sex of individuals, the INQ for a nutrient in a particular serving of food will vary for one person (e.g., a child) compared to another (e.g., a pregnant woman).

Criteria for Assessing the Adequacy of a Diet

Since the adequacy of the diet is a function of the extent to which its contribution of particular nutrients meets our best estimate of the need for those nutrients, it is helpful to calculate a Nutrient Adequacy Ratio (NAR) for each nutrient.

$$NAR = \frac{\text{amount of nutrient in diet}}{\text{RDA for that nutrient}}$$

When NAR is greater than 1, the requirement is met. If it falls below 1 it may still be sufficient, since the RDA is set at the mean requirement of 77 percent RDAs. The farther the NAR falls below 1, the higher the probability that the diet will fail to meet the needs of the individual. Only by determining some biochemical marker of dietary adequacy, however, can a judgment be made as to whether the intake of a particular nutrient is adequate.

An MAR or Mean Adequacy Ratio is used to indicate the overall adequacy of the diet. This is the average NAR for as many nutrients as are of interest, with each NAR truncated at 1 since requirements for nutrients are independent of one another inasmuch as each performs a specific function and they cannot substitute for one another. Thus the highest possible MAR is 1, and again, the higher the overall quality of the diet the closer the MAR will be to 1. An examination of the individual NARs used in calculating the MAR will identify the most limiting nutrients and the extent to which they contribute to levels below 1.

RDAs have not been established for all nutrients and food components. The focus of dietary guidelines has been on fat, saturated fat, cholesterol, sodium, and fiber, for which there are not yet RDAs. Many scientific committees have encouraged dietary practices to modify these food components. The views of the committees have been expressed in *Nutrition and Your Health: Dietary Guidelines for Americans*.[53] The guidelines recommend that total fat provide 30 percent or less of calories, that saturated fat provide less than 10% of calories, that animal fat intake be reduced to lower cholesterol, and that salt and sodium be used in moderation. The guidelines emphasize that these goals are not for children under two years old. Furthermore, they are goals that apply to the diet over several days. The goals should also apply to total diet and not individual foods.

Recent studies suggest that not all long-chain fatty acids raise plasma cholesterol.[54] Stearic acid does not appear to be hypercholesterolemic and may have an LDL-cholesterol lowering effect. Future guidelines may need to reflect the differential impacts of specific fatty acids on cholesterol.

CONCLUSION

Several methods are commonly used to assess diet intake. There is no single perfect dietary method. Methods that require that clients recall intake are dependent upon the respondent's memory. Though an experienced clinician will probably recognize when a client has overall poor recall of food intake, it is much more difficult to account for suppressions and distortions of memory. Reported intakes may be influenced by the respondent's sense of what should be eaten rather than by what is typically consumed. Methods vary in estimating typical intake.

Some of the limitations of dietary assessment are inherent in the methods and cannot be altered easily. For example, by its very nature, the diet history is more time consuming than a 24-hour recall. The 24-hour recall describes the intake of one day, not necessarily for any longer period of time, unless the diet is quite monotonous or when multiple recalls are conducted. Other limitations of dietary assessment relate to respondents themselves—their abilities and willingness to provide data.

A focus on the limitations of dietary methods fails to recognize their importance in studies of diet and health. There has been a lively debate in the past decade on which methods to select for which purposes. The debate continues, as do efforts to decrease errors by improving both data collection and analysis.

REFERENCES

1. Medlin C, Skinner JD. Individual dietary intake methodology: a 50-year review of progress. *J Am Diet Assoc.* 1988;88:1250–1257.

2. Life Sciences Research Office, Federation of American Societies for Experimental Biology. *Nutrition Monitoring in the United States: An Update Report on Nutrition Monitoring.* Washington, DC: US Government Printing Office; Sept. 1989. DHHS Publication No. (PHS) 89-1255.

3. Freudenheim JL. Dietary assessment in nutritional epidemiology. *Nutr Metab Cardiovasc Dis.* 1991;1:207–212.

4. Life Sciences Research Office. *Guidelines for Use of Dietary Intake Data.* Bethesda, Md: Federation of American Societies for Experimental Biology; 1986.

5. Dwyer JT. Assessment of dietary intake. In: Shils ME, Young VR, eds. *Modern Nutrition in Health and Disease.* 7th ed. Philadelphia, Pa: Lea & Febiger; 1988:887–905.

6. Pao EM, Sykes KE, Cypel YS. *USDA Methodological Research for Large-Scale Dietary Intake Surveys. 1975–78.* US Dept of Agriculture, Human Nutrition Information Service; December 1989. Home Economics Research Report No. 49.

7. Block G. Human dietary assessment: methods and issues. *Prev Med.* 1989;12:653–660.

8. Bingham SA. The dietary assessment of individuals: methods, accuracy, new techniques and recommendations. *Nutr Abst Rev.* (series A) 1987;57:705–742.

9. Cameron ME, Van Staveren WA. *Manual on Methodology for Food Consumption Studies.* New York, NY: Oxford University Press; 1988.

10. Derr JA, Mitchell DC, Brannon D, Smiciklas-Wright H, Dixon LB, Shannon BM. Time and cost analysis of a computer-assisted telephone interview system to collect dietary recalls. *Am J Epidemiol.* 1992;136:1386–1392.

11. Fox TA, Heimendinger J, Block G. Telephone surveys as a method for obtaining dietary information: a review. *J Am Diet Assoc.* 1992;92:729–732.

12. Feskanich D, Buzzard IM, Welch BT, et al. Comparison of a computerized and a manual method of food coding for nutrient intake studies. *J Am Diet Assoc.* 1988;88:1263–1267.

13. Gersovitz MM, Madden JP, Smiciklas-Wright H. Validities of the 24-hour dietary recall and seven-day record for group comparisons. *J Am Diet Assoc.* 1978;73:48–55.

14. US Dept of Health and Human Services. *National Health and Nutrition Examination Survey III Data Collection Forms.* Hyattsville, Md: Public Health Service, Centers for Disease Control, National Center for Health Statistics; March 1990.

15. Moss A, Levy AS, Kim I, Park Y. *Use of Vitamin and Mineral Supplements in the U.S.: Current Users, Types of Products, and Nutrients.* Hyattsville, Md: National Center for Health Statistics; 1989. Advance Data No. 174.

16. Radimer KL, Olson CM, Campbell CT. Development of indicators to assess hunger. *J Nutr.* 1990;120:1544–1548.

17. Dwyer J, Krall EA. Coleman KA. The problem of memory in nutritional epidemiology research. *J Am Diet Assoc.* 1987;87:1509–1512.

18. Wiese HJC. *The Diet Interview: A How-to-Guide.* American Dietetic Association Audiocassette Series; 1984.

19. Guthrie HA. Selection and quantification of typical food portions by young adults. *J Am Diet Assoc.* 1984;84:1440–1444.

20. Smiciklas-Wright H, Guthrie HA, Cook RA, Beal VA. *Subjects' Ability to Estimate Portions of Beverages.* University Park, Pa: Pennsylvania State University Agricultural Experiment Station; 1987.

21. Dubois S, Boivin J-F. Accuracy of telephone dietary recalls in elderly subjects. *J Am Diet Assoc.* 1990;90:1680–1687.

22. Bolland JE, Ward JY, Bolland TW. Improved accuracy of estimating food quantities up to 4 weeks after training. *J Am Diet Assoc.* 1990;90:1402–1407.

23. Yuhas JA, Bolland JE, Bolland TW. The impact of training, food type, gender, and container size on the estimation of food portion sizes. *J Am Diet Assoc.* 1989;89:1473–1477.

24. Guthrie HA, Crocetti AF. Variability of nutrient intake over a 3-day period. *J Am Diet Assoc.* 1985;85:325–327.

25. Gibson RS, Gibson IL, Kitching J. A study of inter- and intra-subject variability in seven-day weighed dietary intakes with particular emphasis on trace elements. *Biol Trace Element Res.* 1985;8:79–91.

26. Ervin B, Smiciklas-Wright H, Fosmire G. Intra- and interindividual differences in zinc intake in older women. *Nutr Res.* 1989;9:613–624.

27. Basiotis PP, Welsh SO, Cronin FJ, Kelsay JL, Mertz W. Number of days of food intake records required to estimate individual and group nutrient intakes with defined confidence. *J Nutr.* 1987;117:1638–1641.

28. Larkin F, Metzner HL, Guire KE. Comparison of three consecutive-day and three random-day records of dietary intakes. *J Am Diet Assoc.* 1991;91:1538–1542.

29. Tarasuk V, Beaton G. The nature and individuality of within-subject variation in energy intake. *Am J Clin Nutr.* 1991;54:464–470.

30. St. Jeor ST, Guthrie HA, Jones MB. Variability in nutrient intake in a 28-day period. *J Am Diet Assoc.* 1983;83:155–162.

31. Streit KJ, Stevens NH, Stevens VJ, Rossner J. Food records: a predictor and modifier of weight change in a long-term weight loss program. *J Am Diet Assoc.* 1991;91:213–216.

32. US Dept of Agriculture. *Continuing Survey of Food Intakes by Individuals.* Washington, DC: National Analysts; 1991.

33. Burke BS. The dietary history as a tool in research. *J Am Diet Assoc.* 1947;23:1041–1046.

34. Hankin JH. 23rd Lenna Frances Losper Memorial Lecture: a diet history method for research, clinical, and community use. *J Am Diet Assoc.* 1986;86:868–875.

35. Beal VA. The nutritional history in longitudinal research. *J Am Diet Assoc.* 1967;51:426–432.

36. Sampson L. Food frequency questionnaires as a research instrument. *Clin Nutr.* 1985;4: 171–178.

37. Block G, Hartman AM, Dresser CM, et al. A data-based approach to diet questionnaire design and testing. *Am J Epidemiol.* 1986;124:453–469.

38. Willet W. *Nutritional Epidemiology.* New York, NY: Oxford University Press; 1990.

39. Kristal AR, Abrams BH, Thornquist MD, et al. Development and validation of a food use checklist for evaluation of community nutrition interventions. *Am J Public Health.* 1990;80:1318–1322.

40. Curtis AE, Musgrave KO, Klimas-Tavantzis DA. A food frequency questionnaire that rapidly and accurately assesses intake of fat, saturated fat, cholesterol, and energy. *J Am Diet Assoc.* 1992;92:1517–1519.

41. Zulkifli SN, Yu SM. The food frequency method for dietary assessment. *J Am Diet Assoc.* 1992;92:681–685.

42. Sempos CS, Briefel RR, Flegal KM, et al. Factors involved in selecting a dietary survey methodology for nutrition surveys. *Austr J Nutr Diet.* 1992;49:96–103.

43. Briefel RR, Flegal KM, Winn DW, et al. Assessing the nation's diet: limitations of the food frequency questionnaire. *J Am Diet Assoc.* 1992;92:959–962.

44. Christakis G. Nutritional assessment in health programs. *Am J Public Health.* 1973;63(IIS): 11–17.

45. Beaton GH, Milner J, Corey P, et al. Sources of variance in 24-hour dietary recall data: implications for nutritional study design and interpretation. *Am J Clin Nutr.* 1979;32:2546–2567.

46. Welsh S, Davis C, Shaw A. Development of the Food Guide Pyramid. *Nutr Today.* 1992;27(6): 12–23.

47. Guthrie HA, Scheer JC. Validity of a dietary score for assessing nutrient adequacy. *J Am Diet Assoc.* 1981;78:240–245.

48. Remmell PS, Gorder DD, Hall Y, Tillotson JL. Assessing dietary adherence in the Multiple Risk Factor Intervention Trial (MRFIT). I. Use of a dietary monitoring tool. *J Am Diet Assoc.* 1980;76:351–356.

49. Watt BK, Merrill AL. *Composition of Foods, Raw, Processed and Prepared.* Washington, DC: U.S. Department of Agriculture; 1963. Agriculture Handbook No. 8, rev.

50. Lacey JM, Beal VA, Hosmer DW, et al. *Coder Variability in Computerized Dietary Analysis.* Amherst, Mass: Massachusetts Agricultural Experiment Station; 1990.

51. National Research Council. *Recommended Dietary Allowances.* 10th ed. Washington, DC: National Academy of Sciences, National Research Council; 1989.

52. Jensen HH, Nusser SM, Riddick H, Sands L. A critique of two methods for assessing the nutrient adequacy of diets. *J Nutr Educ.* 1992;24:123–129.

53. US Dept of Agriculture/US Dept of Health and Human Services. *Nutrition and Your Health: Dietary Guidelines for Americans.* Washington, DC: US Government Printing Office; 1990. Home and Garden Bull. No. 233.

54. Kris-Etherton PM, Mustad V, Derr J. Effects of dietary stearic acid on plasma lipids and thrombosis. *Nutr Today.* 1993;28(3):38–46.

Chapter 11

Laboratory Assessment of Nutritional Status

Nicholas H.E. Mezitis and F. Xavier Pi-Sunyer

OVERVIEW

Laboratory tests are a valuable adjunct in nutritional evaluation. Their appropriate use requires understanding of the purpose of each test, awareness of relevant normal values, and knowledge of the conditions contributing to abnormal results. Available tests for nutritional evaluation focus on determination of levels of macro- and micronutrients in body fluids. Generally, only body fluids such as blood and urine are used for sampling. Laboratory techniques utilizing tissue biopsies or hair samples for nutritional analysis are not readily available and are rarely used. They are not discussed in this chapter. The concentration of an essential nutrient in body fluids can be decreased as a result of dietary deficiency, poor absorption, impaired transport, abnormal utilization, or a combination of any of these factors. Further exploration of the patient's dietary and medical history, a more detailed physical examination, and diagnostic testing may be necessary to define the causes or abnormal values more precisely.

TECHNIQUES FOR LABORATORY MEASUREMENTS

Most laboratory techniques assessing nutritional status measure one of the following parameters: (1) nutrient level in the blood, (2) urinary excretion rate of the nutrient, (3) urinary metabolites of the nutrient, (4) abnormal metabolic products in the blood, (5) changes in the blood components or enzyme activities that can be related to intake of the nutrient, or (6) response to a loading, saturation, or isotopic test.[1]

Tests for nutrient status determination vary in diagnostic value. For example, direct tests for water-soluble vitamins in the blood are more sensitive than indirect tests of the excretion of metabolites of these vitamins in the urine. In addition, the precision and accuracy of each test are of vital importance.

Precision in testing refers to the ability to reproduce a value; *accuracy* refers to the closeness of any reported value to the actual value. The four bull's eyes in Figure 11–1 illustrate the difference between precision and accuracy. The bull's eye represents the acceptable range of results for a given sample. The asterisks represent sequential measurements of the given sample. The distance between asterisks corresponds to variability between measurements and illustrates precision. The distance of the asterisks from the bull's eye illustrates accuracy. The precision of a test can be measured by determining the coefficient of variation, that is, the standard deviation of a series of identical samples expressed as a percentage of the mean value of the samples. The smaller the coefficient of variation, the greater the precision of the test. Measures of the deviation between the "true" value of the sample and the measured value are an indicator of accuracy.

CARBOHYDRATE

Glucose is the circulating form of carbohydrate in the blood. It is a monosaccharide with the formula $C_6H_{12}O_6$. It provides fuel for energy to tissues, and it may be stored in liver and muscle as glycogen for later use.

The dietary forms of carbohydrate include two other monosaccharides, fructose and galactose, which share the same structural formula with glucose but have a different three-dimensional structure. They also include disaccharides

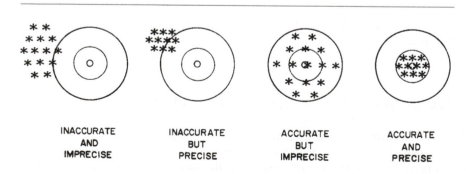

| INACCURATE AND IMPRECISE | INACCURATE BUT PRECISE | ACCURATE BUT IMPRECISE | ACCURATE AND PRECISE |

Figure 11–1 Bull's Eyes Illustrating Difference between Precision and Accuracy

and polysaccharides, which are first digested to monosaccharides in the intestine and then absorbed and converted to glucose in the liver and kidneys. Disaccharides such as sucrose, lactose, and maltose are made up of two monosaccharide molecules. Polysaccharides such as starch and glycogen are made up of hundreds to thousands of glucose molecules.

Glucose concentration can be determined in whole blood, plasma, or serum. Plasma represents blood fluids remaining after all cellular elements have been removed by centrifugation. Serum is the fluid remaining after blood has clotted and the clot containing all cellular elements and certain blood proteins has been compressed and removed by centrifugation. Blood cells contain little free glucose. Therefore processing of blood to yield plasma or serum in effect concentrates glucose in these fluids, and levels tend to be 10 to 15 percent higher than those in whole blood.

Available methodologies to determine glucose may be specific ("true" glucose methods) or nonspecific ("reducing" sugar methods). The latter do not discriminate between glucose and other reducing sugars in the blood and therefore give about 10 percent higher values than "true" methods. The most popular "true" glucose determination used in modern laboratories measures glucose in plasma by using the enzyme glucose oxidase. This is the measurement referred to in subsequent discussions and tables in this chapter. Fingerstick methodologies, which are widely used in modern diabetes management, involve glucose determination in capillary whole blood. These values are lower than those obtained from paired serum or plasma samples.

A variety of tests measure "true" glucose in the urine. Glucose enters the urine if the average renal threshold of 170 mg/dl (9.52 mM/L) is exceeded in the blood.

Healthy individuals maintain their blood glucose levels within a very narrow range. The currently acceptable lower and upper limits in the fasting state for plasma are 60 and 115 mg/dl (3.36 and 6.44 mM/L), respectively.[2] In individual subjects, blood glucose levels are much more narrowly controlled within this range and are very consistent. Excursions below or above these limits are quickly corrected by hormonal adjustments.

After meals, plasma glucose levels in normal individuals usually exceed the upper fasting limit of 140 mg/dl (7.84 mM/L), but then are rapidly corrected and never exceed 140 mg/dl (7.84 mM/L) two hours after the meal. Likewise, in certain conditions such as pregnancy and after prolonged exercise, glucose values may drop below 60 mg/dl (3.36 mM/L), but correct rapidly, particularly after ingestion of carbohydrate.[3]

To check for abnormalities in glucose tolerance, nonpregnant individuals may be tested with a 75-gram glucose load offered as a carbonated drink. For three days immediately preceding the test, the diet must include at least 250 grams of carbohydrate per day to prime the insulin-producing beta cells of the pancreas for optimal function. During the test, blood is drawn before the liquid meal and every half hour thereafter for two hours. The diagnostic criteria for normal, glucose-intolerant, and diabetic individuals are shown in Exhibit 11–1. Specific criteria for pregnant females after a customary 100-gram glucose challenge are also depicted.

Impaired glucose tolerance (IGT) defines a glycemic response to the 75-gram glucose challenge that exceeds normal levels, yet remains below the diagnostic criteria for diabetes. This condition has not been correlated with excess morbidity and mortality, but may progress to frank diabetes.

Hypoglycemia usually reflects plasma glucose values below 60 mg/dl (3.36 mM/L)[4] that are associated with symptoms such as tremors, sweating, confusion, and general distress. It may occur after meals (postprandial) or in the

---

Exhibit 11–1 Criteria for Evaluation of Plasma Glucose Levels (SI Units in Parentheses)

1. Normal Glucose Values—Nonpregnant Adults
    1.1. Fasting plasma glucose (PG) ≤ 115 mg/dl (6.44 mM/L)
    1.2. Oral glucose tolerance test (OGTT) PG values between zero time and 2-hour PG ≤ 200 mg/dl (11.2 mM/L), using 75-g glucose load

2. Diabetes Mellitus—Adults
    Any of the following conditions met:
    2.1. PG ≥ 200 mg/dl (11.2 mM/L) with classic symptoms of diabetes mellitus
    2.2. Fasting PG ≥ 140 mg/dl (7.84 mM/L) on at least two occasions
    2.3. 75-g OGTT PG values (at last one) between zero time and 2-hour ≥ 200 mg/dl (11.2 mM/L) *and* 2-hour value ≥ 200 mg/dl (11.2 mM/L)

3. Impaired Glucose Tolerance (IGT)
    Fasting PG < 140 mg/dl (7.84 mM/L) and 2-hour PG ≥ 140 mg/dl (7.84 mM/L) and < 200 mg/dl (11.2 mM/L), with one intervening value ≥ 200 mg/dl (11.2 mM/L)

4. Gestational Diabetes Mellitus (GDM)
    Two or more of the following PG results on OGTT, using a 100-g glucose load:
    • Fasting PG ≥ 105 mg/dl (5.88 mM/L)
    • 1-hour PG ≥ 190 mg/dl (10.64 mM/L)
    • 2-hour PG ≥ 165 mg/dl (9.24 mM/L)
    • 3-hour PG ≥ 145 mg/dl (8.12 mM/L)

5. Diabetes Mellitus—Children
    Any of the following conditions met:
    5.1. Classic symptoms with random PG ≥ 200 mg/dl (11.2 mM/L)
    5.2. Fasting PG > 140 mg/dl (7.84 mM/L) and 2-hour PG and one intervening value ≥ 200 mg/dl (11.2 mM/L), using 1.75 g/kg to maximum of 75-g glucose load

Source: National Diabetes Data Group. Classification and diagnosis of diabetes mellitus and other categories of glucose intolerance. *Diabetes.* 1979;28:1039–1057.

fasting state. The timing in relationship to meals defines the differential diagnosis. Symptoms correct rapidly after ingestion of carbohydrate.

LIPIDS

Lipids represent a heterogeneous group of water-insoluble nutrients including triglycerides, phospholipids, cholesterol, and fatty acids. Structural formulas of representatives of each of these four groups are shown in Figure 11–2.

Triglycerides account for more than 95 percent of fat ingested in the diet. Phospholipids and cholesterol occur mainly as constituents of cell membranes and nerve tissue myelin and are ingested in small amounts.

In the intestine, lipids are digested to fatty acids, monoglycerides, phosphate, and glycerol. Cholesterol is deesterified. These substances then enter the intestinal mucosa by passive diffusion and are processed. Triglycerides, phospholipids, and cholesterol esters are resynthesized and enveloped by proteins (apoproteins) to promote solubility in water. The resulting complexes are mainly secreted as chylomicrons into the lymphatic system. The intestine also produces some very low-density lipoproteins (VLDL) and high-density lipoproteins (HDL). Shorter chain fatty acids (less than 12 carbons) bypass this packaging process and are absorbed directly into the circulation, to be transported to tissues in association with albumin.

After delivering their triglyceride contents to the tissues, circulating VLDL are transformed into denser particles due to an increase in their protein-to-lipid ratio. This transformation generates intermediate-density lipoprotein (IDL) and low-density lipoprotein (LDL). Figure 11–3 graphically depicts the size relationships between the five major lipoprotein classes and their relative densities. LDL ultimately attach to cell membrane receptors in the liver and other tissues and release their remaining contents, which consist primarily of cholesterol.

Epidemiological evidence indicates that lipoprotein levels are better predictors of coronary artery disease (CAD) than clinical or electrocardiographic examinations. The five lipoprotein fractions mentioned above, which transport cholesterol and triglycerides, influence atherogenicity in different ways.

The level of plasma LDL, which transport 60 to 70 percent of the total plasma cholesterol, is directly related to risk for CAD. In contrast, HDL levels are inversely correlated to the occurrence of atherosclerotic vascular lesions in the coronary vessels. Studies have shown that of all lipids and lipoproteins measured, HDL have the greatest impact on risk for those over 50 years old.

In adults, plasma HDL-cholesterol levels are consistently lower in men than in women (Tables 11–1 and 11–2). A gender difference does not appear until puberty, when the HDL-cholesterol levels in boys begin to decline.

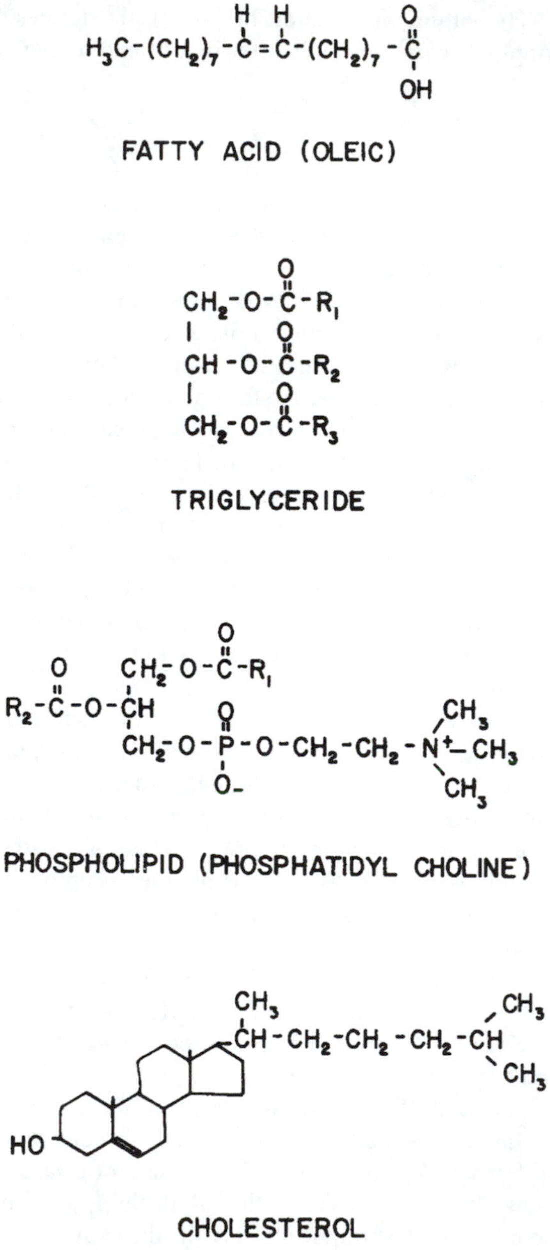

$$H_3C-(CH_2)_7-\overset{\overset{\displaystyle H}{|}}{C}=\overset{\overset{\displaystyle H}{|}}{C}-(CH_2)_7-\overset{\overset{\displaystyle O}{||}}{\underset{\underset{\displaystyle OH}{|}}{C}}$$

FATTY ACID (OLEIC)

$$CH_2-O-\overset{\overset{\displaystyle O}{||}}{C}-R_1$$
$$CH-O-\overset{\overset{\displaystyle O}{||}}{C}-R_2$$
$$CH_2-O-\overset{\overset{\displaystyle O}{||}}{C}-R_3$$

TRIGLYCERIDE

$$R_2-\overset{\overset{\displaystyle O}{||}}{C}-O-\overset{\overset{\displaystyle CH_2-O-\overset{\overset{\displaystyle O}{||}}{C}-R_1}{|}}{CH}$$
$$CH_2-O-\overset{\overset{\displaystyle O}{||}}{\underset{\underset{\displaystyle O-}{|}}{P}}-O-CH_2-CH_2-N^+-\begin{matrix}CH_3 \\ CH_3 \\ CH_3\end{matrix}$$

PHOSPHOLIPID (PHOSPHATIDYL CHOLINE)

CHOLESTEROL

Figure 11–2 Structural Formulas of Four Lipid Groups

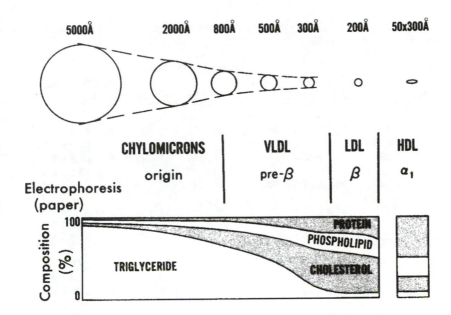

Figure 11–3 Classification of Plasma Lipoproteins by Physical and Chemical Properties. *Source:* Reprinted from Edwin L. Bierman, *Hyperlipoproteinemia*, Scope monograph (Kalamazoo, Mich.: Upjohn Co., 1973), with permission of the author, © 1973.

HDL-cholesterol levels in men and women are in the range of 45.5 ± 9.4 mg/dl and 55.5 ± 12.9 mg/dl, respectively.[5] As HDL levels rise, the risk of CAD declines. Risk for CAD correlates with the total-cholesterol/HDL ratio (Tables 11–3 and 11–4).[6] Factors associated with high levels of HDL are female gender, estrogens, exercise, moderate alcohol consumption, and high fiber intake.[7] Factors associated with low levels of HDL are male gender, progestogens, obesity, consumption of carbohydrates low in fiber,[8] non-insulin-dependent diabetes mellitus (NIDDM),[8] hypertriglyceridemia, cigarette smoking, and familial disorders of lipoprotein metabolism.[7]

Little is known about the functions of HDL or the biochemical mechanisms by which HDL protect against cardiovascular disease. Since LDL-cholesterol and HDL-cholesterol consist of different lipoprotein classes, the apoprotein composition rather than the lipid may be the most important factor for atherogenicity. LDL consist of a single apoprotein known as apo B. HDL, on the other hand, are composed of several apoproteins, the principal ones being apo A-I and apo A-II. Studies suggest that compared to apo-B, total cholesterol, triglycerides, and HDL, apo A-I and apo A-II are the best discriminators of the severity of CAD.[9]

Table 11–1 Means and Percentile Values of Plasma High-Density Lipoprotein Cholesterol (mg/dl) by Age in White Males

Age (Years) Males	n	All Clinics (Mean ± SD)	Percentiles (All Clinics)							Clinic Range* (Mean ± SEM)
			5	10	25	50	75	90	95	
0– 4	17	—	—	—	—	—	—	—	—	—
5– 9	145	55.8 ± 11.5	38	43	49	55	63	70	75	54.8 ± 1.8 56.0 ± 1.1
10–14	298	54.9 ± 12.7	37	40	46	55	61	71	74	53.9 ± 1.0 58.5 ± 2.3
15–19	300	46.1 ± 10.6	30	34	39	46	52	59	63	42.2 ± 1.2 48.6 ± 1.6
20–24	118	45.4 ± 10.7	30	32	38	45	51	57	63	40.0 ± 1.6 48.2 ± 1.8
25–29	253	44.7 ± 10.4	31	32	37	44	50	58	63	39.6 ± 1.8 45.7 ± 1.2
30–34	403	45.5 ± 11.1	28	32	38	45	52	59	63	39.8 ± 1.6 50.2 ± 2.2
35–39	372	43.5 ± 10.8	29	31	36	43	49	58	62	34.6 ± 1.2 48.0 ± 1.8
40–44	385	44.2 ± 12.3	27	31	36	43	51	60	67	35.5 ± 1.7 49.9 ± 2.1
45–49	326	45.5 ± 11.2	30	33	38	45	52	60	64	40.2 ± 2.0 49.3 ± 2.2
50–54	340	44.1 ± 11.3	28	31	36	44	51	58	63	36.5 ± 1.3 50.1 ± 2.1
55–59	261	47.6 ± 13.8	28	31	38	46	55	64	71	41.2 ± 1.6 51.1 ± 3.0
60–64	131	51.5 ± 14.5	30	34	41	49	61	69	74	44.8 ± 2.2 54.6 ± 2.3
65–69	105	51.1 ± 15.4	30	33	39	49	62	74	78	41.2 ± 2.1 56.7 ± 2.1
70+	119	50.5 ± 18.9	31	33	40	48	56	70	75	53.2 ± 2.1 53.2 ± 2.1

Note: Means not given if $n < 25$; 5th and 95th percentiles not given if $n < 100$; 10th and 90th percentiles not given if $n < 75$; 25th and 75th percentiles not given if $n < 50$; 50th percentile not given if $n < 40$.

*Lowest Lipid Research Clinic mean value and highest Lipid Research Clinic mean value.

Source: Lipid Research Clinics, "Visit 2 Survey Examination"; and Gerardo Heiss et al., "Epidemiology of Plasma HDL," *Circulation* 62, suppl. 4 (1980): 124–125; by permission of the American Heart Association, Inc.

Table 11–2 Mean and Percentile Values of Plasma High-Density Lipoprotein Cholesterol (mg/dl) by Age in White Females

Age (Years) Females	n	All Clinics (Mean ± SD)	Percentiles (All Clinics)							Clinic Range* (Mean ± SEM)
			5	10	25	50	75	90	95	
0– 4	15	—	—	—	—	—	—	—	—	—
5– 9	127	53.2 ± 11.8	36	38	48	52	60	67	73	51.1 ± 1.1
										56.5 ± 2.7
10–14	248	52.2 ± 10.3	37	40	45	52	58	64	70	51.3 ± 0.8
										53.0 ± 1.8
15–19	297	52.3 ± 12.3	35	38	43	51	61	68	74	50.2 ± 1.3
										53.7 ± 3.1
20–24	199	53.3 ± 14.3	33	37	44	51	62	72	79	43.6 ± 2.2
										56.9 ± 1.9
25–29	314	56.0 ± 14.1	37	39	47	55	63	74	83	46.9 ± 1.8
										60.4 ± 1.9
30–34	336	56.0 ± 13.2	36	40	46	55	64	73	77	48.5 ± 1.8
										62.7 ± 2.2
35–39	299	55.0 ± 14.5	34	38	44	53	64	75	82	45.5 ± 1.6
										61.7 ± 2.6
40–44	319	57.8 ± 16.3	34	39	48	56	65	79	88	47.4 ± 2.6
										64.0 ± 3.5
45–49	329	59.4 ± 17.4	34	41	47	58	68	82	87	47.3 ± 2.6
										66.5 ± 3.4
50–54	256	62.0 ± 16.3	37	41	50	62	71	84	92	57.0 ± 2.7
										75.6 ± 3.0
55–59	250	62.2 ± 17.5	37	41	50	60	73	85	91	55.3 ± 2.0
										67.4 ± 3.6
60–64	145	63.8 ± 16.6	38	44	51	61	75	87	92	54.6 ± 2.1
										68.2 ± 2.0
65–69	130	63.3 ± 20.0	35	38	49	62	73	85	98	50.3 ± 2.2
										68.6 ± 2.2
70+	143	60.7 ± 17.2	33	38	48	60	71	82	92	53.3 ± 1.9
										66.6 ± 1.9

Note: Means not given if $n < 25$; 5th and 95th percentiles not given if $n < 100$; 10th and 90th percentiles not given if $n < 75$; 25th and 75th percentiles not given if $n < 50$; 50th percentile not given if $n < 40$.

*Lowest Lipid Research Clinic mean value and highest Lipid Research Clinic mean value.

Source: Lipid Research Clinics, "Visit 2 Survey Examination"; and Gerardo Heiss et al., "Epidemiology of Plasma HDL," *Circulation 62*, suppl. 4 (1980): 125; by permission of the American Heart Association, Inc.

Table 11–3 National Heart, Lung and Blood Institute (NHLBI) Guidelines for the Classification of Cholesterol Levels in Adults over 20 Years of Age

Risk Level	Total Cholesterol		LDL Cholesterol	
	(mg/dl)	(mM/L)	(mg/dl)	(mM/L)
Desirable	< 200	< 5.20	< 130	< 3.38
Borderline-high	200–239	5.20–6.21	130–159	3.38–4.13
High	≥ 240	≥ 6.24	≥ 160	≥ 4.16

Source: The Expert Panel: Report of the National Cholesterol Education Program Expert Panel on detection, evaluation, and treatment of high blood cholesterol in adults. *Arch Intern Med.* 1988;148:36–39.

Average reference levels of total cholesterol and triglycerides in the U.S. population are shown in Tables 11–5 through 11–8. These averages are much higher than those in many other countries and thus should not necessarily be interpreted as the universal norm.

At least two plasma lipid analyses should be done two to four weeks apart, with the patient taking an unrestricted diet and abstaining from alcohol the day before the blood sampling. If abnormal lipid levels are discovered, the following causes of secondary hyperlipidemia should be systematically explored:

1. obesity
2. alcohol
3. diabetes mellitus
4. hypothyroidism
5. chronic renal disease
6. obstructive liver disease

Table 11–4 NHLBI Guidelines for Definition of Coronary Artery Disease Risk in Relation to LDL, HDL, and Total Cholesterol

Risk	Men		Women	
	LDL/HDL	Total C/HDL	LDL/HDL	Total C/HDL
½ average	1.00	3.43	1.47	3.27
Average	3.55	4.97	3.22	4.44
2 × average	6.25	9.55	5.03	7.05
3 × average	7.99	13.39	6.14	11.04

Source: The Expert Panel: Report of the National Cholesterol Education Program Expert Panel on detection, evaluation, and treatment of high blood cholesterol in adults. *Arch Intern Med.* 1988;148:36–39.

Table 11–5 Plasma Total Cholesterol (mg/dl) for White Males

Age (years)	n	Mean	SD	5	10	50	90	95
				Percentiles				
0– 4	238	154.6	27.2	114	125	151	186	203
5– 9	1,253	159.9	25.3	121	130	159	191	203
10–14	2,278	157.6	25.6	119	127	155	190	202
15–19	1,980	149.9	26.5	113	120	146	183	197
20–24	882	166.5	28.6	124	130	165	204	218
25–29	2,042	182.2	35.0	133	143	178	227	244
30–34	2,444	192.2	36.8	138	148	190	239	254
35–39	2,320	201.3	36.8	146	157	197	249	270
40–44	2,428	206.5	36.5	151	163	203	250	268
45–49	2,296	212.2	36.0	158	169	210	258	276
50–54	2,138	212.7	37.0	158	169	210	261	277
55–59	1,621	213.9	38.3	156	167	212	262	276
60–64	905	213.0	36.7	159	171	210	259	276
65–69	750	212.6	34.8	158	170	210	258	274
70–74	484	208.2	34.7	154	165	207	250	269
75–79	244	204.9	34.7	151	163	204	249	261
80+	122	206.6	42.9	144	150	202	263	275
Total	24,425							

Note: To convert to SI units (mM/L), multiply values by 0.026.

Source: Lipid Research Clinics Program Epidemiology Committee. Plasma Lipid Distributions in Selected North American Populations: The Lipid Research Clinics Program Prevalence Study. *Circulation* 60: 433, 1979; by permission of the American Heart Association, Inc.

7. chronic pancreatitis
8. dysglobulinemia—autoimmune disease
9. oral contraceptives
10. pregnancy
11. glucocorticoid excess
12. porphyria
13. other causes

Phospholipids

Phospholipids are major components of plasma lipoproteins, but their significance in plasma is unclear. About 70 percent of phospholipids consist of phosphatidylcholine, and about 20 percent consist of sphingomyelin. It is possible that the phospholipids serve as detergents, helping to stabilize less polar lipids such as cholesterol and triglycerides.

Table 11–6 Plasma Total Cholesterol (mg/dl) for White Females Not Taking Sex Hormones

Age (years)	n	Mean	SD	Percentiles				
				5	10	50	90	95
0– 4	186	156.0	26.9	112	119	156	189	200
5– 9	1,118	163.7	24.7	126	134	163	195	205
10–14	2,080	159.6	24.1	124	131	158	190	201
15–19	1,911	156.6	26.4	119	126	154	190	200
20–24	778	164.1	29.6	122	130	160	203	216
25–29	1,329	170.7	29.0	128	136	168	209	222
30–34	1,569	175.4	31.2	130	139	172	213	230
35–39	1,606	184.3	31.7	140	147	182	225	242
40–44	1,583	193.0	34.6	147	154	191	235	252
45–49	1,515	202.5	37.5	152	161	199	247	265
50–54	1,257	217.7	37.8	162	172	215	268	285
55–59	1,112	230.5	39.0	172	183	228	282	300
60–64	723	230.8	39.9	172	186	228	280	297
65–69	593	232.8	40.4	171	183	228	280	303
70–74	411	228.5	45.7	166	181	226	277	293
75–79	207	231.0	37.9	172	181	229	282	291
80+	130	222.1	37.3	165	175	220	271	279
Total	18,108							

Note: To convert to SI units (mM/L), multiply values by 0.026.

Source: Lipid Research Clinics Program Epidemiology Committee. Plasma Lipid Distributions in Selected North American Populations: The Lipid Research Clinics Program Prevalence Study. *Circulation* 60: 433, 1979; by permission of the American Heart Association, Inc.

Triglycerides and Fatty Acids

Triglycerides are esters of glycerol with three fatty acid molecules and function as an energy reserve when stored in adipose tissue. To meet energy requirements, triglycerides may be catabolized to glycerol and free fatty acids. The fatty acids yield energy as they are oxidized in the tricarboxylic acid cycle, while glycerol may be utilized for new glucose production in the liver.

The plasma half-life of fatty acids is very short, and levels fluctuate widely throughout the day, depending on whether the individual is in the fed or fasted state. As a result, fatty acids are not a good measure of lipid status.

PROTEIN

Protein nutritional status is reflected by anthropometric measures (Chapters 7 and 8) and biochemical tests. The latter determine by-products of protein

Table 11–7 Plasma Total Triglyceride (mg/dl) for White Males

Age (years)	n	Mean	SD	Percentiles 5	10	50	90	95
0– 4	238	56.4	24.2	29	33	51	84	99
5– 9	1,253	55.7	22.7	30	33	51	85	101
10–14	2,278	65.6	30.6	32	37	59	102	125
15–19	1,980	78.0	38.1	37	43	69	120	148
20–24	882	100.3	56.4	44	50	86	165	201
25–29	2,042	115.8	104.3	46	54	95	199	249
30–34	2,444	128.3	121.2	50	58	104	213	266
35–39	2,320	144.9	120.8	54	62	113	251	321
40–44	2,428	151.4	146.8	55	64	122	248	320
45–49	2,296	151.7	115.8	58	68	124	253	327
50–54	2,138	151.8	117.8	58	68	124	250	320
55–59	1,621	141.4	88.1	58	67	119	235	286
60–64	905	142.3	94.4	58	68	119	235	291
65–69	750	136.7	142.2	57	64	112	208	267
70–74	484	129.5	70.8	57	68	112	217	258
75–79	244	129.1	69.1	59	65	112	206	267
80+	122	132.1	120.6	55	64	105	182	255
Total	24,425							

Note: To convert to SI units (mM/L), multiply values by 0.0113.

Source: Lipid Research Clinics Program Epidemiology Committee. Plasma Lipid Distributions in Selected North American Populations: The Lipid Research Clinics Program Prevalence Study. *Circulation* 60: 434, 1979; by permission of the American Heart Association, Inc.

catabolism (urea, creatinine) and products of protein synthesis (transferrin, albumin, prealbumin, retinol-binding protein), from which the adequacy of body protein stores can be inferred. Protein stores are rigorously defended and biochemical homeostasis is maintained until late in the process of malnutrition.

Measures of Protein Catabolism

Urea

Urea is produced in the liver as a by-product of the deamination of amino acids. It circulates in the blood and is excreted unchanged in the urine. Urea is the principal nitrogenous constituent of the urine, making up 60 to 90 percent of urinary nitrogen. The mean daily excretion of urea is 15.0 to 49.0 grams. In protein deficiency states, urea values in both the blood and urine decrease.

The normal range for blood urea concentration in the adult population is 7.2 to 22.8 mg/dl (2.57–8.14 mM/L). The range for a given population,

Table 11–8 Plasma Total Triglyceride (mg/dl) for White Females Not Taking Sex Hormones

Age (years)	n	Mean	SD	Percentiles				
				5	10	50	90	95
0– 4	186	63.9	24.3	34	38	59	96	112
5– 9	1,118	60.3	25.3	32	36	55	90	105
10–14	2,080	75.4	30.9	37	44	70	114	131
15–19	1,911	72.4	32.5	39	44	66	107	124
20–24	778	72.4	35.3	36	41	64	112	131
25–29	1,329	74.7	37.0	37	42	65	116	144
30–34	1,569	78.5	40.1	39	44	69	123	150
35–39	1,606	86.2	49.0	40	46	73	137	176
40–44	1,583	98.4	82.0	45	51	81	155	191
45–49	1,515	104.5	69.5	46	53	87	170	214
50–54	1,257	114.8	69.6	52	59	97	186	233
55–59	1,112	125.0	76.7	55	63	106	203	262
60–64	723	126.9	88.5	56	64	105	202	239
65–69	593	131.3	110.1	60	66	112	204	243
70–74	411	133.8	112.1	60	69	113	205	231
75–79	207	127.9	101.0	57	69	106	195	242
80+	130	135.2	103.8	60	70	112	211	242
Total	18,108							

Note: To convert to SI units (mM/L), multiply values by 0.0113.

Source: Lipid Research Clinics Program Epidemiology Committee. Plasma Lipid Distributions in Selected North American Populations: The Lipid Research Clinics Program Prevalence Study. *Circulation* 60: 435, 1979; by permission of the American Heart Association, Inc.

---

particularly regarding the lower limit, is defined by the prevailing dietary intake of protein.

Creatinine

Creatinine is a metabolite of creatine phosphate, which is present principally in muscle in a stable relationship with protein, from which it is derived.

Each day approximately 2 percent of the creatine phosphate is converted to creatinine by an irreversible reaction:

$$\text{creatine phosphate} \longrightarrow \text{creatinine} + \text{HOH}$$

The usual range of serum creatinine values in adults is

	Creatinine	
	(mg/dl)	*(mM/L)*
Men	0.9–1.5	79.6–132.6
Women	0.8–1.2	70.7–106.1

The amount of creatinine excreted by the kidneys and serum creatinine levels are proportional to body muscle mass. The usual ranges for urine creatinine in adults (mg/kg body weight/24 hours) are 20 to 26 for men and 14 to 22 for women. Urinary creatinine excretion (UCE) manifests considerable variability from day to day and may necessitate two or three consecutive 24-hour urine collections for reliable determination. Meat should be eliminated from the diet during the urine collection period. Factors such as protein intake, exercise, age, and renal and thyroid function may influence UCE and should be considered in the interpretation of results.

Urinary Urea/Creatinine Ratio

Urinary urea reflects current protein consumption. Urinary creatinine is more a measure of long-term protein intake. Therefore the ratio of urea/creatinine in the urine will be low if recent protein intake has been restricted but protein stores are adequate. However, chronic protein restriction with significant muscle catabolism may limit the usefulness of this ratio since both total creatinine excretion and the urea level decrease, normalizing the ratio of urea/creatinine (Table 11–9).[10]

Creatinine-Height Index

The combination of a 24-hour urinary creatinine determination with an anthropometric measurement, such as body weight or height, is used to assess chronic protein nutritional status in adults. Height is used as a measurement more often because it remains constant while muscle protein is gradually depleted in

---

Table 11–9 Relationship of Urea to Creatinine on a High- and Low-Protein Diet

Urine	High-Protein Diet Grams/24 hrs	Low-Protein Diet Grams/24 hrs
Total nitrogen	16.80	3.60
Urea nitrogen	14.70	2.20
Creatinine nitrogen	0.58	0.60
Other nitrogen (uric acid, ammonia, undetermined)	1.52	0.78
Ratio of urea/creatinine	14.70/0.58 = 25.3	2.20/0.60 = 3.7

Note: A ratio of 12 or greater is considered normal; less than 12 is low.

Source: Adapted from Allison and Bird. Relationship of Urea to Creatinine High and Low Protein Diet, in Elimination of Nitrogen from the Body in Mammalian Protein Metabolism, ed. Hamish Munro (New York: Academic Press, 1964), p. 488.

long-term protein malnutrition. Creatinine excretion decreases proportionately to muscle mass, decreasing the ratio of creatinine to height.[11,12] Creatinine excretion also decreases with age.[12]

The index is calculated as a percentage of normal:

$$\frac{\text{mg of creatinine/24 hours excreted by individual}}{\text{mg of creatinine/24 hours excreted by reference individual of same height}} \times 100$$

An index below 90 percent is considered abnormal. Tables 11–10 and 11–11,[13] respectively, list expected 24-hour creatinine excretion values in men and women of ideal weight according to height.

Table 11–10 Expected Creatinine Excretion (mg/Day) in Men of Ideal Weight

Height (cm)	Age (Years)						
	20–29	30–39	40–49	50–59	60–69	70–79	80–89
146	1258	1169	1079	985	896	807	718
148	1284	1193	1102	1006	915	824	733
150	1308	1215	1123	1025	932	839	747
152	1334	1240	1145	1045	951	856	762
154	1358	1262	1166	1064	968	872	775
156	1390	1291	1193	1089	990	892	793
158	1423	1322	1222	1115	1014	913	812
160	1452	1349	1246	1137	1035	932	829
162	1481	1376	1271	1160	1055	950	845
164	1510	1403	1296	1183	1076	969	862
166	1536	1427	1318	1203	1094	986	877
168	1565	1454	1343	1226	1115	1004	893
170	1598	1485	1372	1252	1139	1026	912
172	1632	1516	1401	1278	1163	1047	932
174	1666	1548	1430	1305	1187	1069	951
176	1699	1579	1458	1331	1211	1090	970
178	1738	1615	1491	1361	1238	1115	992
180	1781	1655	1529	1395	1269	1143	1017
182	1819	1690	1561	1425	1296	1167	1038
184	1855	1724	1592	1453	1322	1190	1059
186	1894	1759	1625	1483	1349	1215	1081
188	1932	1795	1658	1513	1377	1240	1103
190	1968	1829	1689	1542	1402	1263	1123

Source: Reprinted from Imbembo, A.L., and Walser, M., Nutritional Assessment, in *Nutritional Management: The Johns Hopkins Handbook*, M. Walser, A.L. Imbembo, S. Margolis, et al., eds., pp. 9–30, with permission of W.B. Saunders, © 1984.

Table 11–11 Expected Creatinine Excretion (mg/Day) in Women of Ideal Weight

Height (cm)	Age (Years)						
	20–29	30–39	40–49	50–59	60–69	70–79	80–89
140	858	804	754	700	651	597	548
142	877	822	771	716	666	610	560
144	898	841	790	733	682	625	573
146	917	859	806	749	696	638	586
148	940	881	827	768	713	654	600
150	964	903	848	787	732	671	615
152	984	922	865	803	747	685	628
154	1003	940	882	819	761	698	640
156	1026	961	902	838	779	714	655
158	1049	983	922	856	796	730	670
160	1073	1006	944	877	815	747	686
162	1100	1031	968	899	835	766	703
164	1125	1054	990	919	854	783	719
166	1148	1076	1010	938	871	799	733
168	1173	1099	1032	958	890	817	749
170	1199	1124	1055	980	911	835	766
172	1224	1147	1077	1000	929	853	782
174	1253	1174	1102	1023	951	872	800
176	1280	1199	1126	1045	972	891	817
178	1304	1223	1147	1065	990	908	833
180	1331	1248	1171	1087	1011	927	850

Source: Reprinted from Imbembo, A.L., and Walser, M., Nutritional Assessment, in *Nutritional Management: The Johns Hopkins Handbook*, M. Walser, A.L. Imbembo, S. Margolis, et al., eds., pp. 9–30, with permission of W.B. Saunders, © 1984.

Measures of Protein Synthesis

Plasma protein concentrations reflect the absolute rate of synthesis of each protein and the body's requirement for amino acids. Albumin has the longest half-life (20 days) and is a low-sensitivity measure for acute changes in protein nutrition. Transferrin, with a half-life of eight days and a smaller metabolic pool than albumin, is a measure of intermediate sensitivity for acute protein deficiency. Prealbumin, with a half-life of two days, and retinol-binding protein, with a half-life of 12 hours,[13] are the most sensitive measures for acute dietary deprivation and refeeding.[14]

Albumin

Albumin is synthesized by the liver. Its two main functions are the binding and transport of small molecules in the circulation and the maintenance of intravascular colloid osmotic pressure. Four percent of plasma albumin is catabolized and regenerated daily. With significant restriction in protein nutrition, the body utilizes amino acids from muscle and visceral catabolism to synthesize albumin. Serum albumin levels may thus be maintained in the normal range even when severe protein malnutrition exists (Table 11–12). They then fall precipitously if nutrition does not improve.

Low levels of serum albumin are also encountered in other conditions. In severe liver disease, albumin production is impaired. In kidney disease, albumin may be wasted in the urine. With excessive burns, albumin is lost from the denuded body surface. In chronic inflammatory bowel disease, the damaged gut is the primary source of albumin loss.

Transferrin

Transferrin is produced in the liver and can be measured directly by immunologic methods.

Plasma transferrin levels rise during the first six months of life (1.68 ± 0.60 mg/ml), after which time the adult level (1.80–2.60 mg/ml) is reached and maintained until late in life, when levels decline.[15] These levels are similar in healthy men and women.

Iron deficiency, pregnancy, hypoxia, and chronic blood loss elevate serum transferrin levels. Decreased levels are seen in pernicious anemia, chronic infection, liver disease, iron overload, and protein-losing enteropathies. Since some of these conditions are frequently encountered in protein-calorie malnutrition (PCM), transferrin alone is not a reliable indicator for evaluating protein status.

Prealbumin and Retinol-Binding Protein

Prealbumin (PA) and retinol-binding protein (RBP) travel together in the bloodstream, complexed with retinol, the vitamin A alcohol. Due to this stable

---

Table 11–12 Usual Range of Serum Albumin Levels

Age	Serum Albumin (gm/dl)
10–14	2.8–5.2
15–19	2.5–5.2
20–24	3.9–5.2
55–59	3.8–5.1
65–69	3.7–5.0
75–79	3.5–4.9
85–99	3.3–4.8

Note: The limits define the 2.5 to 97.5 percentile range. To convert to SI units (g/L), multiply values by 10.0.

relationship, serum concentrations of vitamin A, PA, and RBP correlate well. In the serum of normal, healthy adults these levels vary within narrow limits. Mean values of RBP and PA for normal, healthy adults in the American population are approximately 46.2 ± 1.0 µg/ml and 250.0 ± 5.0 µg/ml, respectively,[16] and they are slightly higher in men than in women. These concentrations are age dependent (Figure 11–4), serum levels in children being approximately half those of adults.

In vitamin A deficiency, RBP accumulates in the liver and is low in the serum, suggesting that the vitamin is required for RBP secretion. Likewise, when the liver cannot synthesize RBP, retinol is not released. Therefore low plasma levels of retinol in PCM may be due to the lack of RBP rather than retinol itself.

PA levels may be a more reliable measure of the capacity of the liver to secrete plasma proteins since they are independent of retinol. Serum PA is not a suitable indicator of low protein intake in patients with chronic renal failure who are being treated by dialysis, because it may appear factitiously normal or elevated.

Stress, inflammation, surgical trauma, cirrhosis, and hepatitis decrease serum PA levels. Concentrations of RBP and retinol are also decreased in liver disease, as well as in hyperthyroidism and cystic fibrosis.

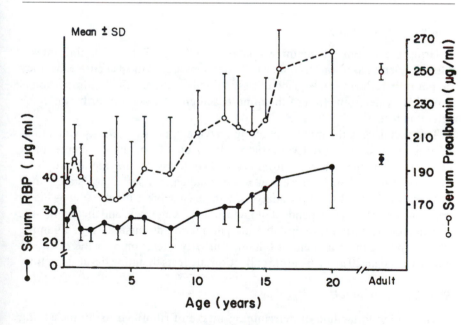

Figure 11–4 Mean Values of RBP and PA in Normal Healthy Adults in the American Population

VITAMINS

Vitamins are complex organic substances essential in very small quantities in the diet for human growth and health. The most convenient way of classifying vitamins is by their solubility, which influences their absorption, mode of action, and disposal.

Water-Soluble Vitamins

All water-soluble vitamins except C are considered B vitamins. With the exception of vitamin B_{12}, water-soluble vitamins are not retained in the body. They are freely absorbed from the diet, circulate widely in body fluids fulfilling their metabolic functions, and are subsequently excreted in the urine. Therefore urinary excretion of these vitamins reflects their intake and is the most commonly used method in assessing nutritional adequacy. Vitamin content of a 24-hour urine collection, a one-hour excretion on fasting, or a random urine sample expressed per gram of creatinine are the usual measures. Expressing urinary excretion per gram of creatinine tends to correct for variations due to body size. Tentative guidelines for the assessment of some of these vitamins are given in Table 11–13.

Thiamine (Vitamin B₁)

Urinary excretion of thiamine relates directly to dietary thiamine intake. Measurements based on 24-hour urine collections are the most accurate, but they do not fully reflect the adequacy of tissue thiamine stores. Such information is provided by determination of thiamine-based enzyme activity or by thiamine retention tests.[17]

Transketolase, a thiamine-containing enzyme, increases activity when thiamine is added to hemolyzed whole blood, the incubation medium. Samples must be kept on ice and analyzed promptly to avoid loss of enzyme activity. An increase of more than 20 percent in activity indicates a deficiency state. Since this test involves split-sample analysis, with each subject functioning as his or her own control, it is independent of factors such as age, sex, and dietary intake.

Thiamine retention tests involve the parenteral administration of thiamine (5 mg) and the measurement of thiamine urinary excretion over the next four hours. Less than 20 µg in the urine collection suggests thiamine tissue depletion.

Riboflavin (Vitamin B₂)

The preferred method of determining intake of riboflavin is by measuring levels of the vitamin in a 24-hour urine collection. Tissue stores are most

Table 11–13 Normal Laboratory Values for Water-Soluble Vitamins

Nutrient and Units/Age of Subject (Years)	Criteria of Status		
	Deficient	*Marginal*	*Acceptable*
Urinary thiamine			
(mcg/g creatinine):			
0–2 years M and F	below 120	120–170	above 170
3–5 years M and F	below 85	85–120	above 120
6–8 years M and F	below 70	70–180	above 180
9–12 years M and F	below 60	60–180	above 180
13–16 years M and F	below 50	50–150	above 150
17+ years M	below 40	40–120	above 120
17+ years F	below 30	30–100	above 100
RBC transketolase-			
TPP-effect (ratio):			
All ages	above 25	15–25	below 15
Urinary riboflavin			
(mcg/g creatinine):			
0–2 years M and F	below 150	150–500	above 500
3–5 years M and F	below 100	100–300	above 300
6–8 years M and F	below 85	85–270	above 270
9–16 years M and F	below 70	70–200	above 200
17+ years M and F	below 30	30–80	above 80
RBC glutathione			
reductase-FAD-effect (ratio):			
All ages	above 1.2	—	below 1.2
Urinary pyridoxine			
(mcg/g creatinine):			
1–3 years	below 90	—	above 90
4–6 years	below 80	—	above 80
7–9 years	below 60	—	above 60
10–12 years	below 40	—	above 40
13–15 years	below 30	—	above 30
16+ years	below 20	—	above 20
Urinary N'-methyl			
nicotinamide			
(mg/g creatinine):			
All ages	below 0.5	0.5–1.59	above 1.6
Pregnant	below 0.8	0.8–2.49	above 2.5
Tryptophan load			
(mg Xanthurenic acid excreted):			
Adults	above 25 (6 hrs)	—	below 25
(Dose: 100 mg/kg body weight)	above 75 (24 hrs)	—	below 75

continues

Table 11–13 continued

Nutrient and Units/Age of Subject (Years)	Criteria of Status		
	Deficient	Marginal	Acceptable
Transaminase index (ratio):			
EGOT*—Adult	above 2.0	—	below 2.0
EGPT**—Adult	above 1.25	—	below 1.25
Urinary pantothenic acid (mcg):			
All ages	below 200	—	above 200
Vitamin C serum (mg/100 ml):			
0–19 years M and F	below 0.2	0.2–0.6	above 0.6
20+ years M and F	below 0.2	0.2–0.4	above 0.4
White cells (mg/100 ml)	0–7	7–15	above 15

* Erythrocyte glutamic oxalacetic transaminase.
**Erythrocyte glutamic pyruvic transaminase.

accurately reflected by determination of riboflavin-dependent enzyme activity, such as that of erythrocyte glutathione reductase levels. The principle of the test is similar to that of the thiamine transketolase test, and an activity coefficient (AC) is calculated after the in vitro addition of flavin-adenine-dinucleotide to chilled red blood cell hemolysates. AC levels above 1.2 suggest riboflavin tissue depletion. Certain drugs such as phenothiazines and tricyclic antidepressants interfere with riboflavin metabolism and may influence test results, but this does not detract from the convenience and reliability that make this test the current method of choice for assessment of tissue riboflavin status.

Niacin

The assessment of dietary intake of niacin is based on urinary measurement of two of its metabolites, N-methylpyridone and N-methylnicotinamide. A ratio of 1.3:4.0 of these metabolites is considered consistent with nutritional adequacy of this important vitamin. Simple direct determinations of niacin reflecting tissue stores are currently unavailable.

Pantothenic Acid

Deficiency of pantothenic acid has not been demonstrated in humans. Urine levels of pantothenic acid reflect dietary intake more accurately than plasma sample determinations, which require special handling in processing.

Pyridoxine (Vitamin B$_6$)

Several useful tests are available for determination of pyridoxine status, including measurements of pyridoxine metabolites in blood and urine and functional tests reflecting pyridoxine-dependent enzyme actions.

The tryptophan metabolic pathway involves several pyridoxine-dependent steps. Inadequate intake of pyridoxine results in increased urinary excretion of xanthenuric acid after an oral tryptophan load (two or five grams). Either a 24-hour or a 6-hour urine collection can be used. Values above 25 mg for the 6-hour collection denote a pyridoxine-deficient state.

A second set of functional tests exploring tissue pyridoxine status involves the measurement of erythrocyte glutamate-oxaloacetate transaminase (EGOT) and erythrocyte glutamate-pyruvate transaminase (EGPT). Due to the variety and simplicity of techniques available for erythrocyte transaminase measurements, these tests lend themselves to mass screening.

Folic Acid

Folic acid is a hemopoietic factor and has also been associated with neural tube development in pregnancy. Its deficiency causes megaloblastic anemia. In pregnancy, deficiency may lead to neural tube defects. Morphological characteristics of megaloblastic anemia, which may also be caused by B$_{12}$ deficiency, include a decreased mean erythrocyte corpuscular volume, oval macrocytes, and neutrophil hypersegmentation. Lactic dehydrogenase levels are elevated, reflecting hemolysis. Since megaloblastic anemia due to B$_{12}$ deficiency may be reversed with folate administration, biochemical clarification of the underlying cause is necessary to avoid missing the diagnosis of pernicious anemia with its devastating neurologic consequences.

Analytical procedures for determining serum folate include sensitive microbiologic assays and radioligand procedures. Serum folate levels are very responsive to short-term changes in dietary intake and do not accurately reflect tissue folate stores. In contrast, red cell folate levels are closely associated with tissue reserves. In the progression of the sequential changes occurring in folate deficiency, low red cell folate levels are seen before megaloblastic marrow and anemia changes but after hypersegmentation and increased urinary excretion of formiminoglutamic acid (FIGLU).

Vitamin B$_{12}$ is required to keep folate in cells; therefore B$_{12}$ deficiency may lead to low red cell folate. For this reason, diagnosis of folate-deficient anemia requires demonstration of low levels of both serum folate (<3 ng/ml) and red cell folate (<150 ng/ml).

Subnormal serum levels of both vitamins may still reflect a primary deficiency of only one, since the megaloblastic state may cause a secondary deficiency of the other. The deoxyuridine (dU) test is useful in making the distinction between the two. Thymidylate synthetase activity, which is dependent on both vitamins, is measured in cultured lymphocytes or bone marrow cells. Deficiency in either vitamin B_{12} or folate or both leads to reduced enzyme activity and suppression of the thymidine pool. Replacement of the deficient principle restores enzyme activity. The dU suppression test on bone marrow measures current status, whereas testing on lymphocytes reflects long-term status. This suppression test is also useful after therapy has begun. Table 11–14 presents a summary of tests for B_{12} and folate deficiency.

Cobalamin (Vitamin B_{12})

Serum B_{12} concentration is most commonly used to assess body cobalamin stores. As depletion of body cobalamin develops, serum levels become subnormal before blood and marrow changes occur. Megaloblastic anemia is a manifestation of rather advanced vitamin B_{12} deficiency. Serum B_{12} levels less than 100 pg/ml are essentially diagnostic of cobalamin deficiency.

Since the metabolism of vitamin B_{12} is closely related to that of folic acid, both nutrients should be evaluated together (see earlier section on folic acid).

Table 11–14 Summary of Tests for B_{12} and Folate Deficiency

	Deficient Value	Normal
Serum B_{12}	<100 pg/ml	>100 pg/ml
Serum folate	< 3 ng/ml	> 6 ng/ml
Red cell folate	<150 ng/ml	>200 ng/ml

FIGLU Excretion in 6-hr urine after 2–5 g 1-histidine load

Deficient Value	Normal
5–10 × normal	5–20 mg FIGLU

Deoxyuridine Suppression Test
(Thymidylate Synthetase Activity)

	B_{12} Deficient	Folate Deficient	Folate and B_{12} Deficient
Add B_{12}	Normalized	Abnormal	Abnormal
Add folate	Abnormal	Normalized	Abnormal
Add B_{12} and folate	Normalized	Normalized	Normalized

Ascorbic Acid (Vitamin C)

Determination of serum or plasma ascorbate levels is the preferred procedure to evaluate dietary intake and body stores of this vitamin. In adults, serum levels below 0.3 mg/dl are considered deficient. Levels in urine are subject to analytical problems and are too variable to be useful in the diagnosis of marginal deficiencies.

Biotin

Little information is available regarding biotin deficiency in humans. Methods exist to determine biotin levels in both blood and urine.

Fat-Soluble Vitamins

Methods for assessing the fat-soluble vitamins should measure total body reserves, which may vary from excess through adequate to marginal states, and on to a deficiency condition.

Retinols (Vitamin A)

The only practical biochemical test currently available to evaluate vitamin A status is plasma retinol determination in serum or plasma. Vitamin A is stored in the liver and transported in the blood predominantly as the alcohol retinol, bound to retinol-binding protein (RBP), with only a minor proportion circulating as the retinyl-ester. Although plasma or serum retinol levels are useful for evaluating long-term intake, they do not reflect liver stores. As long as there are reserves of vitamin in the liver, the blood level remains normal. Because of the transport relationships explained earlier, plasma vitamin A and prealbumin are proportional to RBP. Decreased serum retinol concentration in PCM often reflects a functional impairment in hepatic release of the vitamin rather than hypovitaminosis A. A retinol deficiency, in turn, will block secretion of RBP. Other conditions unrelated to nutrition in which low levels may be seen include chronic infection, liver disease, celiac disease, obstructive jaundice, and cystic fibrosis of the pancreas.

Mean plasma vitamin A values in adults range from 45 to 65 µg/dl, with higher levels in older age groups. Serum retinol levels below 30 µg/dl indicate inadequate intake, with vitamin stores probably being depleted. Levels lower than 10 µg/dl are indicative of depletion and usually are accompanied by clinical signs.[18] Early deficiency symptoms, such as night blindness, make visual function or dark adaptation tests useful adjuncts in confirming suspected deficiencies.[1]

Plasma carotenoids represent the metabolic precursors of the retinoid compounds. Their serum levels, which range from 24 to 216 μg/dl, are poor indicators of vitamin A status because they are more variable and directly reflect dietary intake of carotenoids.[19]

Excess vitamin A is highly toxic. Hypervitaminosis A has been reported acutely in children who were given a single, massive dose of the vitamin, and chronically in food faddists and patients who received large doses as treatment for dermatologic conditions without continued medical supervision.[20] In chronic conditions, elevation of serum vitamin A, but not of RBP or prealbumin, is due mainly to marked increases in the circulatory retinyl-ester form. A positive correlation may exist between plasma retinyl-ester concentration, severity of symptoms, and length of time required to return to normal.

Calciferols (Vitamin D)

The traditional biochemical measures used to assess vitamin D status are determinations of calcium and inorganic phosphate levels and serum alkaline phosphatase activity. Methods for direct measurement of vitamin D do not exist, but assays for the 25-hydroxy derivative and the 1,25-dihydroxy form have been developed for clinical laboratory use. Concentrations of 25-hydroxy vitamin D (25-OHD), the major circulating form, felt by some investigators to be a reasonable index of vitamin D status, vary widely, reflecting degree of solar exposure as well as amount of the vitamin in the diet.[21] Since no disease state exists where the 25-hydroxylation is totally impaired, low assayed values indicate vitamin D deprivation or intestinal malabsorption.

Normal plasma concentration of 25-OHD ranges from 10 to 80 ng/ml (mean 27 ± 12 ng/ml). A level less than 5 ng/ml is regarded as the lower limit of normal and an indication for vitamin D supplementation, even though signs of bone disease may not yet be evident. Blood samples for assessment must be drawn prior to initiation of treatment, since 25-OHD levels will rise within a few days of therapy. Supranormal levels of 25-OHD result only from dietary excess or inappropriate supplementation.[21] Concentrations of about 400 ng/ml have been reported in those developing vitamin D intoxication, but a precise threshold has not been established.

In contrast, 1,25-dihydroxy vitamin D concentrations are difficult to interpret. Levels are lower in renal disease, absent in anephric patients, and elevated with parathyroid hormone. Upper limits are not exceeded regardless of the degree of 25-OHD elevation. Therefore 1,25-dihydroxy vitamin D concentrations are not useful for assessment of vitamin D. These indirect methods are employed because a reliable assay for plasma or urine concentrations of vitamin D or its metabolites is not readily available.

Serum alkaline phosphatase levels (normal: 1.5–4.0 Bodansky units/dl in adults, 5.0–14.0 units/dl in children) rise early with the onset of rickets in children (<20 units/dl) and osteomalacia in adults (<15 units/dl). However, the relationship of enzyme activity to states of subclinical vitamin D deficiency is not clearly established. In addition, alkaline phosphatase is increased above normal in other disease processes, including hyperparathyroidism, Paget's disease, osteomalacia, and metastatic carcinoma, and may be subnormal in PCM.[1]

Some information concerning vitamin D status may be obtained from determination of serum calcium and phosphorus levels. Both are decreased in rickets and osteomalacia, where their product (Ca × P) is decreased below 40. Changes in these minerals, however, are not specific to vitamin D deficiency.

Tocopherols (Vitamin E)

Deficiency of vitamin E generally occurs only in premature newborns and in those with severe, prolonged fat malabsorption or bizarre food habits. Evaluation of vitamin E status remains inaccurate, and blood tocopherol levels do not reflect either level of intake or tissue storage reliably.

Normal adult levels of tocopherol in plasma range from 0.8 to 1.5 mg/dl, with values less than 0.5 mg/dl considered indicative of deficiency. These values have little meaning unless interpreted in conjunction with lipid levels since, in plasma, tocopherols are associated with the lipoproteins and correlate highly with cholesterol or total lipid concentrations. It has been suggested that a ratio of 0.8 mg total tocopherols per gram of total plasma lipids indicates adequate nutritional status.[22,23]

Erythrocyte hemolysis tests are simple and provide indirect information on vitamin E status. The hydrogen peroxide hemolysis test (HPH), which involves incubation of washed erythrocytes, compares the amount of hemoglobin released by the red blood cells during dilute hydrogen peroxide versus distilled water incubations. The result is expressed as a percentage, with levels greater than 20 percent indicating a deficiency. However, this test is a crude estimator of status because variables other than vitamin E intake can affect in vitro hemolysis, and low rates are not necessarily indicative of adequacy of tissue stores.

Phylloquinones and Menaquinones (Vitamin K)

Vitamin K deficiency is rare. It is largely limited to newborns, patients with malabsorption syndromes or bile disorders, patients on total parenteral nutrition, and individuals treated with bowel-sterilizing antibiotics. Deficiency states are accompanied by an increased bleeding tendency and decreased prothrombin levels.

Direct analyses for this vitamin are not available, so indirect measurements are utilized. The Quick one-stage prothrombin time test measures the activities of plasma prothrombin as well as factors VII and X. A normal prothrombin time is considered to be between 11 and 13 seconds, or 70 to 100 percent of normal control, depending on the laboratory. Prothrombin times greater than 25 seconds are associated with major bleeding. Clinical symptoms are unlikely unless prothrombin levels in blood are reduced to less than one-half of normal.[24] Prothrombin time prolongation also occurs in severe liver disease, where normal synthesis of clotting factors does not occur, in bleeding disorders, with anticoagulant therapy, and possibly with large doses of vitamin E. Correction of vitamin K deficiency improves prothrombin time abnormalities related to this cause.

MAJOR MINERALS

Sodium

Sodium enters the diet as the chloride salt or in flavor enhancers, such as monosodium glutamate (MSG). Nutritional sodium deficiency rarely occurs, but sodium depletion may be seen due to hormonal abnormalities, such as cortisol deficiency. Normal levels in serum are 135 to 147 mg/dl.

Potassium

Dietary potassium deficiency and hypokalemia may be seen in conditions promoting excess fluid losses, such as vomiting, diarrhea, and diuretic use, and with hormonal aberrations such as hyperaldosteronism. Normal serum levels are 3.5 to 5.3 mg/dl.

Calcium

Calcium is present predominantly in bone (99 percent of total body calcium) and in the intra- and extracellular spaces. Its concentration is usually determined in serum or plasma, where it is present either as a free ion (46 percent), as a chelated complex with organic acids (7 percent), or bound to protein (47 percent), especially albumin. The ionized calcium fraction is readily available to cells and represents the critical calcium component monitored by the parathyroid and thyroid glands. The concentration of ionized calcium is usually very constant. Particularly important in this homeostasis are parathormone, calcitonin, magnesium, cyclic AMP, and vitamin D. There is no significant difference in ionized calcium concentrations between men and women, nor is there any change with age.

About 80 percent of the calcium-protein fraction consists of calcium bound to albumin; the remainder is bound to globulin. How much calcium is bound to protein (CaPr) can be estimated with the following equation: CaPr (mg/dl) = 0.44 + 0.76 × albumin (mg/dl). When serum albumin is in the normal range, the ratio of percent bound calcium to percent free calcium is constant, and therefore the measurement of total serum calcium is a reliable index of ionized calcium. When the serum albumin is low, however, the total serum calcium will also be low, but the ionized calcium will be normal. Therefore the concentration of serum albumin must always be taken into account when evaluating a total serum calcium. The usual range of serum calcium values for ages 15 to 99 is 8.7 to 10.7 mg/dl.

Phosphorus

Phosphorus is involved in skeletal and soft tissue structure and is essential in intermediary metabolism. The concentration of phosphate varies with age: levels are higher in children and gradually decline in adults. In females, levels rise again after menopause. Phosphorus may be elevated in kidney disease, hypoparathyroidism, with healing fractures, and in poorly controlled diabetes. Phosphorus levels decline after insulin administration, in hyperparathyroidism, rickets, and in some intestinal malabsorptive diseases. Since red blood cells are very rich in phosphorus, hemolysis falsely elevates levels. Phosphorus is usually measured in serum. The generally accepted ranges are 2.0 to 4.5 mg/dl for adults, 4.0 to 7.0 mg/dl for children, and 5.0 to 6.5 mg/dl for infants.

Magnesium

Magnesium is present as an ion in the intracellular space and functions as an activator for a number of enzymes, including alkaline phosphatase and creatine phosphokinase. It is essential for protein synthesis, DNA metabolism, and ribosomal structure. Magnesium is also needed for oxidative phosphorylation and is highly concentrated in mitochondria. At the neuromuscular junction, magnesium decreases the sensitivity of the motor endplate to acetylcholine and impairs its release. Magnesium deficiency causes increased neuromuscular excitability with weakness and tremor, which can progress to tetany, seizures, and coma. Hypomagnesemia often results in hypocalcemia and hypokalemia. This is partly related to the fact that a minimum amount of magnesium is required for an end organ response to parathyroid hormone.

Since 95 percent of magnesium is intracellular, the serum level may not adequately reflect tissue stores. Approximately one-third of serum magnesium is bound to protein; the remaining two-thirds is "free" or "ionic." Usual ranges of magnesium values for adults are:

Serum	*Urine*
1.4–1.8 mM/L	1.5–8.5 mM/24 hrs
1.3–2.1 mEq/L	3–17 mEq/24 hrs
1.6–2.6 mg/dl	36–207 mg/24 hrs

Red cells contain three times more magnesium than does serum, so hemolysis will falsely elevate serum or plasma values.

TRACE ELEMENTS

Iron

Iron is the most abundant trace element in the human body (3–4 grams). The bulk of iron circulates in the erythrocytes in the form of hemoglobin. Much smaller amounts are carried in the blood bound to a specific plasma protein, transferrin. Each molecule of transferrin can accommodate two molecules of iron. The ability of transferrin to bind iron is called the total iron binding capacity (TIBC). Transferrin can be estimated from TIBC by the formula:

$$\text{transferrin (mg/dl)} = \frac{\text{TIBC } (\mu g/dl)}{1.45}$$

Extra iron is stored intracellularly as myoglobin, ferritin, and hemosiderin. Myoglobin is found in muscle cells. The molecule ferritin consists of protein subunits surrounding a micelle of ferric hydroxyphosphate and is found in all cells and in the blood, but primarily in the liver, spleen, and bone marrow. Hemosiderin is a breakdown product of ferritin.

Iron deficiency represents a continuum of stages from marginal depletion of iron stores through deficient erythropoiesis, culminating in anemia. In the initial phase, serum ferritin is the most useful determination. Transferrin saturation and free erythrocyte protoporphyrin levels reflect iron store depletion and iron-deficient erythropoiesis, respectively. In overt iron deficiency, hemoglobin and hematocrit levels are reduced (Table 11–15).

In the anemia of iron deficiency, erythrocyte indices such as mean corpuscular volume (MCV), mean corpuscular hemoglobin (MCH), and mean corpuscular hemoglobin concentration (MCHC) are all low. In a combined iron-folate deficiency, the indices lose their diagnostic selectivity since a mixed population of erythrocytes is in circulation, some with high or normal indices characteristic of folate and B_{12} deficiency and some with the microcytic, hypochromic indices of iron deficiency. These erythrocyte indices are calculated as follows:

Table 11–15 Hemoglobin and Hematocrit Values

Age of Subject (years)	Criteria of Status		
	Deficient	Marginal	Acceptable
Hemoglobin (gm/dl):			
6–23 months	< 9.0	9.0–9.9	10.0+
2–5	<10.0	10.0–10.9	11.0+
6–12	<10.0	10.0–11.4	11.5+
13–15 (M)	<12.0	12.0–12.9	13.0+
13–16 (F)	<10.0	10.0–11.4	11.5+
16+ (M)	<12.0	12.0–13.9	14.0+
16+ (F)	<10.0	10.0–11.9	12.0+
Pregnant			
trimester 2	< 9.5	9.5–10.9	11.0+
trimester 3	< 9.0	9.0–10.5	10.5+
Hematocrit— PCV or Packed Cell Volume (percent):			
Up to 2	<28	28–30	31+
2–5	<30	30–33	34+
6–12	<30	30–35	36+
13–16 (M)	<37	37–39	40+
13–16 (F)	<31	31–35	36+
16+ (M)	<37	37–43	44+
16+ (F)	<31	31–37	38+
Pregnant			
trimester 2	<30	30–35	35+
trimester 3	<30	30–33	33+

Source: Adapted from J.W. King and W.R. Faukner, eds., *Critical Resources in Clinical Laboratory Sciences* (Cleveland, Ohio: CRC Press, 1973), p. 116; and George Christakis, ed., "Nutritional Assessment in Health Programs," *American Journal of Public Health* 63, pt. 2 (1963): 34; with permission of the CRC Press, Inc., Boca Raton, Fla., © 1973, and the American Public Health Association, © 1963.

MCV (normal range: 80–90 fl*):

$$\frac{hematocrit \times 1000}{red\ blood\ cells\ (millions/\mu l)}$$

MCH (normal range: 27–32 pg):

$$\frac{hemoglobin\ (g/L)}{red\ blood\ cells\ (millions/\mu L)}$$

MCHC (normal range: 33–38 g/dl):

$$\frac{hemoglobin\ (g/dl)}{hematocrit} \times 100$$

(* 1 femtoliter = 1 μm^3)

Other characteristics of iron status in the body may be accomplished with more sophisticated tests, such as determination of serum ferritin. A decrease in the serum ferritin level is the first biochemical change occurring during the development of iron deficiency. It reflects depletion of iron stores. The information obtained from a serum ferritin measurement is equivalent to that obtained from a bone marrow iron examination. In the latter, the marrow aspirate is stained for iron. Absence of deposits on microscopic examination is diagnostic of iron deficiency.

In the intermediate stage of iron deficiency, serum ferritin continues to be low, and, in addition, serum iron is low. Transferrin, which is responsible for iron transport to its points of utilization in the marrow and peripheral tissue, increases, thus increasing TIBC. Iron saturation expresses the percentage of TIBC occupied by serum iron and is decreased. Free erythrocyte protoporphyrin levels are increased.

	Normal Range	Suspect Iron Deficiency
Plasma iron	45–150 µg/dl	<45
Plasma TIBC	240–410 µg/dl	>350
Iron saturation	33 ± 15%	<15
Free erythrocyte protoporphyrin	to 100 µg/dl	>100

In summary, the sequence of events in iron deficiency is:

- depletion of iron stores; serum ferritin decreases
- TIBC and free erythrocyte protoporphyrin increase; iron saturation decreases
- serum iron decreases; iron saturation decreases further
- hemoglobin and hematocrit levels decrease (i.e., anemia)
- erythrocyte indices (MCV, MCH, and MCHC) decrease

Zinc

The laboratory criteria for the diagnosis of zinc deficiency are not clearly established. To date, the response to zinc therapy is probably the most reliable index. Clinical manifestations of deficiency include growth retardation and hypogonadism, impaired taste and/or smell acuity, and poor wound healing. Laboratory indices that have been used include plasma or serum zinc levels (normal: 102 ± 17 µg/dl serum), erythrocyte zinc concentrations (14.4 ± 2.7 µg/ml), urinary zinc excretion (400–600 µg/24 hr), salivary zinc levels, activity levels of zinc metalloenzymes (for example, alkaline phosphatase and carbonic anhydrase), and taste acuity testing.[25]

Table 11–16 Other Normal Laboratory Values of Interest in Nutrition Assessment

	Plasma Values
Electrolytes:	
Sodium	136–145 mEq/l
Potassium	3.5–5.0 mEq/l
Chloride	100–106 mEq/l
Carbon Dioxide Content	26– 28 mEq/l
Liver function tests:	
Bilirubin, total	0.7 mg/dl
Bilirubin, direct	0.4 mg/dl
Alkaline phosphatase	
Bodansky units	2.0– 5.0 units (infants to 14U, adolescents to 5U)
King-Armstrong units	8.0–14.0 units (infants to 42 U)
Serum glutamic oxalic transaminase (SGOT)	6–40 μ/ml
Serum glutamic pyruvic transaminase (SGPT)	6–36 μ/ml
5' Nucleotidase	0.3–2.6 Bodansky units
Other minerals:	
Copper	100–200 μg/dl
Chromium	1–5 mg/l
Iodine	> 50 μg iodine/gm creatinine in urine
Zinc	85–120 μg/dl

Although management of plasma or serum zinc is the simplest index, factors such as stress, hypoalbuminemia, infection, and steroids are known to depress circulating concentrations without necessarily affecting total body zinc nutriture. Hair zinc could be anticipated to reflect chronic status, but its concentration depends not only on the delivery of zinc to the hair root but also on the rate of hair growth. Urinary zinc excretion is unreliable since most studies have reported hyperzincuria with hypozincemia and presumed zinc deficiency states. This is because increased urinary excretion of zinc has been generally implicated in the pathogenesis of zinc deficiency. Conflicting results of this nature underline the need to utilize an extensive battery of indices rather than one alone in assessing zinc status.

Copper

Plasma or serum copper levels are the most reliable tests for evaluation of copper stores. Levels may exhibit diurnal variation, with the highest levels occurring in the morning. They may be affected by medical conditions such as pregnancy, malignancy, or inflammation.

Other Elements

Other elements such as selenium, molybdenum, manganese, fluorine, and chromium are known to be essential for the body in trace amounts. Deficiency states have been described and toxic amounts have been identified. The sophistication of the currently available assays limits their use to the research setting and has made the development of acceptable normal ranges difficult.

Other values of interest in nutrition assessment are shown in Table 11–16.

REFERENCES

1. King JW, Faukner WR, eds. *Critical Reviews in Clinical Laboratory Science.* Cleveland, Ohio: CRC Press; 1973.

2. National Diabetes Data Group. Classification and diagnosis of diabetes mellitus and other categories of glucose intolerance. *Diabetes.* 1979;28:1039–1057.

3. Felig P, Lynch V. Starvation in human pregnancy: hypoglycemia, hypoinsulinemia, and hyperketonemia. *Science.* 1970;170:990–992.

4. Merimee TJ, Tyson JE. Hypoglycemia in man, pathologic and physiologic variants. *Diabetes.* 1977;20:161–165.

5. Beaglehole R, Trost DC, Tahir I, et al. Plasma high-density lipoprotein cholesterol in children and young adults. *Circulation.* 1980;62(suppl. 4):83–98.

6. The Expert Panel: Report of the National Cholesterol Education Program Expert Panel on detection, evaluation, and treatment of high blood cholesterol in adults. *Arch Intern Med.* 1988;148:36–39.

7. Levy RI, Rifkind BM. The structure, function and metabolism of high-density lipoproteins: a status report. *Circulation.* 1980;62(suppl. 4):4–8.

8. Vinik AI, Wing RR. The good, the bad, and the ugly in diabetic diets. *Endocrinol Metab Clin North Am.* 1992;21:237–274.

9. Riesen WF, Mordasioi R, Salzman C, Theler A, Gartner HP. Apoproteins and lipids as discriminators of severity of coronary heart disease. *Atherosclerosis.* 1980;37:157–162.

10. Allison, Bird . Relationship of urea to creatinine on a high and low protein diet. In: Munro H, ed. *Elimination of Nitrogen from the Body in Mammalian Protein Metabolism.* New York, NY: Academic Press; 1964.

11. Alleyne GAO, Viteri F, Alvarado J. Indices of body composition in infantile malnutrition: total body potassium and urinary creatinine. *Am J Clin Nutr.* 1970;23:875–878.

12. Satyanarayana K, Naidu AN, Rao SBN. Studies on the effect of nutritional deprivation during childhood on body composition of adolescent boys: creatinine excretion. *Am J Clin Nutr.* 1981;34:161–165.

13. Imbembo AL, Walser M. Nutritional assessment. In: Walser M, Imbembo AL, Margolis S, et al, eds. *Nutritional Management: The Johns Hopkins Handbook.* Philadelphia, Pa: WB Saunders Co; 1984:9–30.

14. Smith FR, Suskind R, Thanangkul O, Leitzman C, Goodman DS, Olson RE. Plasma vitamin A, retinal-binding protein and prealbumin concentrations in protein-calorie malnutrition III: response to varying dietary treatments. *Am J Clin Nutr.* 1975;28:732–738.

15. Igenbleek Y, Vandenschrieck HG, Dehayer P, De Visscher M. Albumin, transferrin and the thyroxine-binding prealbumin/retinal-binding complex in assessment of malnutrition. *Clinica Chimica Acta* 1975;63:61–67.

16. Vahlquist A, Peterson PA, Wilbell L. Metabolism of the vitamin A transporting protein complex I: turnover studies in normal persons and in patients with chronic renal failure. *Eur J Clin Invest.* 1973;3:352–362.

17. Rask L, Arundi H, Bohme J, Eriksson U, Fredriksson A, Nilsson SF, et al. The retinal-binding protein. *Scand J Clin Lab Invest.* 1980;154:45–61.

18. Dewhurst WG, Morgan HG. Importance of urine volume in assessment of thiamin deficiency. *Am J Clin Nutr.* 1970;23:379–381.

19. Smith F, Goodman DS. Vitamin A transport in human vitamin A toxicity. *N Engl J Med.* 1976;294:805–808.

20. Olson J. Letter. *Am J Clin Nutr.* 1981;34:435–436.

21. Mawer EB. Critical implications of measurements of circulating vitamin D metabolites. *Clin Endocrinol Metab.* 1980;9:63–79.

22. Bergen SS, Roels OA. Hypervitaminosis A. *Am J Clin Nutr.* 1965;16:265–269.

23. Bieri JG. Vitamin E. Nutrition reviews' present knowledge in nutrition. *Nutr Rev.* 1975;33(6): 161–167.

24. Horwitt MK, Harvey CC, Dahm CH Jr, Searcy MT. Relationship between tocopherals and serum lipid levels for determination of nutritional adequacy. *Ann NY Acad Sci.* 1972;203:223–236.

25. Almquist HJ. Vitamin K: discovery, identification, synthesis, functions. *Fed Proc.* 1979;38:2687–2689.

26. Solomons NW. On the assessment of zinc and copper nutriture in man. *Am J Clin Nutr.* 1979;32:856–871.

Case Management, Documentation, and Providing Nutrition Services

Chapter 12

Case Management and the Interdisciplinary Health Team

Carla Mariano

OVERVIEW

Society today is facing health and social problems so complex that no one profession or discipline has either the educational or practical background to deal comprehensively with them. Additionally, health care services are provided in multiple care settings and by several care providers. AIDS, substance abuse, domestic violence, homelessness, poverty, chronic illness, adolescent pregnancy, and the growing number of elderly are but a few of the phenomena necessitating comprehensive, coordinated action and skilled management. These crises require that health care professionals collaborate with practitioners in numerous disciplines and relate to a myriad of client/institutional systems. Decreasing fragmentation, improving access to health care delivery, and providing cost-effective health care have become national appeals.

THE CASE MANAGEMENT PROCESS

Definition and Purpose

Case management is a system of client/patient-focused practices designed to coordinate care. It unites "clinical and management skills in providing or arranging for whatever health care a person needs."[1(p71)] It is defined as "a set of logical steps and a process of interaction within a service network which assure that a client receives needed services in a supportive, effective, efficient, and cost-effective manner."[2(p2)] Cohen and Cesta suggest that "such management emphasizes early assessment and intervention, comprehensive care planning, and inclusive service system referrals."[3(p6)]

Case management has emerged as a response to a costly and fragmented health care delivery system. As Bower[4(p2)] notes,

> Health care delivery must be restructured and refocused to attain an effective balance between costs, desired outcomes, and processes for delivery of care. . . . The overall purpose of case management is to advocate for the patient through coordination of care, which reduces fragmentation and, ultimately, cost.

Its goal is to attain intended results for client populations with complex problems needing comprehensive care through organizing and "brokering services across the health care continuum"[4(p3)] and among multiple systems.

Attributes of Case Management

Bower[4] identifies the distinguishing features of case management programs. This approach

- is episode based, focusing on the client care needs across settings and phases for the duration of the episode.
- is longitudinally based, following the client throughout the illness and referring when necessary.
- most often focuses on clients from high-cost, high-risk, or high-volume classifications.
- concentrates on coordination, transitions, and continuity.
- is quality driven, outcome motivated, and fiscally responsive.
- puts clients and their families at the center of the service endeavor.
- focuses on obtaining and enhancing access to services for the client/family.
- is proactive and fosters prevention, health promotion, independence, advocacy, holism, growth, and fulfillment of potential.
- necessitates interdisciplinary collaboration (this area is discussed further in the section on interdisciplinary teams).

Case Management: Process and Roles

Case management is both a system or process of health care delivery and a role or function of health care providers. As a system and process, case management exemplifies particular components. These include a multidimensional assessment (of physical health; mental health; nutrition; personal and community supports; financial resources; and spiritual, legal, environmental, and vocational issues), diagnosis/problem identification, goal setting, planning and decision making, intervention (securing, delivering, referring, and coordinating needed services), monitoring, and evaluating both short- and long-term outcomes. Cohen and Cesta[3] discuss two contemporary models of case management: a "Within-the-Walls" or hospital-based case management model, and a "Beyond-the-Walls" or community-based approach model of case management. Karls and Wandrei[5] describe a strategy for more effective case management, the "Person-In-Environment System for Classifying Client Problems" or PIE system.

Case management affords clients and their families someone who coordinates their care. Whether or not case managers provide direct care to the client, they must possess strong clinical knowledge and competence to know what the client's needs are in order to effectively manage the required care. In addition, case managers must possess broad-based knowledge of resources to accountably relate to, negotiate with, and obtain as necessary multiple service providers.

There has been much discussion regarding who should serve as a case manager. Grau[6(p373)] suggests:

> Most policy makers and practitioners agree that case management is not a profession, but a set of functions to be carried out by persons capable of doing so. . . . For the client, the nature of the case manager's background is important. It influences the kind of direct care the case manager provides as well as other aspects of service delivery and monitoring. The critical factor in determining who fills the case manager role is the nature of the population to be served.

Regardless of the practitioner's discipline, there are primary case manager role functions[4,7] that are closely aligned with the components and process of case management. These role functions are

- c case finding and screening to identify appropriate clients and determine their need and eligibility for case management services
- c assessing comprehensively all areas of the client's functioning and support systems (see above) as well as the client's goals
- c analyzing and integrating all data for generating diagnoses or problem statements
- c developing, implementing, overseeing, and adjusting a plan of care through an interdisciplinary team process, in conjunction with the clients and appropriate caregivers

- identifying and obtaining needed services such as hospitalization or home care
- linking the client with the appropriate institutional or community resources and producing new resources if gaps exist
- coordinating care and services in many models and in a variety of reimbursement sources
- monitoring (1) the client's progress toward goal achievement; (2) the plan, to assure the appropriateness, quality, quantity, timeliness, usefulness, and cost-effectiveness of services provided; (3) the activities, to guarantee that services are being delivered and meet client needs
- evaluating the client and case management program objectives to determine achievement, continuation, or discharge

Throughout these activities, the case manager solves problems; expedites access to care; serves as a liaison; educates the client, family, and community; facilitates communication; documents progress and changes; and continually advocates for the client.

THE NATURE OF INTERDISCIPLINARY TEAMS

Effective case management programs require collaboration. One of the most productive vehicles for implementing the case management approach is the interdisciplinary/interprofessional team.

There is much misunderstanding about exactly what an interdisciplinary team is. Terms such as *interdisciplinary, multidisciplinary, transdisciplinary,* and *crossdisciplinary* are used synonymously and interchangeably. Mariano[8,9] notes that an interdisciplinary team is more than a collection of people. It is a group of highly diverse people and competent professionals who combine their talents, have a unified direction, share a collective purpose and common objectives, and aim toward an integrated outcome. The team entity has a structure, a distinctness, a direction, an identification, and a "group energy." It is an illusion to think that if a group of very skilled professionals is called a team it will in fact operate as a team. Effective teamwork requires time, ability, and a process of development and change.

Another frequently held myth regarding team performance is that there is no discipline-specific activity. Ducanis and Golin[10] identify both individual and team efforts. Individual activities (data collection, data interpretation and reporting, and specific tasks) do exist. However, they must complement team endeavors (problem identification, goal setting, diagnosis, development and coordination of treatment plans, and evaluation of outcomes). The team is the mechanism for organizing and integrating the actions of various professions. It does not eradicate discipline-specific functions and responsibilities. Figure 12–1 outlines the relationship between individual and team activities.

Another crucial consideration is the inclusion of the client as an integral member of the team (see Figure 12–2). We should always remember that the client is the nucleus of the team's venture and the justification for the team's existence. Clients also become empowered through their contribution to treatment goals, decision making, and evaluation. The therapeutic effect of this empowerment cannot be underestimated.

FACILITATORS AND BARRIERS TO INTERDISCIPLINARY FUNCTIONING

Within a team, four factors seem to promote or hinder interdisciplinary endeavors: role and goal definition and conflict, decision making, communication, and institutional variables.[9,11,12]

Understanding Roles

When a group is formed, individuals place themselves or are placed into certain roles. Role definition within the interdisciplinary team is extremely important because disagreement often leads to role conflict. Role conflict arises when (1) there is role ambiguity, (2) there are overlapping responsibilities and competencies among team members, and (3) team members hold stereotypic preconceptions of the professionals in other disciplines and/or of the client.

Newberger[13] cited a number of reasons why different disciplines have difficulty in working together. There may be ignorance of the conceptual base for practice of each other's discipline. Poor communication often exists among members of different disciplines. There may be confusion between disciplines as to who should take what responsibilities. And chauvinistic attitudes, distrust, and lack of confidence in colleagues in other disciplines may be present.

Bruce[14] recognized "social proximity" as a pivotal factor determining whether individuals from different fields can work collaboratively. He noted that differences in social status originating from historical determinants and social distance create barriers to cooperation among various professional groups. This "clearly lies at the root of much of the failure to cooperate which has been observed throughout the health and welfare services."[14(p47)]

Several elements foster role definition and appropriate role development within teams. A thorough awareness of one's own profession is indispensable in communicating that discipline's strengths, limitations, and contributions to the

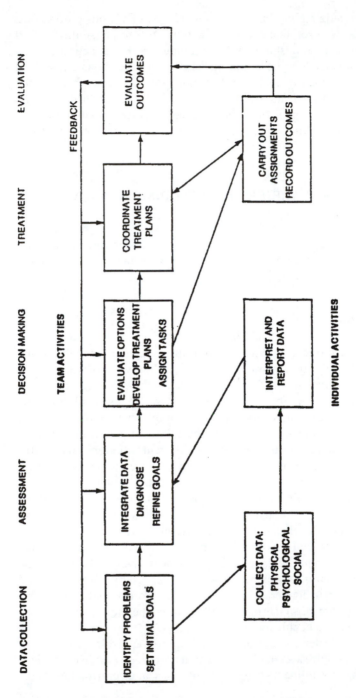

Figure 12–1 Individual and Team Activities. *Source:* Reprinted from *The Interdisciplinary Health Care Team* by A. Ducanis and A. Golin, p. 108, with permission of the authors, © 1979.

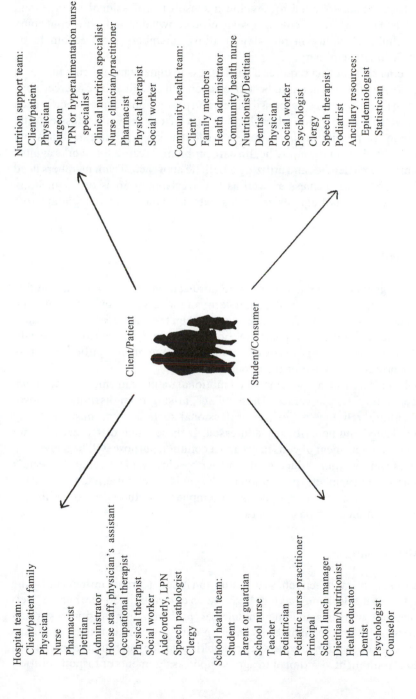

Nutrition support team:
  Client/patient
  Physician
  Surgeon
  TPN or hyperalimentation nurse
    specialist
  Clinical nutrition specialist
  Nurse clinician/practitioner
  Pharmacist
  Physical therapist
  Social worker

Community health team:
  Client
  Family members
  Health administrator
  Community health nurse
  Nutritionist/Dietitian
  Dentist
  Physician
  Social worker
  Psychologist
  Clergy
  Speech therapist
  Podiatrist
  Ancillary resources:
    Epidemiologist
    Statistician

Client/Patient

Student/Consumer

Hospital team:
  Client/patient family
  Physician
  Nurse
  Pharmacist
  Dietitian
  Administrator
  House staff, physician's assistant
  Occupational therapist
  Physical therapist
  Social worker
  Aide/orderly, LPN
  Speech pathologist
  Clergy

School health team:
  Student
  Parent or guardian
  School nurse
  Teacher
  Pediatrician
  Pediatric nurse practitioner
  Principal
  School lunch manager
  Dietitian/Nutritionist
  Health educator
  Dentist
  Psychologist
  Counselor

Figure 12–2 Team Interaction in Various Health Care Settings

team effort. Members need to develop a sense of professional security and competence in order to articulate how specific knowledge and skills contribute to the whole. Certainty in one's field allows members the freedom to be genuinely interdisciplinary.

Reducing role conflict requires a willingness to understand the role that each discipline plays. There needs to be a discussion and clarification of perceptions regarding members' roles, responsibilities, and professional competencies; each other's values; expectation of each other and of one's own profession; and overlapping responsibilities. It is imperative that no single discipline thinks that it "owns" the client or the entire health care problem, because this works against combining competencies and utilizing a holistic approach. Team members need to recognize the uniqueness as well as the overlapping areas of various disciplines. And all participants must learn to negotiate and renegotiate role assignments.

Goal Conflict

Several goals must be considered by interdisciplinary teams: client, professional, and organizational goals; short-term and long-term goals; and task and maintenance goals.[10] Goal conflict can arise when the team goals are unclear or nonspecific, when the team goals are too complex and no priorities are established, or when goals proposed by one or more team members conflict with those of other professionals and/or the client.

Goal conflict of a very personal and emotional nature can emerge when team members hold different values. These values, arising from dissimilar philosophies, culture, religious beliefs, or professional socialization, must be openly communicated and noncritically addressed. If these value differences are not discussed, achievement of consensus and a common purpose will be subverted.

Teams can avoid or reduce goal conflict by clearly identifying the team's goals, assessing members' perceptions of the goals, reaching agreement as to the priorities and plan of action to be taken. emphasizing the *union* of skills and expertise, and focusing on *outcomes*.

Decision Making

Interdisciplinary effectiveness or disruption is considerably influenced by the process used for decision making. Ingredients contributing to ineffectual decision making in teams include an unclear problem, imprecision regarding members' roles and accountability in the process, insufficient data, consideration of only one option, disallowing risk taking, lack of attention to timeliness, and no commitment to action or to agreed-upon assignments or responsibilities.

Five questions should be addressed for productive decision making[15]:

1. What needs to be decided?
2. Who should be involved in the process?
3. What decision-making process should be used?
4. Who will be responsible for carrying out the decision?
5. Who needs to be informed of the decision?

Fruitful decision making must begin with a clearly defined problem. Once it is agreed upon, the team members must gather sufficient and relevant data about the problem, generate numerous alternatives, and test options.[16] The team needs to specify responsibilities, and individuals must then commit themselves to identified actions.

There should be regard for each member's contributions and expertise, including the client's. All members, again including the client, must share responsibility for the ultimate result. Unanimous agreement is not the goal. Rather the opportunity is there for each member to *influence* the final outcome. Leadership of an interdisciplinary team may rotate among members depending on the needs and particular focus.

> The team should also consider that in certain situations, interdisci-
> plinary planning and implementation may require both a different time
> span and different people. Emphasis, however, is always on coordina-
> tion of specialized knowledge versus dilution of expertise and compre-
> hensive outcome versus duplication of members' activities.[9]

Communication

Communications that cultivate interdisciplinary functioning include sharing within a climate of candor but safety, sincere listening to each person's opinions and feelings, thoughtful consideration of differences, and feedback that is frank, constructive, and issue oriented rather than personal or retaliatory. Openness, trust, and negotiation should prevail versus power struggles, tyranny, control, and unspoken personal agendas. These attitudes and patterns can be maintained if team members are willing to trust, respect, and value each other and themselves. Team members must also take risks and confront each other (in a professional manner) when necessary. To develop and preserve this milieu, the team must regularly evaluate its own process and operations.

Organizational Factors

> In human service, the organization acts as a host to the team. . . . The
> organization also determines overall purpose and policy, is responsible

for executive decisions about how these policies shall apply to the team, and generally defines the nature and extent of team participation in organizational matters. The manner in which the organization carries out these tasks creates a climate that markedly affects the functioning of the team.[17(p111)]

It is obvious that the institution plays a major role in the success or failure of collaborative functioning. Interdisciplinary teams are very complex entities. They require fiscal resources and support services to sustain their comprehensive operations. Collaboration demands time for exchanging information, dealing with group decision making, and exploring and resolving group and practice issues. Team members should be allowed to make sufficient time commitments to team efforts. This is often not possible if the members' interdisciplinary duties are over and above their discipline-specific or departmental obligations.

Consideration must also be given to space and physical location. Proximity of members can facilitate both formal and informal communication. And there needs to be adequate and neutral space for team activities. When all disciplines on the team share the same or comparable space, status becomes less of an issue, and conflict may be reduced.

Legitimization of team activity within the larger organization is vital lest the relevance of team undertakings be overlooked or dismissed as nonessential. Is the team an integral part of the organization's formal authority, communication, and policy-making structure? Does the institution have a well-designed, integrated record-keeping system that incorporates all essential client information as opposed to discipline-specific documentation? Is success judged on a long-term or short-term basis? Because of the comprehensive nature of interdisciplinary intervention, long-term results should be measured and the team given the opportunity to demonstrate progress over time. Answers to these questions often indicate the institutional climate toward interdisciplinary teams.

Finally, institutional recognition and reward of collaborative endeavors play a pivotal role in cooperative ventures. If the organizational reward system is such that only competition and individual- and discipline-specific achievements are recognized and valued, collaboration will not occur and the team system will not function.

CHARACTERISTICS OF EFFECTIVE INTERDISCIPLINARY CASE MANAGERS

A number of attributes promote practitioners' skills in collaborating with others. These include[11,18]

- an ability to conceptualize, to think critically, to pull things together and synthesize one's *discipline* role with one's *team* role
- a sense of curiosity and interest in other than one's own field; a sense of discovery and creativity and the need to understand things that are not quite understood
- a willingness to remain a student and to learn from others what their skills, competencies, and values are; a broad interest in a variety of topics and perspectives
- an ability to wait without instant gratification, to use knowledge toward long-range holistic outcomes
- appreciation of interdependence and needing others to enhance one's own effectiveness
- a capacity to share one's self, expertise, ideas, successes, and disagreements
- a sense of humor
- a comfort with and ability to speak up in groups
- maturity and open-mindedness, being goal directed but not having to win every point
- an awareness of one's own needs, style, strengths, limitations, and aspirations. Self-knowledge enhances one's capability for contributing to the whole.

The role of case manager requires additional knowledge and skills. A case manager must possess in-depth knowledge of health care financing, including financial and delivery systems (HMOs, DRGs, PPOs), guidelines and requirements of third-party payers and government agencies, insurance arrangements, and cost-containment efforts and trends. Clinical expertise is necessary because the case manager attends to the care needs of clients across the care continuum. Knowledge of inpatient, home, and rehabilitative care is essential, as are skills in assessment, mutual goal setting, and evaluation.

The case manager needs to be integrally aware of both institutional and community resources and how to access them efficiently. Discharge planning, management skills, networking, consultation, advocacy, delegation, negotiation, teaching, counseling, and quality improvement strategies are further areas in which the case manager must be proficient.[4] In addition, there are both advocacy and ethical issues related to case management with which the case manager must be familiar.[19,20]

OUTCOMES AND ADVANTAGES OF INTERDISCIPLINARY CASE MANAGEMENT

There are many benefits to using an interdisciplinary team/case management approach.[4,11,21,22] These include

- *Management of complexity.* There is a focus on the full spectrum of client needs and the breadth of resources available to meet those needs.

- *Quality decisions.* The health care problems that society is facing today have numerous ethical considerations and life and death implications. An interdisciplinary approach removes the burden of total responsibility from one person, thereby minimizing the potential for a wrong decision.

- *Member support.* Interdisciplinary teams provide the opportunity for members to explore and vent their feelings with peers. Feelings of frustration, anger, helplessness, discouragement, and disillusionment are not uncommon among health professionals. Mutual support can minimize the possibility of burnout, which is so prevalent among clinicians.

- *Cost-effectiveness.* Interdisciplinary case management minimizes fragmentation, optimizes coordination, and assists client movement through the health system. It reduces or eliminates duplication and overlapping of care, tests, and treatments through coordination of care activities. Furthermore, it can decrease or avoid delay in required tests or treatments. Team members also develop an enhanced knowledge of financial aspects of care.

- *Motivation.* Through collaborative efforts, all members can learn from other disciplines, gain different insights, develop an appreciation for various perspectives, become familiar with the array of resources needed to deal with multidimensional needs, and experience the value of a comprehensive approach.

- *Collective strength.* This model of care maximizes and organizes the expertise and contributions of all disciplines. It also improves communication among professionals as well as with clients and families. Working together, both professionals and consumer clients can facilitate system changes to improve quality care and control costs.

- *Outcome orientation.* The aim of interdisciplinary case management is to move the client/family progressively toward desired care outcomes. This approach is antithetical to the traditional health care system, which tends to be self-serving and bureaucratic. Accountability for achieving identified outcomes becomes paramount and is the responsibility of all team members.

- *Proactive versus retrospective response.* Interdisciplinary teams are capable of responding quickly and thoroughly. With early identification of potential client problems and impediments to care services, plans can be developed to address real and potential barriers before they occur. This capacity lends itself to primary prevention, a focus so important to today's health problems.

- *Client empowerment.* Case management enhances communication with and education of clients/families. This allows them to better plan for their needs and to make more informed decisions about care. Knowing that they have an identified practice care team to whom they can turn promotes a sense of security and satisfaction.

CONCLUSION

"The provision of outcome-oriented, cost-effective health care is no longer a goal—it is a mandate. To accomplish this mandate, the relationship between the costs of care, the desired outcomes of care, and the processes involved in providing care must be reexamined."[4(p1)] There is a national urgency to provide optimal care at reduced cost to the consumer. In order to accomplish this end, professionals must exercise mutual respect and foster cooperation among themselves.

Through case management and interdisciplinary collaboration, health providers can participate in transforming today's increasingly specialized and fragmented health care system. Modern societal health problems make it almost irrefutable that comprehensive, collaborative health care delivery will become increasingly important in the future.

REFERENCES

1. Schoor T. Case management companies run by nurses? *American Journal of Nursing.* 1990;90(10):71.

2. Weil M, Karls J. *Case Management in Human Service Practice.* San Francisco, Calif: Jossey-Bass Publishers; 1985.

3. Cohen E, Cesta T. *Nursing case management from concept to evaluation.* St. Louis, Mo: CV Mosby Co, 1993.

4. Bower K. *Case management by nurses.* Kansas City, Mo: American Nurses Association; 1992.

5. Karls J, Wandrei K. The person-in-environment system of classifying client problems. *Journal of Case Management.* 1992;1(3):90–95.

6. Grau L. Case management and the nurse. *Geriatric Nursing.* 1984;5(8):372–375.

7. Weil M, Karls J. Historical origins and recent developments. In Weil M, Karls J, eds. *Case Management in Human Service Practice.* San Francisco, Calif: Jossey-Bass Publishers; 1985:1–28.

8. Mariano C. *Interdisciplinary/interprofessional collaboration in education and practice.* Presented at the American Academy of Nursing 1992 Conference; October 1992; St. Louis, Mo.

9. Mariano C. The case for interdisciplinary collaboration. *Nursing Outlook.* 1989;37(6):285–288.

10. Ducanis A, Golin A. *The Interdisciplinary Health Care Team: A Handbook.* Gaithersburg, Md: Aspen Publishers, Inc; 1979.

11. Mariano C. Interdisciplinary collaboration: a practice imperative. *Healthcare Trends and Transitions.* 1992;3(5):10–12, 24–25.

12. Mariano C. Facilitators and barriers to interdisciplinary collaboration in child abuse and neglect. In: Mauro L, Woods J, eds. *Building Bridges: Interdisciplinary Research in Child Abuse and Neglect.* Philadelphia, Pa: Temple University Press; 1991:171–181.

13. Newberger E. A physician's perspective on interdisciplinary management of child abuse. *Psychiatric Opinion.* 1976;2:13–18.

14. Bruce N. *Teamwork for Preventive Care.* Chichester, UK: Research Studies Press, John Wiley & Sons, Ltd; 1980.

15. Baldwin D, Tsukuda R. Interdisciplinary teams. In Cassel C, Walsh J, eds. *Geriatric Medicine, Vol 2: Fundamentals of Geriatric Care.* New York, NY: Springer-Verlag; 1984.

16. Conley A, Mariano C. Group participatory decision making: issues and guidelines. *J NY State Nurses Assoc.* 1991;22(2):4–8.

17. Brill N. *Teamwork: Working Together in the Human Services.* Philadelphia, Pa: JB Lippincott Co; 1976.

18. Mariano C. A qualitative study of interdisciplinary/interprofessional collaboration. In: *Proceedings of the Thirteenth Annual Interdisciplinary Health Care Team Conference.* Indianapolis, In: Indiana University School of Medicine, Division of Allied Health Services; 1991:165–175.

19. Dubler N. Individual advocacy as a governing principle. *Journal of Case Management.* 1992;1(3):82–86.

20. Browdie R. Ethical issues in case management from a political and systems perspective. *Journal of Case Management.* 1992;1(3):87–89.

21. Mariano C. Interdisciplinary collaboration in the treatment of addictions. *Addictions Nursing Network.* 1989;1(4):7–10.

22. Francis D, Young D. *Improving Workshops: A Practical Guide.* San Diego, Calif: University Associates; 1979.

Chapter 13

Documentation of Nutrition Care

Judith A. Gilbride, Joan Castro, and Isabelle A. Hallahan

OVERVIEW

Documentation and accountability for health and nutrition services are mandated by law and accrediting bodies with increasing frequency. Documentation of nutritional care provides not only proof of care but is the basis for audit to ensure and monitor quality care. Providers of nutritional care should strive to develop a system for clear, concise communication of both interdepartmental and intradepartmental activities focused on the holistic approach to improving client/patient care. Coordination of care and cost containment can be promoted through sharing appropriate, precise, and accurate data. Facility policies may determine the who, where, and what of record maintenance, but the responsibility for proper and sufficient accounting for use of time and resources that will withstand audit and external review lies with each member of the health care team.

RATIONALE FOR DOCUMENTATION

The passage of P.L. 92-603 in October 1972 established professional standards review organizations for health care facilities and agencies supported by Medicare, Medicaid, and Maternal and Child Health funds. This legislation identified the need to develop criteria for judging services, audits of service provided, and written documentation to justify all pertinent decisions on client/patient care. Quality control was the chief objective, along with expected cost containment. The Joint Commission on Accreditation of Healthcare Organizations (Joint Commission) published standards requiring that dietitians perform proper recording in the patient's medical records.[1] The guidelines were revised in 1980 by a joint committee of dietitians from the American Dietetic Association and the American Hospital Association.[2] The 1994 *Accreditation Manual for Hospitals* further modified these standards, and the completion of "an initial assessment/screening of each patient's physical, psychological and social status to determine the need for care or treatment, the type of care or treatment to be provided, and the need for any further assessment"[3(p.13)] is now required. It is also necessary to give a reason for assessing the patient's nutritional status.

Nationally established requirements for documentation are augmented by numerous local and institutional requirements. In addition, there are obvious motivations for recording data that can be grouped under five major headings:

1. Client/patient service
   - Documentation of nutritional care is an instrument for sharing appropriate, pertinent data with members of the health care team. Scientific knowledge of the importance of nutrition in preventive, diagnostic, curative, restorative, and rehabilitation health care services is expanding. It is therefore essential that nutritional care data be communicated both interdepartmentally and intradepartmentally to assist in the coordination of services.
   - Such documentation becomes a part of the patient's health care history. Included are progress reports of care, the patient's status at the time of termination of care in the facility, and recommendations for continued care in another environment.
   - The documentation is used in referral systems to ensure an appropriate continuum of care.
   - Documentation helps to distinguish the need for therapy from the need for patient education or nutrition counseling.
   - Documentation creates a system for establishing, measuring progress toward, and modifying patient care goals.
2. Continuous quality improvement
   - Documentation of nutritional care becomes a reference and the database for comparing decisions and actions to criteria and standards of care.
   - Following an audit, such documentation is useful in developing a plan for continuing education for the staff.
   - Documentation also assists in the evaluation of the continuing effectiveness of both the process and the provider used to change the outcomes of care.

- Discharge planning is required by the Joint Commission as a component of a hospital quality assurance program and is a condition of participation for Medicare and Medicaid. Dietary data that should be documented in the medical record include description or copy of a diet forwarded to another institution, counseling provided to a patient on a modified diet, patient's comprehension of a diet instruction, and counseling related to potential drug–food interactions.[4]

3. Economics/cost containment
   - The documentation of nutritional care can save time and money for the patient and the provider by giving access to data required to process with care, to make recommendations to that effect, to prevent unneeded repetition of services, and to assist in providing uninterrupted optimal care.
   - Documentation allows for medical record coding of diagnosis and treatment of malnutrition to obtain optimal reimbursement for care provided, to identify nonroutine nutrition services, and to establish billing procedures for inpatient nutrition services.
   - Documentation is a management tool for establishing and maintaining efficient use of available resources and time and for planning and implementing departmental budget and personnel requisitions.
   - Documentation can also justify discharge care, cost of equipment, supplies (supplements/tube feedings), and follow-up care.

4. Legal issues
   - Patients have the right to see their hospital records. Informed consents are included in medical records showing the consent of patients for a variety of procedures. Natural death acts authorize the use of living wills to give directions concerning care and often include specific instructions on artificial feeding and hydration.
   - Although classified as confidential, health care records may be subpoenaed, along with the recorder, during litigation over the appropriateness of the care rendered or the lack of care. The possibilities for malpractice claims accelerate as the responsibilities of the provider escalate. Registered dietitians are not exempt from malpractice claims. This process may take a number of years; therefore all documentation must be clear to the future reader and must not force the author to rely on memory.
   - Documentation of compliance with physician's orders and preestablished criteria for professional decisions and judgments are essential to provide proof of quality and quantity of care. Evidence of compliance with the standards for dietetic services developed by the Joint Commission is recognized as authoritative when records are presented to support appropriate care.

- Documentation of provision of care and of recommended continued care becomes the basis for insurance claims, third-party reimbursement, and financial or food assistance when needed to justify recommended nutritional requirements.
- Documentation of nutritional care is required for an audit of the care. Any feeding decisions involving ethical and legal issues should be documented accurately and appropriately in department and patient records.
5. Professional integrity
   - The documentation of services provided with a subsequent audit is a stimulation for self-improvement.
   - Such documentation establishes guidelines for evaluating personal competencies, complying with established policies and procedures and standards of practice or practice guidelines, managing time and resources, and planning continuing education strategies.
   - Documentation is also a medium for job satisfaction. Excessive or nonspecific documentation is cumbersome for clinicians, and incorporating simple charting tasks, approved forms, or computerized medical records into the job description of support staff can be very motivating.

PROCEDURES IN DOCUMENTATION

The procedural aspects of documentation are concerned with the traditional questions of who, what, where, when, and how. The goals of developing a set of records designed to be mutually beneficial to patients and members of the health care team should have an immediate objective of deciding what kinds of records best meet this goal. Because of the mandated requirements noted previously, the absence of some documentation of nutritional care would be rare. Thus critical review of records for possible revision is the first step in moving toward better accountability of nutrition care services.

The exact kind of record to use and the location of data to be recorded vary from institution to institution, agency to agency, and, in the case of sole practice, from individual to individual. The question to be addressed in developing and evaluating a record is: Does it contribute to the system for improving the quality of care?

DIET MANUAL

A diet manual approved by representatives of staff from nutrition, medicine, nursing, and pharmacy or by a patient care policy committee should be made available to all appropriate staff. Some small facilities adopt a diet manual from another organization or institution with approval from a nutrition or medical committee. The diet manual should be a guide for all those responsible for translating diet orders into nutritionally adequate, palatable meals and should serve as a basis for staff and client education. The manual is an adopted standard that is designed to be useful to the prescriber of the diet. It represents what the facility agrees to provide in food to fulfill the prescription; it is both a reference and a communication channel for those who are serving the patient.

The Joint Commission mandates that an up-to-date diet manual be available in facilities that it accredits. Thus the diet manual becomes a criterion for judgment and accountability and the vehicle for establishing precise terminology related to diet and procedures. It provides guidance for consistent nomenclature in communication initiated by nutrition care staff. The manual is, however, only a guide, and thus must allow for adaptation of the prescribed diet to acceptable meal patterns of individuals and groups.

CARDEX FILE

A cardex or kardex, a file kept in the department of nutrition and dietetics, is the most accessible source of client information for the nutrition staff and should thus be developed in a format to meet the needs of the staff. Depending upon department and facility policy, as well as available resources, the cardex file may be kept on cards, one for each client, or on individual computer printouts. In either case, the file contains a reiteration of the client profile found in the medical record; the diet order (unless this is recorded and maintained separately); the client's food preferences, intolerances, and allergies; and the nutritional care plan. Again, depending upon resources, the cardex file may include screening and assessment data: pertinent laboratory, anthropometric, and psychological data. Some or all of the information may be obtained via computer from either the nursing department, the admitting office, or the physician's office.

MEDICAL RECORD

The American Hospital Association (AHA) Bulletin points out that "the patient's medical record serves as an information-sharing tool that promotes and assists in coordinating the activities of all health team members involved in the patient's care. As such, it should reflect the health team's ultimate goal of high-quality care and optimal cost effectiveness."[2] Frequently referred to as the "chart," the medical record contains entries that are referred to as "charting," "progress notes," or "continuation notes."

How the recording is done and by whom are determined by the policies governing the standards for practice in a facility. Some institutions have developed protocols that combine process and outcome standards. One inpatient diabetes treatment program designed a protocol with a documentation record as an abbreviated method of charting a patient's response to diabetic teaching.[4] The documentation record included three columns: one for the date of teaching, one for the initials of the instructor, and one measuring patient and/or caregiver's level of understanding, on a scale from 1 to 5, in six content areas: physiology, medications, blood glucose monitoring, diet, complications, and general health follow-up. Each content area emphasized preestablished outcome criteria with goals; content highlighting of key words and phrases; and plan, a listing of tools and methods used as teaching aids. A comments section allowed additional space to explain any follow-up teaching that was necessary.[4]

The Source-Oriented Medical Record

The source-oriented medical record (SOMR) is the traditional form of charting patients' progress from admission to discharge from a facility, with records of the course of action taken in their behalf during their stay. The term *source-oriented* describes the content of the individual's file. The file is composed of separate records from each of the health disciplines that is a source of care—for example, medicine, laboratory, nursing, social service, and nutrition. In this format, the progress notes become a chronological narrative of the provider's observations and plans that is maintained in each provider's file. Each of these separate accountings is consulted for information to plan and coordinate care for the patient and to complete departmental documentation of pertinent data.

The progress note section of a medical record is considered to be the most appropriate location for recording dietetic information and nutritional care plans. Both the source- and problem-oriented systems of medical records provide for such recording, commensurate with the policies of the particular facility. In any event, regardless of where the data are kept, there should be an assigned responsibility for documenting sufficient information to support the nutrition assessment, to justify the nutritional care plan and its implementation, and to conduct an audit for ensuring the quality of nutritional care.

The Problem-Oriented Medical Record

The problem-oriented medical record (POMR) is a system of charting care that supports the holistic approach. This type of record is viewed by its proponents as a vehicle for improving the quality of care by coordinating the services of all members of the health care team who serve the client. In the POMR, data pertinent to the disposition of a client's identified "problem" are recorded. The problem is a condition requiring action by a member or members of the health care team to obtain more information, treat, and/or educate. The problem is considered to exist as long as any of these three components is present. A client may have more than one problem: for example, with diabetes mellitus (a diagnosis and a problem), accompanying obesity is a problem, not a diagnosis. In the POMR system, action is focused on the client, with emphasis on all factors contributing to the client's discomfort or condition rather than merely on a single diagnosis.

Becoming problem oriented requires defining the client's conditions as accurately, thoroughly, and precisely as available information permits during the course of intervention. Once defined, the problem appears prominently on the record, so that all members of the provider team may give due consideration to its resolution. The database for recording in the client's medical record and the format for the nutritional care plan should be developed according to the *Guidelines for Recording Nutritional Information in Medical Records.*[2]

The format of POMR promotes recording in consistent, precise language with uniform acronyms and abbreviations. The POMR database includes the physician's admission note; client's name, age, sex, and race; referral source; place of primary care; a brief profile of pertinent socioeconomic factors; a review of systems; and the medical history. Supplementing this is a list of all precisely identified problems, numbered consecutively, on the POMR's first page. This is followed by an initial plan of action for each problem, including diagnostic, therapeutic, and patient education. In effect, this list of data becomes the table of contents of the POMR.

Following the establishment of the initial formulation and plan for treating the patient's problems, the progress sheets function as a flow sheet of the activities surrounding the patient's treatment and progress. The providers are responsible for documenting problems associated within their scope of practice, incorporating those outlined by the initial and primary caretakers. Progress notes should contain the patient's medical record or admitting number and name, the date, health care team service, the nature of the problem, the interaction, and the signature, credentials, and title of the caretaker. Policy may require that duplicate copies of POMR entries be kept in each department. In hospitals where documentation is computerized, a standard record-keeping process can be more efficient and less time consuming, and simplifies monitoring of care.

The initial note from each service may be on a consultation form or an assessment form or in a SOAP format (subjective data, objective data, assessment, plan of approach). Assessment forms are preprinted, are usually specific to the service, and should comply with the institution or regulatory agency requirements. Such forms provide consistency in charting procedures as well as a format for quality assurance. These forms are often used when formal nutrition consultations are requested and also by students or entry-level practitioners who may need assistance with formatting their notes.

Progress notes in the SOAP format are designed to guide the professional in providing well-rounded information in a brief and concise manner (Exhibit 13–1). The note is divided into the following sections:

- S: *Subjective data* are obtained from patients, family, or significant others; what the patients say about their condition, appetite, intake, weight, eating problems, digestion, and elimination; information that usually cannot be verified, often intangible.
- O: *Objective data* include measurable data or facts perceived by the care provider to represent signs and symptoms of the disease; and relevant and verifiable clinical information obtained from the chart, such as diagnoses, medication, laboratory, and anthropometric data that affect nutritional status.
- A: *Assessment* is an analysis of the patient's nutritional status and needs based on the subjective and objective data and is supported by professional expertise and knowledge.
- P: *Plan* of approach for nutrition intervention is divided into three sections: (1) diagnostic—the plan or recommendation to obtain needed data or clinical information to complete the evaluation; (2) treatment/therapeutic actions to be taken that will address identified problems or recommendation of such action; and (3) education to be taken for patient instruction and follow-up counseling, stated in terms of objectives or outcome measures.

Regulatory bodies have mandated that planning for discharge be initiated at the onset of care. This information may be incorporated into discharge planning rounds or placed in each discipliner's chart note as a subsection of the plan or in addition to the note. The records should be in a consistent format and coordinated with other health care providers.

Other Charting Formats

Alternative charting styles have been developed to improve communications, to minimize replication of information, and to identify the care provided and the outcomes of nutrition intervention. Focus, a charting method, was developed for documentation of care by nurses given in accordance with the patients' nursing care plan.[6] This format, when used by nutrition services, clearly identifies nutrition diag-

Exhibit 13–1 Sample SOAP Format

DATE   *NUTRITION ASSESSMENT*

S.   Patient reports frequent thirst and hunger throughout the day, UBW 185 lb

O.   Dx: New onset NIDDM, PMH: HTN, 68-year-old male

Diet: Diabetic Diet; Ht: 5'9", Wt: 198 lb, DBW: 160 lb +/– 10%

Lab: (date) glucose, BUN, creatinine, cholesterol, albumin

Med: Diabinese

No known allergies, diet history taken

A.   1. Patient is an overnourished male (125% of his DBW), approximately 124% of his IBW, with a history of wt gain, 13 lb in 6 mos.

2. Diet history reveals patient consumed approximately 2,700 kcal/day, from 3 meals and 2 snacks prepared by spouse or consumed in fast food facilities, intake high in saturated fat, cholesterol, sodium (>4 g/day), and low in fiber, adequate in protein and essential nutrients. Estimated kcal need for weight loss are 1,800 kcal/ day (25kcal/kg DBW), protein needs are 64 g/day (0.8gm/kg DBW). Present diet is nonspecific; calorie and sodium restriction for weight loss indicated in view of diagnosis, medications, and need to reduce cardiovascular risk factors.

3. Most laboratory data WNL, glucose and cholesterol elevated, laboratory data consistent with anthropometric and dietary information indicating need for dietary intervention.

4. Patient and spouse in need of diet education on diet in relation to disease states (diabetes, HTN), weight loss, and meal pattern for home use. Patient and spouse appear receptive to diet instruction (written and verbal), as evidenced by questions and request for further discussion.

P.   Rx:

1. Request MD order lipid profile and weekly weights for future nutritional intervention

2. Recommend change of diet to 3 g Na, 1,800 kcal diabetic diet

Pt. Ed:

Will begin education on basic diabetic/dietary principles on (date), with patient and spouse, will review exchange groups, meal preparation, dining out, and sources of hidden sodium and simple sugars, and instruct on specific meal pattern upon clarification of diet order.

Discharge plan:

Complete diet instruction with written materials, so that patient is able to determine food choices based on meal pattern and calorie level to promote glycemic control and 1–2 lb wt loss/wk.

NAME, RD, LD

Key: NIDDM = noninsulin dependent diabetes mellitus; PMH = past medical history; HTN = hypertension; BUN = blood urea nitrogen; UBW = usual body weight; DBW = desirable body weight; WNL = within normal limits.

noses, the nutrition care process, and the response to nutrition care. This allows the dietitians to chart on nutrition issues and avoid replication of medical or non-nutrition problems. Once nutrition care guidelines are established for various diagnoses, these can be individualized and incorporated into the Focus note according to each patient's needs (Exhibit 13–2). The format of a Focus chart is:

- Focus: statement of the identified nutrition diagnosis
- Data: subjective and objective information related to the diagnosis
- Action: actions taken to resolve the problem
- Response: patient's reaction to treatment

PIE/O (problems, intervention, evaluation/outcome) is another charting style that can be used for an initial nutrition assessment note or for follow-up documentation.[7] This format again emphasizes nutrition-specific problems, services rendered, and the patient's response. Preprinted or computerized forms or adhesive labels are also used for nutrition documentation. These forms facilitate the transcription of information and standardize the format used while assuring compliance with the institution and legal standards.

Regardless of the charting format used, certain guidelines are generally recommended:

1. Use black ink and write legibly.
2. Place only pertinent facts in the medical record; avoid any personal opinions, criticisms, or opinions of the patient or other professionals.

Exhibit 13–2 Sample Focus Note

F: Patient requires diabetes nutrition education.

D: Patient usually consumes 2,700 kcal/day, high in sodium and saturated fat. Current diet order nonspecific, patient requires specific guidelines for weight loss (125% UBW) and improved glycemic and hypertension control as seen by elevated glucose (value) and cholesterol (value).

A: Request MD change diet to 1,800-kcal diabetic diet 3 g Na. Provided rationale for dietary intervention and synopsis of exchange system used for menu selection. Plan to continue diabetes education with patient and wife on (date) with specific exchange patterns and meal planning in various settings and how to decrease weight and cholesterol values. Will provide listing of alternative resources available upon discharge.

R: Patient able to select daily menu in accordance with meal pattern, expect 1–2 lb weight loss/week and reduced fasting blood glucose to acceptable values.

NAME, RD, CDE

Quotations from patients, when appropriate, should be noted as such or placed in the subjective section of the note.

3. All entries are dated and time noted, and all notes are in chronological order, leaving no blank lines or blank spaces.
4. Use only institution- or agency-approved abbreviations.
5. To void any information, draw a single line through it and write "error/void" and initial and date.
6. Do not go back and insert information; you may write an addendum if indicated.
7. Document as soon as care is given.
8. Date (use calendar dates, not days) and sign all entries with name and credentials.

ACTIVITY LOGS

Nutrition staff maintain a daily record of the activities performed in order to allow for the evaluation of productivity and collection of data used by intradepartmental quality assurance programs. This information is also used for time studies and accountability of activities that can assist with staff justification (Exhibit 13–3).

BEDSIDE CHARTING

The dietitian can make recommendations about nutrition care in the computer at the patient's bedside. The Food and Nutrition staff at Valley Hospital in Ridgewood, New Jersey has embarked on a streamlined method for charting in the computerized medical record in every patient's room. The model for their bedside computer charting is based on the Department of Nursing, which instituted a project in 1987 for writing nursing notes in the medical record. After the success of the Nursing Department, the Food and Nutrition Services Department went on-line.

The Nursing Department estimates that approximately one-half hour per nurse per shift can be saved via computerized documentation, allowing more time for patient care and an emphasis on patient and family education. Additionally, a critical care computer system is used in the Intensive Care Unit.

The Food and Nutrition Department staff developed their own screens containing words, phrases, and descriptors, with eight sections, that are essential to nutrition intervention. They include Observation, Interview, Diet, Height and Weight, Medications, Laboratory Data, Assessment, and Plan. The Assessment section is further broken down into Weight, Diet Intake, Diet History, Diet Teaching, and TPN/PPN. The Medications section was devised based on food and drug interactions. Besides the established descriptors on each screen, the

Exhibit 13–3 Sample Activity Log

Dietitian/Technician: _____

Month: <u>June 1994</u>

Clinical Nutrition Activity Log

DATE	PATIENT NUMBER	DIAGNOSIS	SCREEN	ASSESSMENT	DIET INSTRUCTION	FOLLOW-UP NOTE	CALORIE COUNT	ROUNDS
6/6	111111	Diabetes		✓	✓ (basic)			
6/6	222222	MI		✓ (basic)		✓	✓	
6/6	333333	AIDS						✓ (Oncology unit)
6/6	444444	Lymphoma		✓				

Exhibit 13–4 Sample Food Nutrition Services Report

THE VALLEY HOSPITAL 2W

<u>FOOD NUTRITION SERVICES REPORT</u>   TEST PATIENT 2

                                                    Adm. Date: 05/05/94
Room/Bed: 500B   Birth Date: 06/07/1944   age 49
Hosp. Days: 1   Post Op: ---   Sex: F   MR# 222222   Acc # 222222
Diagnosis: DIABETES MELLITUS   Doctor:

<u>Nutritional Interview</u> Pt states appetite improving, dissatisfied w/diet, NKA

<u>DIET HISTORY</u> Diet PTA: regular, Pt lives alone, no interest in following diet

<u>DIET</u> Calories ADA 1800

<u>Height and Weight:</u>

| | | Usual | Adm. | IBW |
Ht. inches	Wt. lbs	Wt. lbs	Wt. lbs	lbs.
69.0	220.0	220.0	200.0	180.0

| IBW | IBW |
% above	% below
22	

<u>Medications:</u> Current meds: Oral hypoglycemic antihyperlipemic
   glucotrol, lopid

<u>Lab Data</u> most recent accucheck: cholesterol elevated

<u>Assessment: Weight</u> unintentional Wt gain

<u>Assessment: Diet History</u> Pt's diet Hx reveals high kcalories intake excess CHO 2
   meals/day

<u>Assessment: Diet Intake</u> Pt may benefit from change in diet

<u>Assessment: Diet Teaching</u>

   Pt not familiar with ADA meal plan and exchanges—Pt does not appear motivated at
   this time to adhere to meal plan, will need continual reinforcement and review, may
   benefit from diabetic education team referral

<u>Plan</u> provide Pt w/meal plan menu options, RD phone number

<u>Recommendation-General</u> 1,800 cal ADA cholesterol fat restricted discharge diet recommended

<u>Pt Education</u> initiated diet teaching w/Pt, reviewed basic principles of diet, provided diet
   guidelines, will instruct Pt prior to D/C

   referred diabetic ed

   glucotrol—food/med interaction discussed—fact sheet provided—understanding
   fair—Pt may benefit from review

Key: CHO = carbohydrate; ADA = American Dietetic Association/American Diabetes
Association; D/C = discharge; NKA = no known allergies; IBW = ideal body weight; PTA
= prior to discharge; Hx = history.

Source: Food and Nutrition Services Department, The Valley Hospital, Ridgewood, New Jersey.

dietitian can add specific comments on a patient at the terminal in the nursing station. One drawback is that the nutrition notes are separate from the other progress notes, but a nutrition note "alert" is available to inform the staff. An example of a Food and Nutrition Service Report is shown in Exhibit 13–4. Time savings have not been investigated since the dietitians have been on-line for only six months and are revising the screens to meet the dietitians' charting needs. They report greater interaction with the team, easier chart reviews, and more consistency in interpreting nutrition care.

CONCLUSION

Documentation in medical records continues to evolve and adapt to the changing needs of health care. Important facts to consider are that nutrition notes be consistent, accurate, brief, succinct, and timely. Quality patient care and communication among health providers are the ultimate outcomes of established documentation procedures and legislative mandates.

REFERENCES

1. American Hospital Association. 1976. *Guidelines for Recording Nutritional Information in Medical Records.* Chicago, Ill: AHA.

2. American Hospital Association. 1981. *Guidelines for Recording Nutritional Information in Medical Records.* Chicago, Ill: AHA.

3. Joint Commission. 1994. *Accreditation Manual for Hospitals.* Chicago, Ill: Joint Commission on Accreditation of Healthcare Organizations (Joint Commission), Dietetic Services Section.

4. Huyck NL, Rowe MM. Interfacing with discharge planning. In: *Managing Clinical Nutrition Services.* Gaithersburg, Md: Aspen Publishers, Inc; 1990:258–259.

5. Hansen-Peters I, Connor D, Savadelena G. A simplified approach to documentation of inpatient diabetes education. *Diabetes Educator.* 1992;18(5):431, 434, 435, 437.

6. Lampe SS. Focus charting. *Nursing Manage.* 1985;16(7):43–46.

7. Maillet JO. Improved documentation as easy as PIE. *Diet Nutr Support News.* 1989;xi(3):6–7.

Chapter 14

Nutrition Assessment in a Pediatric Ambulatory Care Setting

Doris Goldberg

OVERVIEW

An ambulatory primary care setting is the best place to assess and address the nutritional needs of children. This setting allows children to be seen over time as they develop in the context of their family and community, through bouts of illness as well as critical periods when health supervision is needed. Such a setting provides the best opportunity to maximize a child's health and growth into adulthood. Children who have special health and nutritional needs can also benefit from a comprehensive ambulatory care clinic because this type of primary care setting provides for a system of multidisciplinary consultation and referral.

INTRODUCTION

The visits of children in pediatric health maintenance programs provide important opportunities for nutrition assessment, counseling, education, and referral. Nutrition is a cornerstone of preventive health care, especially regarding growth and energy needs as well as food selection and preparation. Nutrition assessment and counseling can provide tangible ways to (1) promote health and growth; (2) strengthen the body's defenses against illness; and (3) compensate for chronic disease problems.

Health education that fits the biologic and psychosocial needs of family members as well as the family's culture can empower both children and caretaking adults to become more responsible for their own health.

NUTRITION FOR CHILDREN

The subject of nutrition is a positive starting place to create an awareness regarding health for both children and their adult family members. Insights into food selection, preparation, and eating can provide both immediate satisfaction and enlightenment for future behavior. The image of Popeye downing his can of spinach when he needed strength transmitted the message that eating the right food can make you feel good and make you powerful at the same time. Nutrition has traditionally been a core concern of ambulatory pediatrics, in comparison to adult medical supervision, where it has largely been ignored. This has been true because of the special growth requirements of infants and children, their physiologic vulnerability, and the development of infant formulas and special foods.

In private pediatric practice, nutrition assessment and counseling have usually been conducted by the physician, with a large part of the medical history covering descriptions of food intake and elimination. In clinics that serve large populations, different aspects of nutrition assessment and counseling have often been divided among a team of professionals that may include nutritionists, physicians, nurses, laboratory technicians, and social workers. Newer public health approaches specify standards of quality of care as well as the evaluation of process and outcome measures (Exhibit 14–1).[1]

PUBLIC HEALTH CONCERNS

Equality of access to quality health care has become an important political issue and pediatric health maintenance systems are being designed to address culturally diverse population groups as well as socioeconomic populations. Public health has broadened its purview to consider how best to serve a large public and address health care needs rather than design clinical systems to serve only the poor and medically indigent. The mission of public health is to identify health needs of populations as well as to find effective strategies to promote health and prevent disease for both individuals and large groups.

The direction of public health programs in the United States is being guided by the document *Healthy People 2000*, a comprehensive set of national health promotion and disease prevention objectives.[2] The objectives stated that are particularly relevant to the current nutritional status of infants and young children include:

1. Increase to at least 75 percent the proportion of mothers who breast-feed their babies during the early postpartum period and to at least 50 percent

Exhibit 14–1 Summary of Contents of NYS C/THP Evaluation (Ages Birth–5)

AGE	Weeks	Months								Years		
	2–4	2–3	4–5	6–7	8–10	12–13	14–15	16–19	22–26	2	4	5
HISTORY												
Initial/Interval	•	•	•	•	•	•	•	•	•	•	•	•
MEASUREMENTS												
Height & Weight	•	•	•	•	•	•	•	•	•	•	•	•
Head Circumference	•	•	•	•	•	•			•			
Blood Pressure										•	•	•
SENSORY SCREENING												
Sight	GROSS SCREENING →									•	•	•
Hearing	GROSS SCREENING →									•	•	•
Developmental Appraisal	•	•	•	•	•	•	•	•	•	•	•	•
Physical Exam	•	•	•	•	•	•	•	•	•	•	•	•
Discussion & Counseling	•	•	•	•	•	•	•	•	•	•	•	•
Dental Care Assessment	GROSS SCREENING →									•	•	•
Dentist's Exam									•	•	•	•
Nutritional Assessment	•	•	•	•	•	•	•	•	•	•	•	•
Immunization Assessment	•	•	•	•	•	•	•	•	•	•	•	•
PROCEDURES												
Tuberculin Test						•					•	
Hematocrit or Hemoglobin					•			•		•	•	•
Urinalysis										•	•	•
Newborn Screening	•											
Sickle Cell					•							
Lead Screening						•			•			

Note: The periodic matrix displayed generally follows the recommendations of the Committee of Standards of Child Health Care of the American Academy of Pediatrics. The contents of the exam are the recommended standard for the specific age and should not preclude providers from performing additional tests if indicated. A bullet indicates the age at which the component of the exam should be performed.

Source: Adapted from American Academy of Pediatrics Committee on Practice and Ambulatory Medicine. Elk Grove Village, Ill: American Academy of Pediatrics; 1991.

the proportion of mothers who continue to breast-feed until their babies are five to six months old.

2. Reduce growth retardation among low-income children age five and under to less than 10 percent.

3. Reduce dietary fat to an average of 30 percent of calories or less for persons two years of age and older.

4. Reduce iron deficiency anemia to less than 3 percent among children one through four years of age.

5. Increase to at least 75 percent the proportion of primary care providers who provide nutrition assessment and counseling and/or referral to a trained nutritionist or dietitian.

6. Increase to at least 90 percent the proportion of school lunch and breakfast service and child care food service with menus consistent with the nutrition principles in the *Dietary Guidelines for Americans*.[3]

7. Increase to at least 75 percent the schools that provide nutrition education from preschool through 12th grade.

Other goals are to reduce overweight and promote moderate to vigorous physical activities. These objectives have been chosen to reduce risk of coronary heart disease in a national effort to reduce mortality that is excessive or preventable. Other nutrition objectives are more traditional in their relevance to specific dietary deficiencies, such as reducing the prevalence of iron deficiency anemia. (See Appendix D.)

IDENTIFYING CHILDREN AT NUTRITIONAL RISK

Children who are at risk for nutrition-related problems require more detailed nutrition assessments, observation, and counseling. It is therefore useful to consider ways to screen for risk of nutrition problems as an efficient means of focusing attention on individuals who need risk reduction strategies.

Risk from the Social Setting

Since children are dependents, they are particularly susceptible to hazards from the social context of their care as well as from the adults who care for them. Very limited family income and lack of education of adult caretakers to make informed choices lead the list of factors that place children at nutritional risk. Recent immigration from a different climatic and cultural setting can also present difficulties in children's obtaining adequate amounts of nourishing food. Health providers must be alert to the fact that they can be most helpful to the adults in such families by guiding them in navigating a new system of food purchasing and preparation. This may involve finding out about the purchasing ability and shopping habits of a family as well as the culture/belief system that places value on certain foods, attributes, and behaviors.

Children who have been living without a stable home, whether they have been in an overcrowded apartment or a shelter, or have recently been placed in foster care, are also at risk for poor nutrition. Children in families that are under great stress because of illness, unemployment, or emotional dysfunction may also be in double jeopardy, with nutritional risk being secondary to situational factors.

Individual Growth Pattern

A child's history of growth (height, weight, and head circumference) may provide clues for nutritional risk. Beginning with pregnancy weight gain, birth weight, and gestational age at birth, indicators of normal and abnormal growth may be evident. One infant may be born three months prematurely, be very low birth weight (birth weight of less than 1,500 grams), and then quickly "catch up" to the height and weight considered normal for his or her age and genetic endowment by two years of age.[4,5] Another infant may be born full term and have a slightly depressed birth weight of five pounds and a small head circumference. Such an infant has experienced intrauterine growth retardation and may not experience a "catch-up" to the expected norms of height, weight, and head circumference by age two years even if optimal nutrition is provided, and therefore will have a poorer prognosis for future growth and development.

A physical examination provides an opportunity to inspect the body for any visible evidence of organ system malfunction, palpate for organ enlargement or area tenderness, and observe the overall strength, vigor, and coordination of the child. It is important to determine if there are any impediments to a full range of motion or special limits to physical exertion.

Growth Measurements

The physical examination is often begun with measuring height and weight. This provides a prime teaching opportunity to discuss with the parent and child the child's growth pattern and show them how it compares with that of other children of the same age. After discussion of the significance of the child's growth measurements, it is useful to put the data on a parent-held medical record as well as to document it in the clinic's medical record. A parent-held record documents the child's growth for the parent as well as for providers who may see the child on an emergency basis for special conditions.

Growth data also provide clues to nutritional status even though the rate and pattern of growth are strongly determined by genetic inheritance. Continuity of health supervision in an ambulatory care setting is a very important component of primary pediatric care, and ideally health providers will have many notations of height, weight, and head circumference over time on each individual child. The child's growth record will allow a comparison to be made of that child's growth at different points in time. For example, if a child is consistently in the 50th percentile for height and weight from birth to five years of age, there is no problem evident in that child's rate of growth or size. If that child were to drop to the 20th percentile for weight at six years of age, the situation would require follow-up. The sudden break in consistency would demand that a cause be found, whether it is biological, psychological, or environmental, for the change in the child's weight gain. Such a pattern has been observed in children who have been physically abused and neglected as well as those with organic illness. If this child were to maintain the 50th percentile in height but gain sufficient weight to place him or her above the 75th percentile for weight, this also would be cause for investigation. Risk, then, can be inferred from a sharp change in the child's growth pattern.

Since obesity is a major risk for chronic disease as well as quite prevalent among American children, nutrition assessments are invaluable in monitoring children in order to develop appropriate strategies of intervention. A disproportion between height and weight, where weight is 25 percentiles greater than height-for-age, can also be considered to put a child at nutritional risk for being overweight in the present and at potential risk for chronic disease in the future.[5-8]

Height or linear growth is particularly susceptible to protein deficiency as well as endocrine abnormalities. A child must be considered at nutritional risk if he or she does not maintain consistent linear growth.

Head circumference is an indicator of brain size although abnormal conditions, such as hydrocephalus, may cause a rapid increase in head size that is not due to an increase in brain tissue. Full-term infants are estimated to have completed two-thirds of their brain growth by two years of age, and therefore careful measurement of head circumference is particularly important during this early period.[4,9] Since brain growth is sensitive to caloric requirements, a child's caloric intake should be closely questioned if accurate head circumference measurements or the rate of head size growth is slow.

Medical Assessment

A medical history may reveal evidence of nutritional risk that is not apparent on casual observation or even on physical examination. Metabolic disturbances, serious food allergies, or congenital problems, for example, may only be revealed by a complete history. Thorough history taking also includes a medical history of family members, which may reveal relevant conditions such as diabetes, congenital anemias, or inherited metabolic conditions that are relevant to the child who is being seen. On the other hand, casual observation may classify the child with spastic cerebral palsy and speech difficulties as being at nutritional risk because of problems coordinating chewing and swallowing.

Methodical physical examination is a way to detect clues of acute and chronic illness, both of which may place a child at nutritional risk. A child with repeated ear infections may be iron deficient due to the repeated infections or may be vulnerable to repeated infections because he or she was iron deficient. An infant with exzema may need careful monitoring and an elimination diet to discover the precipitating allergens. Skin and oral lesions may provide clues to specific vitamin deficiencies. Dental problems may indicate dietary or feeding problems. Elevations in blood pressure may indicate kidney problems or endocrine dysfunction.

Laboratory screening of blood and urine is advised periodically for preschool children and less frequently for school age children (see Exhibit 14–2).[10] Iron deficiency anemia is still too prevalent an occurrence among children in the United States, and the target for the year 2000 is to reduce its prevalence to 3 percent among children one to four years of age.[2] Lead poisoning presents a prevalent nutritional risk to young children. New standards from the Centers for Disease Control have lowered the acceptable lead level to 10 micrograms per deciliter. At low blood lead levels, iron supplementation is advised because of the competitive relationship between iron and lead to form hemoglobin. At higher levels, in addition to iron supplementation, environmental inspection and abatement of lead hazards is advised, and chelation is prescribed for children with lead toxicity.

Urinalysis provides an important method of detecting kidney abnormalities and the possibility that protein is being excreted. The presence of sugar in the urine is a clue to test blood sugar and rule out diabetes mellitus.[11]

Developmental Assessment

Developmental assessment is an evaluation of a child's functioning in the areas of social behavior, thinking and problem solving, ability to speak and communicate feelings, and coordination of motor activities. In the context of assessing a child's nutrition, this information is relevant because the child's development can determine daily activities, caloric requirements, appropriate feeding, and the child's ability to participate in food selection and preparation. Although in-depth developmental assessment is usually reserved for children

Exhibit 14–2 Recommendations for Preventive Pediatric Health Care, Committee on Practice and Ambulatory Medicine

Each child and family is unique, therefore these Recommendations for Preventive Pediatric Health Care are designed for the care of children who are receiving competent parenting, have no manifestations of any important health problems, and are growing and developing in satisfactory fashion. Additional visits may become necessary if circumstances suggest variations from normal. These guidelines represent a consensus by the Committee on Practice and Ambulatory Medicine in consultation with the membership of the American Academy of Pediatrics through the Chapter Presidents. The Committee emphasizes the great importance of continuity of care in comprehensive health supervision and the need to avoid fragmentation of care. A prenatal visit by the parents for anticipatory guidance and pertinent medical history is strongly recommended. Health supervision should begin with medical care of the newborn in the hospital.

	INFANCY						EARLY CHILDHOOD					LATE CHILDHOOD					ADOLESCENCE			
	Months						Months			Years		Years					Years			
AGE	<1	2	4	6	9	12	15	18	24	3	4	5	6	8	10	12	14	16	18	20+
HISTORY																				
Initial/Interval	•	•	•	•	•	•	•	•	•	•	•	•	•	•	•	•	•	•	•	•
MEASUREMENTS																				
Height & Weight	•	•	•	•	•	•	•	•	•	•	•	•	•	•	•	•	•	•	•	•
Head Circumference	•	•	•	•	⊙	•														
Blood Pressure										•	•	•	•	•	•	•	•	•	•	•
SENSORY SCREENING																				
Vision	S	S	S	S	S	S	S	S	S	S	O	O	O	O	S	O	O	S	O	O
Hearing	S	S	S	S	S	S	S	S	S	S	O	O	S	S	S	O	S	S	O	S
Devel/Behav Assessment	•	•	•	•	•	•	•	•	•	•	•	•	•	•	•	•	•	•	•	•
Physical Exam	•	•	•	•	•	•	•	•	•	•	•	•	•	•	•	•	•	•	•	•
PROCEDURES																				
Hered/Metabolic Screening	◄•																			
Immunization	•	•	•		◄	•	•			◄	•	►			◄	•	►			
Tuberculin Test					•	►				•	►				•	►				
Hematocrit or Hemoglobin	◄			•	►	◄	•		►	◄	•	►	◄	•	►	◄	•	►		
Urinalysis	◄	•		►	◄	•	►	◄	•	►	◄	•	►							
Anticipatory Guidance	•	•	•	•	•	•	•	•	•	•	•	•	•	•	•	•	•	•	•	•
Initial Dental Referral										•										

Note: • = To be performed; S = Subjective, by history; O = Objective, by a standard testing method.

Source: American Academy of Pediatrics, Committee on Practice and Ambulatory Medicine. *Recommendations for Preventive Pediatric Health Care.* Elk Grove Village, Ill: American Academy of Pediatrics; 1991.

who exhibit special needs, some form of developmental screening or appraisal is standard practice within good pediatric care.

Observing the child's spontaneous behavior in the clinic and the interaction with family members and strangers has become an established means of obtaining more information about a child's functional level of development as well as providing clues as to how he or she characteristically acts. In recent years there has been new interest in incorporating semistructured development assessment techniques within an office visit (such as "Draw Your Family") as well as using developmental screening or assessment tools.[5,6] Comparisons from baseline information over time are valuable.

A developmental evaluation involves finding out what motor activities the child can perform and what language and communication abilities exist. A child's concept of self as well as understanding of his or her world will also affect how the child functions in both his or her familiar environment and new situations. All this information is relevant to nutrition assessment. Children who are developing normally should be guided toward nutritional independence and maturity by developmentally appropriate feeding. Their growing independence should be supported by encouraging increasing participation in food selection, in food preparation activities, as well as nutrition education about food.[5] Examples of developmentally appropriate feeding and participation in food selection and preparation activities are shown in Exhibit 14–3.

Exhibit 14–3 Developmental Milestones of Feeding Skills

MONTHS				
One	Six	Twelve	Eighteen	Twenty-Four
Exclusively breast-fed and/or bottle fed with adult support of infant's head and body	Introduction of single strained foods when infant is in a sitting position	Drinks from a cup Holds own bottle Eats family foods Finger feeds	Lifts cup to drink Feeds self with a spoon Indicates food preferences	Holds small glass in one hand Begins to select foods when shopping with adult

YEARS			
Three	Four	Five	Six
Helps to mix foods with a spoon and mash foods with a fork	Pours from a pitcher Washes fruits and vegetables	Helps to set table Feeds self well Begins to measure with a measuring cup	Turns over pancakes with a spatula Peels potatoes and fruit with a peeler

Children who have developmental impairments sometimes require compensatory methods and dietary management to adjust to their special needs. An extreme example of this would be a child with spastic cerebral palsy who requires head support and positioning as well as pureed food to aid his or her feeding.

In addition to assessing a child's developmental performance, nutrition assessments must rely on qualitative and quantitative assessment of food intake. A 24- to 48-hour food recall may be appropriate or a child/parent log book. There are benefits to having both child and parent work together keeping track of what foods are consumed. Logs and workbooks can be structured so that parents with low literacy skills can check off food types and portion sizes, and young children can use stickers to indicate types of food eaten and their amounts. Since school-age children may frequently take two meals and snacks outside their home, children and parents must become aware of what they are consuming and learn about what they are eating. An activity log may also be useful for a child to keep because lack of physical exercise contributes to the prevalence of overweight problems in American children.

With adolescence there comes a dramatic spurt in linear growth as well as the appearance of secondary sex characteristics that are not under control of the child.[5,8] Sometimes unhappiness with these changes will be associated with extremes in eating habits ranging from anorexia and bulimia to overeating and huge weight gain. This is but another example of the need for health professionals to be cognizant of the client's developmental stage and address nutrition within that context. Questions to adolescents about their desired weight, shape, and future activities, rather than assuming what they should ideally be like, can be particularly useful.

STRATEGIES FOR NUTRITION INTERVENTION

Nutrition interventions for children and their parents or caretaking adults are concerned with imparting the basic concept that balanced nutrition can promote health and energy and decrease the possibility of chronic illnesses such as cardiovascular disease and cancer. A family history can be used to reveal familial risks for specific chronic diseases.

Feeding a young child (under six years of age) provides the special opportunity to shape later, lifelong eating preferences and habits. Parents should be made aware of this "imprinting window" and the benefits of providing the young child with a range of foods that are nutritious; not overly refined; not heavily sugared, salted, or seasoned; and not deep fried.

REFERENCES

1. American Academy of Pediatrics Committee on Standards of Child Health Care. Elk Grove Village, Ill: American Academy of Pediatrics; 1992.

2. *Healthy People 2000: National Health Promotion and Disease Prevention Objectives.* Washington, DC: US Dept of Health and Human Services, Public Health Service; 1990.

3. *Nutrition and Your Health: Dietary Guidelines for Americans.* Washington, DC: US Government Printing Office, 1990.

4. Fomon SJ. *Infant Feeding.* St. Louis, Mo: Mosby-Year Book, Inc.; 1993.

5. Ekvall SW. *Pediatric Nutrition in Chronic Diseases and Developmental Disorders.* New York, NY: Oxford University Press; 1993.

6. Scott BJ, Altman H, St. Jeor S. Growth assessment in children: a review. *Top Clin Nutr.* 1992; 8:5–26.

7. Frisancho AR. *Anthropometric Standards for the Assessment of Growth and Nutritional Status.* Ann Arbor, Mich: University of Michigan Press; 1990.

8. Queen PM, Lang CE. *Handbook of Pediatric Nutrition.* Gaithersburg, Md: Aspen Publishers, Inc; 1993.

9. Shils ME, et al. *Modern Nutrition in Health and Disease.* Vol 2. Philadelphia, Pa: Lea & Febiger; 1994.

10. Committee on Practice and Ambulatory Medicine. *Recommendations for Preventive Pediatric Health Care.* Evanston, Ill: American Academy of Pediatrics; 1987.

11. *Pediatric Nutrition Handbook.* Elk Grove Village, Ill: American Academy of Pediatrics; 1993.

Chapter 15

Nutrition Care for the Acute Care Patient

Peter L. Beyer

OVERVIEW

The practice of applied, clinical nutrition has always required a broad combination of knowledge and skills. Recently, however, major changes in the philosophy, technology, products, and practices in health care have resulted in even more challenges to clinical nutrition practitioners and managers.[1] New developments and the fascinating problems and opportunities they create appear to spring up almost daily. Hospitals will continue to compete for health care dollars, patients, and resources. Programs and services that do not increase revenue, improve outcomes, or have market value will be curtailed.[2] At the same time, hospitals must continue to improve quality, sophistication, and scope of patient services to increase patient satisfaction and advance accepted standards of health care.

TRENDS IN ACUTE CARE AND NUTRITION SUPPORT

More patients are being treated as outpatients for a wider variety of medical and surgical problems. Only those who require more intensive care and monitoring are admitted to acute care facilities. As a result, patients admitted to today's acute care facilities are typically more critically ill, require more immediate evaluation and attention to their needs, and require more resources from a wider variety of specialists than patients admitted to hospitals just a few years ago. More of the beds in the hospital are for ICU or critical care purposes, and more patients are treated with specialty care protocols. Skill levels of health care workers must be higher at entry into the acute care workplace and must be constantly upgraded.

Despite increased acuity of hospitalized patients, however, the acute phase of medical and surgical management is becoming more efficient and effective. Advances in diagnostic procedures, medical and surgical management, pharmacology, and nutrition care have provided the opportunity to improve quality of care while dealing with more complicated patient care problems. Because of the continued increase in costs associated with increased acuity level and new technologies, attention to continuous quality improvement and cost-effectiveness will continue to be stressed.[3]

As a result of the shortened length of stay, less time is available to identify, assess, provide for, and document patient needs. The need for preadmission and admission screening, discharge planning, and after-discharge communications is greater than ever before. The practitioner in the acute care setting must recognize early in the patient's hospital stay the need to arrange for chronic care. Prolonged stay in acute care settings is often the result of inability to arrange for after-discharge care in a timely manner.[4]

When patients are moved from acute care hospitals to other facilities, communications must be provided regarding (1) what has been done, (2) what still needs to be done, and (3) precautions to be observed. Communication must be clear enough to allow continuation of treatment plans and prevent duplication of treatments and diagnostic procedures. Insufficient or delayed discharge planning often results in poor outcomes or readmissions for the same or more severe problems and increased overall health expenditures.[5]

Patients dismissed from acute care facilities tend to require more care and follow-up than in years past.[6] The result is a trickle-down effect—as the acuity levels required to enter and remain in the hospital rise, so do the intensity of care requirements for patients prior to and after acute care hospitalization. Besides the increase in acuity of illness, the population continues to grow older. Particular concern has been directed to care of the infirm elderly, who often leave acute care facilities requiring considerable rehabilitation and support.

Evidence of the trickle-down effect is seen in an increasing acuity level of patients treated in extended care facilities such as nursing homes and home health agencies. In many areas of the country, shortages of skilled nursing facilities and home health resources are occurring.

New emphases and new methods have emerged in measuring the overall acuity of hospital populations and clinical and cost-effectiveness. Although not always directly translated into improved productivity, a new mind-set regarding cost control, efficiency, and documentation of services has evolved.[7-12] The future emphasis will be to:

- continue to evaluate clinical effectiveness of health care therapies, technologies, surgical procedures, managed care systems, and other health care delivery systems
- study ways to accurately define and categorize acuity of care and predict service requirements
- identify characteristics and predictors of complications, and increased costs; continue to improve utilization review performance, productivity, and documentation of services provided
- improve discharge-planning activities and communications; study after-discharge outcomes
- improve transfer of information to and from extended care and outpatient facilities

Challenges for Clinical Nutrition in Acute Care

The same compression of activity holds true for nutrition screening, assessment, planning, and interventions. The time available in the acute care setting to provide for patients' needs is shorter. The need to evaluate, provide for, and teach patients and their families about nutritional aspects of care is more important than ever. Although inpatient nutrition education is still considered an important aspect of care, only a limited amount of time is available in the acute care setting for teaching, counseling, and practicing new nutrition behaviors.

The science and clinical practice of nutrition, including the areas of enteral and parenteral nutrition, are far more sophisticated and are now more routinely incorporated into standards of medical and surgical care. The list of options for enteral and parenteral nutrition products alone has exploded. In the 1960s and 1970s acute care facilities typically had two or three types of tube feedings, and parenteral nutrition was in its infancy. Nutrition care protocols and quality assurance for these procedures had just begun to evolve.

Nutrition screening and assessment practices have also improved and have become part of standard operating procedure. Early recognition of nutrition risk and preexisting malnutrition has led to earlier interventions and improved outcomes. Because nutrition-related research is booming, new specialty products and new approaches to diet therapy applications are likely to continue to be introduced to hospital practice at an unprecedented pace.

Innovations in the nutritional aspects of patient care management are likely to further improve the overall effectiveness of care in areas such as oncology, infectious disease, gastrointestinal disorders, trauma, and surgery. Although the important role of nutrition in illness and patient care is finally being recognized, nutrition professionals will have to continue to demonstrate the value of nutrition care practices.

The practitioner certainly needs sufficient scientific knowledge and clinical skills to understand and practice nutrition, but in reality, the practitioner must have other skills. Delivery of nutrition care must also be efficient, effective, and targeted for the specific patient/client mixture of the institution. Legal and ethical issues, human and public relations matters, marketing strategies, cost-benefit ratios, priorities, and productivity must all be considered as part of everyday practice. Because of the ever-increasing requirement for knowledge and skills in clinical nutrition, the need is great for not only sound preprofessional education but also continuous professional development.

ROLE OF THE NUTRITIONIST IN ACUTE CARE

Even when confined to the acute care clinical setting, the role of the nutritionist is quite diverse. Recent role delineation studies for entry- and advanced-level dietetic practitioners have pointed out the need for many skills in accomplishing the various nutrition care tasks. The roles involve not only the clinical skills used in assessment and treatment of nutrition-related problems but also knowledge and skills in organization and management communications, counseling, and research.

The basic, all-encompassing role of the nutritionist in acute care is to provide for the nutritional needs of the patient. The practice is guided by guidelines and standards developed by the professions involved in nutrition care, institutional standards of care, goals, and objectives. The practice is improved by studying and applying new approaches to nutrition care.

Examples of the typical roles of the dietitian/nutritionist in the acute care setting follow. More advanced roles are taken as the individual gains in experience, education, and position.

Entry Level	*Advanced Level*
• Screens and assesses clients	• Develops screening and assessment systems
• Adheres to standards of care in carrying out patient care	• Develops standards of care and nutrition care protocols
• Offers suggestions and contributes to nutrition care	• Takes leadership in providing nutrition care
• Teaches and counsels clients, caretakers in therapeutic diets	• Determines the type and characteristics of therapeutic diets
• Selects appropriate teaching materials for patient education; uses reference books, current literature to guide practice	• Develops and improves teaching materials; performs, presents, publishes research to improve practice
• Serves as preceptor and role model for students, provides outreach services, serves as guest lecturer in formal classes	• Teaches courses, serves as guest speaker in interdisciplinary courses
• Attends continuing education and professional development events, joins professional organizations	• Makes scholarly presentations at educational events, holds offices in professional organizations

Nutrition care is usually accomplished through a series of tasks that are performed in a stepwise order using combinations of patient screening and assessment data, patient care protocols, department policies and procedures, and practitioner knowledge and skills. The decisions made and the subsequent actions taken are driven by the data available, the combination of nutrition care problems, and the patients' response to interventions.[13–18]

SCREENING

Nutrition departments in acute care settings can no longer afford to wait for a specific request to evaluate or assess patient needs. Without an admission screening program, the department finds itself in constant crisis, with patients getting inappropriate diets and insufficient nutrient intake, depleted patients not being recognized, and poor discharge and transfer instructions given at discharge. Figure 15–1 is an example of an algorithm that illustrates a nutrition care model. Table 15–1 gives examples of screening information that might be collected; it also lists services, assessment activities, and interventions that could be utilized in the nutrition care process.

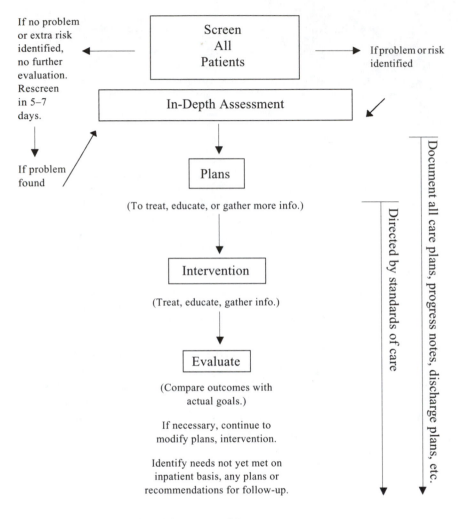

Figure 15–1 Algorithm of Nutrition Care Model

Simply stated, the purpose of screening is to identify early in the hospital stay patients who should be further evaluated. Screening should take only a few minutes, should be done for all patients admitted, and should be designed to identify the patients who are likely to need nutrition intervention. The screening can include input from technicians and clerical staff, the admitting department, computerized databases, nurses, and/or the patients themselves. The number and complexity of the screening process depend on the desired outcomes, the resources available, and the number of services to be offered. In many intensive

Table 15–1 Nutrition Care Processes

Examples of Screening Information— Check For:	Nutrition Care Services Provided for All Patients	When Indicated in Screening: Assessment Activities	Nutrition Care Services/ Interventions when Indicated by Assessment
Modified Diet Order	Selective Menu and Information Regarding Services	Gather Pertinent Medical History/Lab Data	Develop Meal Pattern
Nutrition-Related Diagnosis			Modified Diet Menu Selector and Instruction
Albumin < 3.5 gm/dl	House Menu and Selection Instructions, General Guidelines	Diet History	Snacks/Special Food Services
Wt./Ht. < 90% Normal or Significant Wt. Loss		In-depth R.D. Interview	For Patient on Modified Diet, Monitor Selections Daily for Compliance
		Observe Performance of Patient (Selections, Feeding Skills, Responses)	
Food Allergy/ Intolerance	Serve Meals at Appropriate Times		R.D. Communication with Team Members
Physical Disability			R.D. Interview/Observation(s)
Adequacy of Intake During Hospitalization	Cursory Review of Menu Selection	Continue Record of Weight and Height	Reevaluate Status Due to Changes in Diet Order, Intake, or Diagnosis
	Monitor and Record Acceptance of Diet	Body Composition Measurements	Write Chart Notes
	Reevaluate Status within Seven Days	Calculation of Energy and Nutrient Needs	Formulate or Adjust Special Feeding
			Explain Rationale or Review Modified Diet or Nutrition Therapy
		Calculation of Nutrient Intake	Provide Diet Instruction/ Counseling
			Evaluate Diet Instruction
			Discharge Plans and Goals

Source: Courtesy of the University of Kansas Medical Center, Kansas City, Kansas.

care and "specialty" care settings, such as renal or cardiovascular units, screening is bypassed and all patients are assessed immediately.

The goals of screening are usually to identify at admission, or shortly after, patients who

- have diagnoses or surgical procedures that will require special diets, schedules, or nutrition support formulas and/or will need instruction and counseling prior to discharge
- have medical problems or diagnoses that often lead to malnutrition, such as gastrointestinal obstruction, malabsorption, alcoholism, trauma, or burns
- are admitted with malnutrition
- may have special needs, such as special foods, diets, or prosthetic devices

- have particular allergies or intolerances
- have been on special or unusual diets or feeding programs, or on harmful diets
- might want additional, nonroutine services on a fee-for-service basis

The earliest screening protocols tended to concentrate on screening for patients who might or might not be at high risk for malnutrition. However, because considerable resources may be required in many other areas of nutrition practice, most screening protocols now include more comprehensive indicators. Typical screening indicators include data such as

- weight loss over time
- percent desirable body weight
- diagnosis or problem
- diet (current and past)
- food allergies or specific tolerances
- laboratory indices, such as albumin or cholesterol
- cursory evaluation of how well the patient is eating/was eating prior to admission
- number of days NPO or receiving hypocaloric fluids
- general questions of the patient/family as to whether the patient needs or would like additional dietetic services/assistance

The next step is to
the information at hand. If the patient's situation simply requires provision of basic services and monitoring, no further evaluation will be required as long as the patient's status remains acceptable. If the results of the screening indicate that the patient is at nutritional risk or may require nutrition intervention, the dietitian can perform a nutrition assessment based on the screening data provided.
Screening indicators

- are not diagnostic; serve only as red flags
- should not be used as the basis for planning or intervention
- provide direction for nutrition assessment
- are done for all patients
- are inexpensive, cost-effective, not labor intensive
- make use of as many available resources as possible
- assure that all who need further evaluation are not missed

Typical screening programs are designed to pick up potential nutrition-related problems that might otherwise be missed or delayed. Screening is a justifiable patient care management process that can be designed for any setting. The nature and number of screening factors and the sophistication of the program depends on the type and the mission of the facility.[13–15,17] See Exhibits 15–1 and 15–2 for examples of screening tools that also include nutrition assessment data collection sections. See Exhibit 19–1 for an example of an initial screening tool that includes a sample guideline for care.

NUTRITION ASSESSMENT

A primary role of the nutritionist is to evaluate patients who may have special needs or nutrition-related problems. Screening information tells the nutritionist which patients need further attention and provides the direction for the nutrition assessment. Assessment is usually concluded with a summary as to the degree and extensiveness of the problems or needs identified, and a plan for nutrition intervention and further evaluation or monitoring. Responsibility for nutrition care or monitoring of patients requiring more routine or basic nutrition care is often delegated to technician positions.

Key pieces of information in screening direct the specific kind of assessment data to be collected. On an internal medicine service, for example, the nutritionist may be greeted with four new admissions. One patient may have been admitted with weight loss and short bowel syndrome; another admitted with angina and hyperlipidemia; another admitted with diabetic ketoacidosis; and the last admitted to the medicine ICU with liver failure secondary to alcohol and acetaminophen overdose. In each case the diagnosis and other screening data dictate: (1) a specific (unique) set of data to gather for the nutrition assessment, (2) a different timetable to accomplish the assessment, and (3) different forms of nutrition intervention and subsequent evaluation.

For the patient with short bowel syndrome and weight loss, for example, the nutrition assessment would probably include information regarding the nature and extent of bowel resected and a diet history concentrating on foods that might enhance or slow GI transit and fluid balance; whether the patient was taking appropriate nutrient supplements; enteral or parenteral nutrition; and whether the laboratory test results indicated that malabsorption was a likely reason for the patient's weight loss. The extensiveness and duration of the patient's weight loss would probably be evaluated. Technical staff would be asked to monitor as part of the assessment, what foods the patient chose while in the hospital and how well he or she was able to select and consume appropriate foods.

The nutrition assessment for the patient admitted with diabetic ketoacidosis would require the collection of a different set of data. The nutrition assessment protocol for diabetes would require the collection of a specific series of

Exhibit 15–1 Sample Nutrition Screening Tool—Food Intake

University of Kansas Hospital
39th & Rainbow Blvd.
Kansas City, Kansas 66103
Department of Dietetics & Nutrition

Screening Form Passed out by   Date   Collected by   Date

F.H.Q. Initiated   F.H.Q. Passed out by   Date   Assessed by   Date

Food Groups (adequate # servings/day)	Low	Adequate	High	NOTATIONS AND GUIDELINES FOR DIETETIC TECHNICIANS
Milk and Milk Products (2–5 servings)				
Meat and Meat Substitute (2–5 servings)				
Breads and Cereals (4–12 servings)				
Fruits and Vegetables (4–8 servings)				

SIGNIFICANT FINDINGS,

Date	B N E	Diet Order	One Meal Orders	Menu Presented (Initials)	TECHNICIAN'S OBSERVATIONS; PATIENT'S INTAKE, ACCEPTANCE, UNDERSTANDING, ETC.

Initialed Entries made by:

Dietetic Technicians   Dietetic Intern(s) & Dietitian(s)

Nutrition Care Plan I

Source: Courtesy of the University of Kansas Medical Center, Kansas City, Kansas.

Exhibit 15–2 Screening, Assessment, and Planning Tool

University of Kansas Hospital
3901 Rainbow Boulevard
Kansas City, Kansas 66160-7250
Department of Dietetics & Nutrition

SCREENING   Date   Diagnosis/Problem

Ht.   Wt.   IBW   % IBW   Usual Wt.   % Usual Wt.

Gain/Lost   Wks/Mos   Albumin

Past Diet   Allergy/Intolerance

ASSESSMENT   Labs/Wt. Data

	✔	Dates	Results/Comments
Medical History			
Brief/In-depth Interview			
Observe Performance			
Anthropometric			
Calc. Kcal/Pro Req.			
Calc./Record Intake			
Medications			
PLANS & SERVICES			
Provide Basic Care			
Re-Evaluate In 7 Days			
Re-Evaluate Status Change			
Visit > 1 ×/Week			
Review Modified Diet			
Explain Rationale			
Provide Diet Instruction			
Evaluate Instruction			
Develop Meal Plan			
Snacks/SP Service			
Communicate with Team			
D/C Plan or Goal			
Enteral/Parenteral Feeding			
Drug-Nutrient Instruction			
Chart Notes			

Initialed Entries made by:

Dietetic Intern(s)   Dietitian(s)

Nutrition Care Plan II

Source: Courtesy of the University of Kansas Medical Center, Kansas City, Kansas.

laboratory data (e.g., fasting glucose levels, glycosylated hemoglobin, lipid profile); computing the patient's calorie and protein needs; checking the amounts and types of insulins used; evaluation of the patient's knowledge, willingness, and ability to select appropriate meals and foods; and sufficient psychosocial data for tailoring a plan to the patient's needs.

In each case, the assessment is directed by the initial database and logical algorithms. Nutrition assessment ends with summary of the meaning or significance of the nutrition-related data in the overall care of the patient. The assessment may take the form of

- a summary of the degree to which dietary habits, indiscretion, lack of nutrition information, or nutrition neglect may have contributed to a patient's problem
- an assessment of the patient's understanding or ability to select or limit certain foods
- the type and severity of various forms of malnutrition
- the ability (or inability) of a patient to meet needs through oral, enteral nutrition, or parenteral support

NUTRITION INTERVENTION

The completed assessment tells the dietitian/nutritionist what types of interventions should be provided. Interventions typically include

- treating the patient (with specific foods, different textures, meal patterns, supplements, enteral and parenteral nutrition)
- arranging the timing, schedules, or size of meals or nutritional products
- explaining the rationale and mechanics of therapeutic diets
- providing counseling and guidance toward new dietary practices
- performing further evaluations to see how the patient responds to therapeutic interventions

The nutritionist generally performs direct interventions in response to specific requests or diet prescriptions. Once the prescription is delegated, the interventions are under the control of, and are carried out by, the nutritionist and/or supporting personnel. Other kinds of interventions typically include modifying the quantity or concentration of foods, beverages, and oral supplements; limiting foods that cause discomfort or adverse reactions or interfere with medical, surgical, or diagnostic treatment; and providing foods in different forms, combinations, or flavors that may facilitate feeding.

Physicians still prescribe diets but, depending on the role and relationships of the dietitian with the health care team, diet prescriptions may take a more categorical or general nature, as in the case of high- or low-fiber or cholesterol-lowering diets. The dietitian then takes more responsibility to see that the diet meets the nutritional needs of the client and translates it into a plan tailored to the patient's needs.[18]

Specific diet patterns may also be driven by protocols worked out previously among physicians and several health care departments so that a consistent approach can always be used despite rotations of personnel or students. For diabetes, for example, the physician might prescribe a "diet for diabetes" and use the calorie level computed by the dietitian. The dietitian would have considered not only the patient's current needs but also needs for weight gain or loss, usual activity, and days with concentrated exercise. The diet would be divided into appropriate meals and snacks, with consideration given to the desired levels of carbohydrate, lipids, protein, fiber, sodium, and so forth, so that it would be consistent with recently accepted guidelines for diet and diabetes. Similar standards of care or dietary protocols might be worked out for problems such as cardiovascular disease, liver failure, renal disease, malnourished tube-fed patients, inflammatory bowel disease, refeeding syndromes, or nutrition care for the HIV-positive patient.

Diet counseling is a form of nutrition intervention that is still performed to a significant degree in the acute care setting. In theory and in practice, dietary counseling is best performed in a quiet, uninterrupted setting when the client has had the time to accept and appreciate the value of the dietary change and is ready to work toward a plan to establish new dietary behaviors. The nature of the acute care setting makes dietary counseling difficult at best, but because of the frequency with which patients are dismissed who still require dietary interventions, diet counseling and instruction are more necessary, expected, and apparently attempted. A real gap exists in what needs to be accomplished in diet counseling and what can realistically be done in the acute care setting. Counseling and instructions can usually be started in the hospital, but too often patients receive little or no follow-up after discharge even though the majority of the education and counseling is yet to be completed.

EVALUATION OF NUTRITION CARE

After nutrition care plans have been implemented, the dietitian, in cooperation with the physician and other health care personnel, evaluates how well the nutritional aspects of care are progressing.[19] As in the assessment, nutritional evaluation is directed toward specific indicators. In the case of the patient with diabetes, for example, the dietitian would evaluate how well the patient was able to make appropriate selections, how well the patient was eating, and whether the diet was achieving goals of weight gain, blood glucose control, control of blood lipids, blood pressure, and so forth. If any aspect of nutrition care was not working, appropriate adjustments—for example, in the meal plan, education, or the timing of food and activity with insulin—would have to be made.

For the malnourished patient receiving TPN, the dietitian might watch specific electrolyte levels, blood glucose levels, CO_2:O_2 ratios, changes in transport protein levels, and changes in weight and body composition.

In practice, evaluation of nutrition care may be the role that is the least consistently achieved and documented of all categories of nutrition care. Time constraints and priorities for intervention are typical reasons for lack of performance. Since this stage deals with the identification of the outcomes and effectiveness of nutrition interventions, the importance of documenting the value of nutrition care must be emphasized.

DISCHARGE SUMMARIES, AFTER-DISCHARGE CARE, AND REFERRALS

One of the roles of the dietitian seldom discussed in acute care settings is after-discharge communications and referrals. Patients leaving acute care facilities today tend to need higher levels of all types of care, including nutrition, than ever before. Many of the same interventions begun in the hospital need to be continued, evaluated, and modified as indicated. Discharge planning includes summarizing care provided, identifying what still needs to be done, and offering referrals to outpatient facilities for support and evaluation.

Diet counseling, for example, is typically only begun in the hospital, and significant dietary changes are best achieved with multiple sessions in small stages. Lack of follow-through leads to poor understanding, poor compliance, and poor outcomes. Inadequate transitions to home care or extended care facilities often lead to continuation or reoccurrence of the same or worse problems, duplication of efforts, and unnecessary patient suffering. Lack of reimbursement for many outpatient nutrition services often leads to little or no outpatient follow-up. Lack of appropriate nutrition counseling and interventions often leads to compromise in patient well-being and considerably higher health care expenditures in the long run.

DOCUMENTATION/RECORD KEEPING

Documentation of services provided is necessary to be able to justify use and expenditure of resources and charges made. The old adage is that if it was not documented, it was not done. Many of the hospitals that improved profits in the early days of prospective, fixed-payment reimbursement systems were successful, in part, because they were able to improve the documentation of the patients' diagnoses, complications, and service requirements.

Recording the results and significance of nutrition screening and assessment data both documents the provision of a nutrition service and provides a measure of severity of illness. Documenting severity or acuity, then, further justifies actions taken and resource expenditures. For example, improving the documentation of malnutrition as a comorbidity has been shown to increase allowable reimbursement and increase the chances that appropriate nutrition therapy will be provided.

In the cycle of quality improvement, appropriate standards of care are developed and the processes used in the provision of care and outcomes (results) of that care are evaluated. Documenting provision of appropriate standards of care is critical in being able to demonstrate quality of care.

Outcomes of nutrition interventions can serve as indicators of the success, or lack thereof, of traditional and new nutrition therapies. Attempts to evaluate improvements in quality, effectiveness, and efficiency of care are futile if results are not recorded. In the early attempts to study and demonstrate effectiveness of nutrition care, lack of documentation of services provided and outcomes often was the weak link.

Summarizing the results of nutrition interventions (e.g., changes in food textures, use of enteral or parenteral nutrition solutions, diet counseling) tells the next provider what has been done, to what degree, and with what level of completeness or success, and explains what is still to be accomplished, monitored, or evaluated. In documenting the outcomes of care, noting lack of success is just as important as noting successful interventions.

Documentation should be placed in the appropriate stream of data. Information that affects or qualifies the patient's overall care or progress should be in the history and progress section of the medical record. Supportive data, questionnaires, copies of instructions, and so forth can be placed in more peripheral sections of the record.[17]

LEVELS OF NUTRITION CARE AND MEASURES OF ACUITY

Levels of dietetic care have been used to categorize units of patient nutrition service requirements, much like acuity scores or categories of severity of illness and resource requirements. Levels of nutrition care, however, were traditionally assigned shortly after admission, using information found in the initial screening and assessment. Usually three to four levels of care were used, such as basic, intermediate, and in-depth care. In some systems, subgroups or modifiers were added.

Level 1 (basic care) typically included

- collection of screening information
- standard house diets (regular, liquid, soft, etc.)
- selective or nonselective menu
- cursory review of patient's intake, tolerance to house diets
- orientation to food service system, menu selection
- technician visit

Level 2 (intermediate care) typically included Level 1 activities plus

- patient interview
- nutrition assessment
- diet history
- provision of modified diet
- observation of performance (selections, feeding skills, etc.)
- review of rationale, basic dietetic teaching
- documentation of services, recommendations
- evaluation and recommendations

Level 3 (in-depth care) typically included Levels 1 and 2 activities plus

- records of nutrient intake
- nutrition counseling
- in-depth diet teaching/counseling
- follow-up assessment and evaluation
- calculation of complex diet schedule, pattern, parenteral or enteral formula

Levels of care categories were helpful in (1) delineating which patients were likely to need additional resources; (2) deciding which patients might be assigned to technician level care; (3) defining which patients should be referred to dietitians or dietitian specialists; (4) prioritizing activities; (5) predicting units of service required (labor, supplies, and other resources); and (6) determining productivity.

The problem with prospective or concurrent assignment of levels of care, however, was similar to that found when hospitals tried to use the admitting diagnosis to reimburse for care. The appropriate care actually provided the patient during the hospitalization may have had little relationship to what was predicted from the admitting information. A patient with an admission diagnosis of shortness of breath secondary to pneumonia, for example, may have turned out to have congestive heart failure, pneumonia, and profound malnutrition. The intensity of care and the service requirements are quite different.

As was the case with diagnosis-related groups (DRGs), nutrition related levels of care, severity of illness indicators, and/or acuity measures are more accurate if based on the mixture of services and products appropriately provided during the hospitalization. Acuity scores can be assigned concurrently or retrospectively and are based on the mixture of the patient's nutrition-related problems, the services provided, and the resources used. Acuity levels would serve better than fixed levels of care to predict costs, staffing (number and level), and other resource requirements. Knowledge of acuity levels would also allow better comparisons of productivity among different facilities and opportunities for studying the value of new products or interventions. Acuity levels or severity of illness can be calculated by assigning units of labor, time, and/or dollars to the services required to meet nutritional needs of the patient. For example, a nutrition assessment for protein-calorie malnutrition might be assigned 0.4 hours, and the cost would be based on the resources needed to provide and document the assessment. Once all the dietetic services were identified and coded, overall acuity levels, service requirements, and cost could be established for any single nutrition care problem or mixture of problems.

A patient with a new onset of diabetes might require, for example, a diet history, a review of medical, surgical, and laboratory profile, a meal pattern, and one or two in-depth diet counseling sessions. Each service provided would have a time requirement, a cost, and an associated description. If a dietitian had three patients with newly diagnosed diabetes, the overall acuity score, time requirement, and cost for providing the service could easily be computed. If one of the patients with diabetes also had sepsis and malnutrition, the patient would have a higher dietetic acuity score because he or she would require additional assessments and interventions. Methods for calculating acuity levels and the terminology employed may vary in different settings and in different fields. Efforts are under way to study, categorize, and standardize units of service, acuity scores, and other "intensity" measures in medicine, nursing, dietetics, and other professions.

CLINICAL PRODUCTIVITY

Productivity has to do with the ratio of products and services produced (outputs) to the amount of resources required (inputs), such as equipment, supplies, labor, and facilities. Incentives to curtail costs of health care and at the same time provide more services to more acutely ill patients have made efforts at increasing efficiency and productivity a priority for acute care hospital management. Estimates and comparisons of hospital productivity can be made in a number of ways, such as the ratio of admissions to full-time-equivalent employees; amount of labor required to produce a mix or specific set of services; or combinations of wages paid, number of FTEs, staff per bed, number of patient days, and/or profit margins. In each case, comparisons of productivity among hospitals have to be controlled or adjusted for severity of patients' illnesses or acuity of care provided.[6,8,20–23]

Products and services (units of service) provided by clinical nutrition departments include nutrition screening and assessments, consultations and chart notations; calorie counts, meal plans, patterns, or tailored parenteral and enteral nutrition regimens; patient education and counseling sessions; classes provided to students and staff in nutrition and other disciplines; and supportive teaching materials for clients and students. As in the case of overall hospital productivity, comparison of productivity of nutrition departments has to take into account the nature of the cases and the services required/desired in each setting.[24–27]

Methods of improving efficiency and productivity—doing more with less— include use of technological advances (e.g., computers and computer systems, communication devices, automated methods for abstracting data and documenting services); changing work schedules, patterns, or locations to conform with service requirements and improve access to data; increasing the capacity or efficiency of equipment; or increasing the skills, experience, knowledge, and incentives of employees.[26–28]

In the clinical nutrition setting, the timing of some tasks, such as extracting data from medical records, conferring with surgeons, or counseling patients and families, is difficult, if not impossible, to accomplish at certain times of the day. Efforts at trying to accomplish them at the wrong times would be inefficient and unproductive. Scheduling activities to times when efforts are more likely to be successful can have a big impact on productivity.[29]

In some settings, use of practitioners with advanced-level credentials might be justified in that they can accomplish more complex tasks in a shorter amount of time. Appropriate use of and access to nutrition and medical reference materials, patient scheduling systems, computerized nutrition assessment systems, and nutrient, laboratory, and medical databases can improve productivity. Organized, protocol-driven, systematic approaches for nutrition screening, intervention, and documentation of care, and good interdisciplinary cooperation also have the potential to enhance productivity.

HOW NUTRITION DEPARTMENTS CAN REDUCE COSTS AND IMPROVE QUALITY OF CARE

If the departments in an acute care facility are efficient in the evaluation and treatment of patients, complications will be minimized, the hospital will spend less money than is reimbursed by third party payers, and the hospital is likely to make money.

Many complications can either prolong hospital stay or increase the expenditure of resources.[30-33] Malnutrition is one example of a complication that has several implications. The following are examples of how the nutritionist can improve care and reduce the patient's cost of hospitalization.

1. Identify malnutrition when it exists. Malnutrition is a legitimate complication that, under certain conditions, results in increased reimbursement for patient hospitalizations.
2. Treat malnutrition when it exists. If malnutrition is appropriately treated, the results are several appropriate outcomes: the patient benefits from decreased risk of morbidity and mortality from both the malnutrition per se and nutrition-related complications of other medical/surgical problems, such as decubitus ulcers, infections, and electrolyte disorders. The hospital benefits because (1) malnutrition is in many cases a complication that increases reimbursement, (2) unnecessary length of stay and expensive complications related to untreated malnutrition do not occur if the malnutrition is recognized and treated promptly, and (3) patients and their families recognize and appreciate the efforts to identify and treat nutritional problems.
3. Prevent malnutrition from becoming a complication in patients who are adequately nourished at admission.
4. Be certain that nutritional aspects of medical and surgical care are timely, appropriate, effective, and efficiently delivered. Appropriate or inappropriate nutrition care for problems such as congestive heart failure, diabetes, or renal disorders can have a significant impact on the quality, cost, and effectiveness of the patient's overall care. Nutrition and therapeutic nutrition formulas themselves may be major components of patients' care. In the case of parenteral and enteral nutrition, the costs involved in the solutions themselves, in admixture costs, and in laboratory tests used in monitoring patients make nutrition support therapies appropriate subjects for studying the effectiveness and appropriateness of nutrition care. Errors, complications, and under- and overutilization of specialized nutrition support can have an even bigger impact on patient care and hospital costs.

5. Provide appropriate nutritional care in the form of standardized test diet protocols, such as diets used prior to radiologic, diagnostic, and surgical procedures and postoperative and transitional feeding schedules.
6. Promote interdisciplinary nutrition care policies, procedures, and quality improvement activities.
7. Provide supportive, timely nutrition care that is tailored to individual needs. Nutrition care in all forms improves the likelihood that overall care will be successful.

Nutritionists can also use data on frequency of patient diagnoses, acuity scores, and complications to improve nutrition care systems.

1. Target the development of department standards of nutrition care to the most frequent and most important nutrition problems. Use current nutrition care literature, position papers, and practice guidelines.
2. Share nutrition standards of care, protocols, and so forth with other disciplines. The result is improved understanding of the role of nutrition and nutrition practices in overall care, increased cooperation and communication, increased referrals, "automatic consults," and improved efficiency.
3. Study how well those standards of care are being documented and achieved, and with what outcomes.
4. Direct quality improvement efforts to the most frequent and significant diagnoses and complications.
5. Determine whether screening and assessment processes are picking up the appropriate nutrition care problems, whether specific types of patients are missed, whether too many or too few services are provided, and whether resources are used based on patients' profiles and acuity levels.
6. Help identify professional qualifications, location, and number of staff required to provide for the needs of patients. Allocate other resources as needed to meet appropriate care requirements.
7. Determine the appropriateness of services provided—whether services were necessary, adequate, or overkill, and whether they were provided to the targeted patients.
8. Plan clinical effectiveness studies for specific nutrition care issues to evaluate new treatments, products, or methods of education.
9. Determine whether discharge planning, transfer of information necessary for continuity of care, and patient education needs are being met effectively. Survey extended care facilities and discharged patients to determine whether nutrition care information received at discharge was sufficient for continuity of care. Examine readmissions for problems in which nutrition is a key issue.

10. Establish overall nutrition care productivity for the department (services provided per staffing level), with acuity as an adjustment factor.
11. Help identify and justify billable charges for services provided.

REFERENCES

1. A decade of change: AHA's annual survey traces national trends. *Hospitals.* 1991;65:32–33.

2. Chirikos TN. Quality competition in local hospital markets: some economic evidence from the period 1982–88. *Soc Sci Med.* 1992;34:1011–1021.

3. Franks P, Clancy CM. Gatekeeping revisited—protecting patients from overtreatment. *N Engl J Med.* 1992;327:424–429.

4. Schwartz WB, Mendelson DN. Hospital cost containment in the 1980s: hard lessons learned and prospects for the 1990's. *N Engl J Med.* 1991;324:1037–1042.

5. Munoz E, Goldstein J, Lory MH, et al. The DRG hospital payment system, surgical readmissions and cost containment. *Ann Surg.* 1990;56:683–687.

6. Lave JR. The effect of the Medicare prospective payment system. *Annu Rev Public Health.* 1989;10:141–161.

7. Phelps CE. The methodologic foundations of studies of the appropriateness of medical care. *N Engl J Med.* 1993;329:1241–1245.

8. Thorpe KE, Gertler PJ, Goldman P. The resource utilization group system: its effect on nursing home case mix and costs. *Inquiry.* 1991;28(4):357–365.

9. Tresch DD, Duthie EH, Newton M, Bodin B. Coping with diagnosis related groups: the changing role of the nursing home. *Arch Intern Med.* 1988;148:1393–1396.

10. Fillit H, Howe JL, Fulop G. Studies of hospital stays in the frail elderly and their relationship to the intensity of social work intervention. *Soc Work Health Care.* 1992;18:1–22.

11. Hirsch CH, Sommers L, Olsen A, et al. The natural history of functional morbidity in hospitalized older patients. *J Am Geriatr Soc.* 1990;38(12):1296–1303.

12. Kenney GM, Dubay LC. Explaining area variation in the use of Medicare home health services. *Med Care.* 1992;30(1):43–57.

13. Kane M, Estes C, Colton D, Eltoft C. *Role Delineation Study for Entry-Level Registered Dietitians, Entry-Level Dietetic Technicians and Beyond Entry-Level Registered Dietitians,* Vols 1–3. Chicago, Ill: American Dietetic Association; 1989.

14. Bradley RT, Ebbs P, Martin J, Young WY. *Role Delineations for Advanced-Level and Specialty Practice in Dietetics: Results of an Empirical Study. Technical Report,* Vol 1. Chicago, Ill: American Dietetic Association; 1992.

15. American Dietetic Association. Position paper on clinical dietetics. *J Am Diet Assoc.* 1982; 80(3):256–260.

16. Franz MJ. Practice guidelines: roadmaps for nutrition care. *J Am Diet Assoc.* 1992;92(9):1136.

17. Gilmore CJ, Beyer PL. Developing and implementing a nutrition screening program. In: Fox MK, ed. *Reimbursement and Insurance Coverage for Nutrition Services.* Chicago, Ill: American Dietetic Association; 1991;80–88.

18. Insull W. Dietitians as intervention specialists: a continuing challenge for the 1990's. *J Am Diet Assoc.* 1992;92(5):551–552.

19. Lohr KN. Outcome measurement: concepts and questions. *Inquiry.* 1988;24(1):37–50.

20. Ashby JL, Altman SH. The trend in hospital output and labor productivity, 1980–1989. *Inquiry.* 1992;29(1):80–91.

21. Mezzich JE. Architecture of clinical information and prediction of service utilization and cost. *Schizophr Bull.* 1991;22(3):469–474.

22. Wong DT, Knaus WA. Predicting outcome in critical care: the current status of the APACHE prognostic scoring system. *Can J Anaesth.* 1991;38(3):374–383.

23. McMahon LF, Billi JE. Measurement of severity of illness and the Medicare prospective payment system: state of the art and future directions. *J Gen Intern Med.* 1988;3(5):482–490.

24. Hannaman K, Penner SF. A nutrition assessment tool that includes diagnosis. *J Am Diet Assoc.* 1985;85:607.

25. McManners MH, Barina SA. Productivity in clinical dietetics. *J Am Diet Assoc.* 1984;84(9):1035–1041.

26. Lutton SE, Baker MM, Billman RV. Levels of patient nutrition care for use in clinical decision making. *J Am Diet Assoc.* 1985;85(7):849.

27. Halling JF, Lafferty L, Feller KS. *Productivity Management for Nutrition Care Systems.* Chicago, Ill: American Dietetic Association; 1986.

28. Gobberdiel L. A new strategy for cost-effective care: clinical dietetic staffing by diagnosis. *J Am Diet Assoc.* 1986;86(1):76–79.

29. Diabetes Control and Complications Research Group. The effect of intensive treatment of diabetes on the development and progression of long-term complications in insulin-dependent diabetes mellitus. *N Engl J Med.* 1993;329:977–986.

30. Economic impact of malnutrition: a model system for hospitalized patients. *J Paren Enter Nutr.* 1988;12:371–376.

31. Smith AE, Smith PE. Reimbursement for clinical nutrition services: a 10-year experience. *J Am Diet Assoc.* 1992;92:1385–1388.

32. Robinson G, Goldstein M, Levine GM. Impact of nutritional status on DRG length of stay. *J Paren Enter Nutr.* 1987;11:49–51.

33. Weddle DO, Schmeisser D, Barnish M, Kamath SK. Inpatient and post discharge course of the malnourished patient. *J Am Diet Assoc.* 1991;91:307–311.

Chapter 16

Nutrition Assessment in Critical Care

Marion Feitelson Winkler

OVERVIEW

Nutrition assessment of the critically ill patient presents a unique challenge to the practitioner because traditional methods of assessing nutritional status are often of limited value in the critical care setting. Anthropometric measurements are not sensitive to acute changes; biochemical parameters are affected by infection, stress, and hemodynamic instability; and there are complex metabolic alterations associated with injury and sepsis that affect nutrient utilization. Furthermore, the presence of preexisting chronic disease and the potential for multiple system organ failure during treatment may affect nutritional management. A thorough understanding of the metabolic response to injury and critical illness is essential for the practitioner who is involved in the assessment and the provision of nutrition support to these patients.

The response to critical illness, injury, and sepsis characteristically involves both the ebb and flow phases.[1] The ebb phase occurs immediately following injury and is associated with hypovolemia, shock, and tissue hypoxia. Typically this phase is manifested by decreased cardiac output, oxygen consumption, and body temperature. The flow phase that follows fluid resuscitation and restoration of oxygen transport is often prolonged and associated with increased morbidity and organ failure in critically ill patients. It is characterized by an increase in cardiac output, oxygen consumption, body temperature, and basal metabolic rate. There is a marked increase in glucose production, free fatty acid release, circulating levels of insulin, catecholamines, glucagon, cortisol, and insulin

285

resistance. The magnitude of the response appears to be associated with the severity of the injury.

MEASUREMENT OF NUTRITIONAL STATUS IN CRITICAL CARE

The standard components of the nutrition assessment are often difficult to apply in the critically ill patient. The severely injured patient is typically unable to provide information on previous dietary intake, food allergies, or change in body weight. Values for weight may be erroneous following fluid resuscitation, and interpretation of plasma protein concentrations is affected by the stress response independent of nutritional status. The altered requirements for and utilization of energy substrates and other nutrients related to the stressed state must also be considered.

An objective evaluation of nutritional status is needed to establish the presence or absence of malnutrition or specific nutrient deficiencies and to monitor the response to nutritional intervention. Subjective global assessment that utilizes clinical history and physical examination is a rapid, inexpensive, noninvasive tool that correlates well with traditional objective anthropometric and laboratory measures, prediction of postoperative infection, and increased morbidity and mortality.[2,3] The technique identifies patients who are well nourished, at risk to be malnourished, or severely malnourished.

Anthropometric measurements, including arm circumference, triceps skinfold thickness, and body weight, though generally a good index of body protein and energy reserves, are insensitive to nutritional repletion over a relatively short period.[4] The critically ill patient is typically in an intensive care unit with numerous indwelling catheters to quantify body fluid losses, and multiple intravenous lines for invasive hemodynamic monitoring and delivery of blood products and fluid. Obtaining accurate anthropometric measurements under these conditions is impractical. In addition, rapid changes in body weight in these patients are probably more reflective of alterations in total body water than that of changes in lean body mass or body fat.

To date there is no single, reliable laboratory marker for moderate malnutrition or for evaluating the short-term response to nutrition therapy. In the critically ill patient, interpretation of serum albumin concentrations is affected not only by its long half-life and large body pool with intercompartmental fluid shifts but also by stress and inflammation, and the provision of exogenous albumin products.[5,6] Stress and inflammation have also been shown to affect the concentration of rapid turnover proteins in critically ill patients.[7] Intensive care unit patients with sepsis have been shown to have significantly lower levels of retinol-binding protein and prealbumin than nonseptic patients.[8] However, when compared to serum albumin and transferrin, prealbumin and retinol-binding protein concentrations offer the advantages of a rapid and persistent response to nutrition therapy and a direct correlation with nitrogen balance.[9–11] A number of acute-phase reactant proteins such as C-reactive protein, α-1 antitrypsin, ceruloplasmin, and α-1 acid glycoprotein are potential protein parameters for nutrition assessment of critically ill patients. These proteins have a high priority for synthesis in the post-trauma or -stress period. Table 16–1 compares the function, half-life, and size of available laboratory markers of protein status.

Nitrogen balance studies are best used not as a nutrition assessment tool but as a means of documenting effectiveness of nutritional therapy. The data indicate whether nutrition support has been sufficient to prevent net catabolism or to promote anabolism. Ideally, total urinary nitrogen measurements should be made; however, estimations of nitrogen loss can be obtained from urinary urea nitrogen (UUN) excretion and an approximation of nonurinary nitrogen losses. In the critically ill patient, abnormal nitrogen loss from burn wound exudate, fistula drainage, gastrointestinal fluid loss, diarrhea, or dialysis should be considered before interpreting data. Measurement of 24-hour UUN excretion has also been used to evaluate the degree of hypermetabolism. When used to determine degree of stress, the most sensitive and specific measure of nitrogen excretion is obtained in the fasting state, where a UUN value of 0 to 5 corresponds with normometabolism, 5 to 10 with mild hypermetabolism, 10 to 15 with moderate hypermetabolism, and greater than 15 with a severe hypermetabolic state.[12]

NUTRITION INTERVENTION IN CRITICAL CARE

Because of the difficulties in applying standard nutrition assessment techniques in the critical care setting, clinical judgment must play a major role in decisions about when to offer nutrition support. The ability to predict the clinical course and the resumption of adequate oral food intake are key components of this process.[13] In a previously well-nourished patient, it may be prudent to wait five to seven days before initiating enteral or parenteral nutrition support; however, in persons with preexisting malnutrition or postoperative complications that preclude oral intake, nutritional intervention must be initiated early if a period of prolonged limited intake is foreseen. In burn and high-risk surgical patients, there is some evidence that initiation of early nutrition support, within 48 hours, may be beneficial.[14–16]

Typically the critically ill patient enters an intensive care unit setting because of a cardiopulmonary diagnosis; multiple trauma, burn injury, or sepsis; or postoperative or intraoperative complications. As part of the nutrition assessment, the following questions should be considered: What was the nutritional

Table 16-1 Laboratory Markers of Protein Status

Protein	Binding Function	Half-Life	Molecular Weight	Response to Stress
C-reactive protein	Bacteria, platelets, lymphocytes	5 hours	120,000	Very strong, rapid increase
Retinol-binding protein	Vitamin A	12 hours	21,000	Negative acute phase reactant
Transthyretin (Prealbumin)	Thyroxine, retinol-binding protein	2 days	55,000	Negative acute phase reactant
α2-Macroglobulin	Endopeptidases, proteases	2–4 days	820,000	Neutral
Ceruloplasmin	Copper	5–7 days	150,000	Weak acute phase reactant
α1-Acid glycoprotein	Drugs	6 days	41,000	Strong positive acute phase reactant
Transferrin	Iron	8 days	77,000	Negative acute phase reactant
α1-Antitrypsin	Proteases	16 days	55,000	Strong positive acute phase reactant
Albumin	Anions, drugs, free fatty acids	20 days	66,000	Negative acute phase reactant

Source: Adapted with permission from Konstantinides FN. Nitrogen Balance Studies: A Special Monitoring Requirement for the Critically Ill Patient. Used with permission of Ross Products Division, Abbott Laboratories, Columbus, OH 43216, from *Laboratory Utilization for Nutritional Support: Current Practice, Requirements, Expectations. Fourteenth Annual Ross Roundtable on Medical Issues,* © 1994 Ross Products Division, Abbott Laboratories.

status of the patient prior to admission, injury, or surgery? What is the diagnosis, type of medical or surgical intervention, and extent of disease or injury? Is there need for initiation of early nutrition support? Is there an ability to predict gastrointestinal function? Can enteral access be achieved? If enteral feeding is contraindicated, will total parenteral nutrition (TPN) be considered? A thorough review of systems may help answer many of these questions. Table 16–2 outlines factors affecting nutritional care that need to be considered in the planning of nutritional intervention.

Energy requirements can be measured directly or estimated using published regression equations. The most widely used predictive equation to approximate resting metabolic expenditure (RME) is that of Harris and Benedict.[17]

RME for males (kcal/day) = 66.5 + (13.8 × weight in kg) + (5 × height in cm) - (6.8 × age)

RME for females (kcal/day) = 655 + (9.6 × weight in kg) + (1.8 × height in cm) - 4.7 × age)

Body weight is the most significant determinant of the results obtained using the Harris and Benedict equation. For patients with weight loss, the usual body weight or the ideal body weight should be used to calculate energy expenditure; for obese patients, the midpoint between actual and ideal body weight can be used. A corrective stress factor is often added to account for the increased metabolic requirements of the critically ill patient. The most widely applied stress factors are those of Long, et al.[18]: 1.35 for skeletal trauma, 1.6 for major sepsis, and 2.1 for severe thermal injury. Shanbhogue and colleagues[19] recommend using 1.05 to 1.25 for peritonitis and 1.3 to 1.55 for severe infection. Energy calculations specific to the adult burn patient can be made using the Curreri formula[20]: (25 kcal × weight in kg) + (40 kcal × percent of total body surface area burn). Predictive energy equations have also been developed for surgical intensive care unit patients receiving mechanical ventilation[21] and for obese patients with and without mechanical ventilation.[22] The presence of obesity was a factor in the spontaneously breathing patients, but the presence of obesity did not significantly affect the energy expenditure of ventilator-dependent patients.[22]

Studies have found that energy expenditure measured by indirect calorimetry closely approximates the predictions of the Harris and Benedict equation[23,24]; however, patients with closed head injury may demonstrate elevated energy expenditure in the absence of barbiturate therapy.[25] Likewise, patients in the intensive care unit receiving routine care (physical exam, dressing change, moving of body or limbs, chest x-ray) or chest physical therapy have significant elevations in measured energy expenditure compared to resting.[26] In practice we have found no consistent increase in metabolic rate when evaluating measured energy expenditure on the basis of disease (pancreatitis or cancer) or sepsis. Trauma patients, in our experience, have significantly greater elevations in measured energy expenditure than nontrauma patients; however, the magnitude

Table 16–2 Review of Systems and Factors That Affect Nutritional Care

System	Factors To Consider
Cardiovascular	Fluid restriction often necessary in congestive heart failure.
Endocrine	Hyperglycemia may necessitate use of insulin.
Gastrointestinal	Presence of ileus, prolonged nasogastric drainage, gastrointestinal bleeding, or severe diarrhea may preclude use of enteral nutrition support.
Hematologic	Anemia
Hepatic	Protein intolerance occurs with severe liver disease and encephalopathy. Formulas high in branched-chain amino acids and low in aromatic amino acids may be necessary.
Immune	Energy and protein requirements are higher in sepsis. Long-term antibiotic therapy may be associated with diarrhea.
Musculoskeletal	Increased protein requirements for wound healing and treatment of pressure ulcers.
	Daily surgical debridement of extensive wounds may interfere with ability to provide adequate oral or enteral nutrition.
Neurologic	Postpyloric tube feeding placement may be beneficial in situations where there is an increased risk of aspiration.
Renal	Fluid restriction may be a limiting factor in providing adequate nutrition in the nondialyzed patient.
	Dialysis patients have increased protein requirements secondary to protein loss from the dialysate.
	Diets high in essential amino acids may be beneficial.
Respiratory	Requirements for prolonged ventilation may necessitate enteral feeding.
	Gastrostomy or jejunostomy tube placement can be recommended at the time of tracheostomy for patients in whom prolonged enteral nutrition support is anticipated. Avoid excessive caloric delivery in the presence of carbon dioxide retention.

Source: Adapted from Silverman D.W. Assessment and Nutrition Management of the Patient with Multiple Organ Dysfunction Syndrome, *Suggested Guidelines for the Nutrition and Metabolic Management of Adult Patients Receiving Nutrition Support* by M.F. Winkler and L.K. Lysen with permission of the American Dietetic Association, © 1993.

of increase rarely exceeds 30 percent of predicted.[27] In critically ill patients with severe trauma, sepsis, or presumed hypermetabolism, energy expenditure can be determined from data obtained with a Swan-Ganz catheter.[28,29]

Recommendations for protein prescription for critically ill patients vary considerably but are generally higher than for the nonstressed individual. There appears, however, to be no clinical advantage to feeding excessive protein to critically ill patients. Studies have shown no gain in net protein synthesis in adult burn patients when they were fed 40 kcal/kg/day and when protein intake was increased from 1.4 to 2.2 g/kg/day.[30] Nitrogen balance was not significantly different in septic patients receiving 1.2 g/kg/day or 2.3 g/kg/day.[31] Similarly, there were no obvious advantages in terms of protein sparing when protein was provided in amounts exceeding 1.5 g/kg/day to septic patients on TPN.[32] In acutely head-injured patients, there was no difference in nitrogen balance when protein was provided as 14 percent or 22 percent of the total calories.[33] In general, recommendations for energy requirements can be made by increasing calculated values by 20 to 30 percent while providing protein at levels of 1.2 to 1.5 g/kg/day.

Electrolytes and other minerals should be individually determined and adjusted according to the needs of the patient, organ function, and gastric, intestinal, urinary, and stool losses. Vitamins and trace elements can be provided based on the RDAs or from published guidelines for intravenous use.[34,35] There is some evidence that vitamin requirements of critically ill, stressed patients may be higher than for the nonstressed individual[36]; however, it is not known to what extent specific disease, fever, or stress may affect requirements or the balance between plasma concentration and tissue stores.

TYPES OF NUTRITION SUPPORT

An oral diet is the preferred route for nutrient delivery. The critically ill patient is often unable to eat because of endotracheal intubation and the need for mechanical ventilation. Patients who are breathing spontaneously and are able to take food by mouth may not be able to meet the increased energy and nutrient requirements of stress without use of oral meal replacements or supplemental enteral tube feedings.

Enteral Nutrition Support

Enteral nutrition should be prescribed whenever oral intake is inadequate for patients who have a functional gastrointestinal tract. Enteral nutrition can be provided through nasogastric, nasoenteric, gastrostomy, or jejunostomy tubes. The use of gastric feeding tubes may be limited in the critical care setting because of the higher risk of aspiration in patients with compromised pulmonary function, gastric ileus that frequently occurs after abdominal surgery, or impaired peristalsis in patients receiving morphine. Gaining access to the duodenum or jejunum can be accomplished via fluoroscopy, endoscopy, or surgery. When a critically ill patient undergoes an endoscopic gastrointestinal workup, surgical placement of a tracheostomy tube, or an abdominal operative procedure, the practitioner should consider recommending placement of a feeding tube at the time of the procedure if the patient is expected to be unable to take food by mouth for a prolonged period of time. The use of a combined gastrostomy-jejunostomy tube offers significant advantages to the critically ill patient since the gastric port can be used for drainage or medication delivery while feedings can be administered through the jejunal limb.

The selection of an enteral nutrition product should be made on the basis of the patient's fluid, energy, and nutrient requirements, and gastrointestinal function. Most patients receiving gastric or enteric feedings can tolerate a standard polymeric diet—formulas containing nutrients in the form of glucose polymers, intact protein, and long- and medium-chain triglycerides that require complete digestion. Critically ill patients may have some evidence of maldigestion or malabsorption and an impaired ability to tolerate large amounts of fat; likewise, patients who may have intestinal or pancreatic insufficiency may benefit from a formula containing hydrolyzed protein and a lower content of fat. A wide variety of disease-specific enteral products containing glutamine, short-chain peptides, arginine, structured lipids, and omega-3 fatty acids are available and should be used on a selective basis.

Much has been written about the benefits of enteral nutrition support. Aside from convenience and moderate expense, enteral nutrition when compared to TPN has been shown to prevent gastrointestinal mucosal atrophy, attenuate the injury stress response, maintain immunocompetence, preserve normal gut flora, and reduce septic morbidity rates in high-risk surgical patients receiving early postoperative feedings.[37-40] The renewed attention on enteral nutrition support stems from the recognition that the gastrointestinal tract serves as a barrier to microorganisms, endotoxins, and other bacterial products. It is suggested that in critical illness this barrier is impaired, thereby allowing bacterial translocation to occur and inducing sepsis and multiple organ failure.[41-43]

Total Parenteral Nutrition

The use of TPN in the critical care unit is reserved for the patient who cannot be fed enterally because of ileus or gastrointestinal intolerance, or because of markedly increased energy requirements. A number of important factors must be considered when prescribing and monitoring TPN in this setting.

Hyperglycemia may be encountered in patients with stress-related glucose intolerance. Poor blood glucose control results in glycosuria, fluid losses, and hyperosmolar dehydration. Insulin therapy is often required. High glucose intake has also been shown to result in excess carbon dioxide production, which may precipitate respiratory failure or prevent weaning from mechanical ventilation in patients with pulmonary disease.[44] When patients are provided with adequate calories and 20 to 30 percent of the daily energy intake as fat, the syndrome of carbon dioxide retention and respiratory failure induced by TPN has been infrequent.[13] It is not the glucose concentration in the parenteral infusate that increases carbon dioxide production, but the actual carbohydrate intake; thus moderate caloric intake appears to be more important in avoiding nutritionally related increases in carbon dioxide production in stable mechanically ventilated patients.[45]

Fluid overload secondary to water and sodium retention accompanying refeeding has been described in patients with cardiac disease and in severely malnourished patients.[46] The fluid retention can be controlled by reducing the amount of sodium and water provided while delivering adequate calories. Acute oliguric renal failure is a complication sometimes seen in the critically ill patient. Medical management often includes restriction of fluid, protein, and minerals to avoid or delay the onset of hemodialysis. Parenteral nutrition support can be accomplished by increasing the caloric density of the nutrition formulation within the fluid allowance, while restricting protein to the minimal amount necessary to provide the essential amino acid requirements. This results in a high calorie-to-nitrogen ratio and improved net protein utilization. The patient undergoing hemodialysis should have protein intake liberalized to 1.2 to 1.5 g/kg/day to account for amino acid losses in the dialysate. Patients with chronic liver disease and hepatic encephalopathy also have limitations to parenteral nutrition support because of fluid and sodium retention and protein intolerance. Use of a disease-specific, branched-chain enriched amino acid solution that is low in aromatic amino acids has enabled practitioners to deliver adequate protein with marked improvement in the plasma amino acid profile. In many clinical studies, however, there has been little or no reduction in the severity of encephalopathy or survival.[47-49]

Glutamine-supplemented parenteral nutrition is an active area of research. The addition of glutamine to TPN in patients undergoing major abdominal surgery has been associated with improved nitrogen balance.[50,51] Similarly, bone marrow transplantation patients who received glutamine-supplemented parenteral nutrition have improved nitrogen balance, a diminished incidence of infection, and shortened length of hospitalization when compared to patients receiving standard TPN.[52] The use of human growth hormone as an adjuvant to traditional nutrition support has also been studied. The metabolic effects of human growth hormone include promotion of protein conservation and stimulation of lipolysis and fat oxidation. Decreased levels of human growth hormone were noted during the acute stage of injury in trauma patients when compared to volunteers.[53] Nutrition support with daily administration of human growth hormone improved protein and fat metabolism but could not reverse it to the normal state. Growth hormone administration was also well tolerated and significantly enhanced nutrient retention compared to standard parenteral feeding alone in stable patients with gastrointestinal and pancreatic disease.[54] Growth hormone administration in conjunction with TPN may potentially enhance recovery of patients with illnesses requiring specialized metabolic and nutritional care.[55]

ROLES AND RESPONSIBILITIES OF THE NUTRITION SUPPORT TEAM

The nutrition support team is a multidisciplinary group usually consisting of a dietitian, nurse, pharmacist, and physician. Most teams typically provide clinical patient care through inpatient consultation, nutrition and metabolic assessment and management, and daily rounds. Other functions include the provision of medical education; quality assurance, including development of policies and procedures and standardized ordering forms; research; and home care. A successful team is dependent on cooperation among team members. This often leads to overlap in roles when caring for the patient receiving nutrition support. Although all members of the team share responsibility for design, implementation, and monitoring of parenteral and enteral nutrition therapies and for education of patients, families, and health care professionals, there are specific role-related functions.

The functions and responsibilities of the dietitian include identification of patients at nutritional risk via screening and assessment, maintenance of the enteral nutrition formulary, assurance of trouble-free and nutritionally complete transitional feedings, and documentation of nutrition care plans.[56] The dietitian obtains the dietary history and provides detailed information on nutrient intake or causes of decreased food intake and intolerances. This information is used to determine the most effective approach to meet the patient's energy and nutrient requirements. Initially the dietitian works with the patient to improve oral food intake through fractionated meals, dietary modification, increased caloric density of the diet, and use of high-calorie liquid beverages.

The nurse member of the team assists with central line placement and catheter site care, serves as an educational resource on tools and techniques for administering nutrition support, coordinates discharge planning, and provides emotional support to patients and families prior to and during nutrition support therapy.[57] The pharmacist is responsible for compounding the intravenous nutrition solutions. Pharmacists also provide expertise on parenteral solution incompatibilities, drug admixture, aseptic solution preparation, drug–nutrient interactions, drug dosage form alterations, and drug-induced feeding intolerance.[58] A physician usually directs the nutrition support team and is responsible for overall team activities. In addition to providing direct patient care and, in some cases, surgically placing the central venous catheters, the physician represents the interests of the team to the medical and hospital staff.[59] Due to the complexity and cost of specialized nutrition support, multidisciplinary teams have been established to minimize complications, improve outcomes, and improve overall efficiency in providing nutrition support.[60]

QUALITY ASSURANCE AND IMPROVEMENT

Quality improvement is the means by which an organization continuously monitors opportunities to improve patient care processes. Unlike quality assurance, in which action is initiated only when a problem is identified, quality improvement emphasizes ongoing monitoring and evaluation, with immediate intervention in situations where care can be improved. Benefits of quality improvement include providing timely feedback to practitioners in terms of performance and educational needs and allowing rapid identification of the need for nutritional intervention or the correction of problems related to nutrition therapy.

Dietitians have a unique opportunity to develop, implement, and coordinate quality improvement programs. Specific areas that can be monitored include nutrition assessment; indications for nutrition support; provision of optimal nutrition therapy; prevention, identification, and management of complications; determination of the endpoint of therapy; patient education; and patient satisfaction.

A useful tool for monitoring important aspects of patient care is the clinical indicator. The Joint Commission on Accreditation of Healthcare Organizations defines a clinical indicator as a quantitative measure that can be used as a guide to monitor and evaluate the quality of important patient care activities.[61] Multiple types of indicators have been identified. A comparative rate-based indicator can continuously evaluate trends in certain rates for which acceptable goals are predetermined. It is usually expressed with a numerator and denominator. The numerator represents the number of patient events of interest, and the denominator refers to the number of patients for which the event of interest could have occurred. An example of a comparative rate-based indicator is:

$$\frac{\text{number of critical care patients at high nutritional risk receiving nutrition intervention}}{\text{number of critical care patients screened at high nutritional risk}}$$

A rate of 100 percent in this case would be ideal; that is, all patients screened at high nutritional risk should receive nutritional intervention. If a particular institution consistently finds rates of 50 percent or less, this should prompt an evaluation to determine why patients at high nutritional risk are not receiving nutritional intervention, or whether the screening parameters are identifying patients who in fact are not actually at high risk.

An indicator can also describe a rare but serious adverse outcome. This type of indicator, termed a *sentinel event indicator*, requires that every occurrence be reviewed. An example of a sentinel event indicator in the critical care setting is respiratory arrest secondary to hypophosphatemia of refeeding.[62] Other complications that warrant further review include tube feeding aspiration or TPN-catheter-associated sepsis. Ideally a sentinel event indicator should have 0 percent occurrence.

Indicators can also monitor structure, process, or outcome. Structure relates to organizational and staff functions. An example of a structural indicator might be that all dietitians in the critical care unit have specialty nutrition support certification. Process indicators relate to activities performed in giving and receiving care. They can be developed to monitor assessment, treatment, and planning activities, or indications for therapy. Nutrition-related process indicators may include examples such as: patients screened at nutritional risk receive nutrition assessment within 24 to 48 hours; nutrition assessment is properly performed; the components of the assessment meet departmental standards; critical care patients receiving nothing by mouth or clear liquids for greater than seven days have documentation of such in the medical record; goals of therapy are documented; or an appropriate enteral or parenteral formula is recommended. Process indicators usually relate back to standards of care or practice guidelines; they measure whether care was delivered according to a protocol.

An outcome-oriented clinical indicator measures the effect of care on the health status of patients and typically relates to complications, adverse events, results of procedures and treatment, patient health, well-being, and functional status. Examples of outcome measures include change in the patient's clinical status and the effect on feeding method and tolerance, improvement in nutritional status or achievement of therapeutic goals, abnormal laboratory values such as hyperglycemia in a patient receiving TPN, change in body weight, adequacy of intake, compliance to diet, or patient knowledge. Outcome assessment helps the practitioner identify what, if anything, in the structure or process of care was responsible for positive or negative findings. When care is suboptimal and the desired outcomes are not achieved, a change in practice is required to promote a better outcome.

Dietetic departments have traditionally monitored processes as part of the overall quality assurance plan. To facilitate the transition to quality improvement, practitioners must reexamine these processes and identify potential outcome indicators. For example, a typical dietetic process indicator states that calorie-count data should be complete and accurate. A more clinically appropriate outcome measure might be developed to monitor whether patients with documented inadequate intake by calorie count receive appropriate nutritional supplementation. Indicators of the end result that nutrition care is expected to achieve, either positive or negative, must be measurable. The most clinically relevant indicators are those that have a definite link between nutrition intervention and outcome. Table 16–3 provides additional examples of clinical indicators that can be adapted to the patient receiving enteral or parenteral nutrition support in the critical care setting.

CONCLUSION

Nutrition support of the critically ill patient is an essential aspect of patient care. An understanding of the hypermetabolic response to illness, injury, and sepsis is critical in the interpretation of nutrition assessment data and for the selection of the appropriate modality for nutrition support. Careful monitoring of nutritional status, tolerance of substrate and nutrient delivery, fluid status, and organ function by the multidisciplinary team should be part of the nutrition care plan.

Table 16–3 Clinical Indicators for Parenteral and Enteral Nutrition Support

Indicator	Type of Indicator
Prescription for tube feeding or total parenteral nutrition (TPN) meets calculated nutritional needs within ± 10%.	Process
Tube feeding or TPN is initiated within 72 hours post burn injury for patients with burns exceeding 25% total body surface area.	Process
TPN is not discontinued until patient tolerates at least 50% of the nutritional goal by enteral tube feeding or oral diet for 3 consecutive days.	Process
Blood glucose during continuous parenteral nutrition support <80 mg% or >250 mg%.	Outcome
Change in pCO_2 over baseline during enteral or parenteral nutrition support.	Outcome
Weight gain over longest dialytic interval > 4 kg.	Outcome

Source: Adapted from *Suggested Guidelines for Nutrition and Metabolic Management of Adult Patients Receiving Nutrition Support* by M.F. Winkler and L.K. Lysen with permission of the American Dietetic Association, © 1993.

REFERENCES

1. Cuthbertson DP. The metabolic response to injury and its nutritional implications: retrospect and prospect. *J Paren Enter Nutr.* 1979;3:108–129.

2. Detsky AS, McLaughlin JR, Baker JP, et al. What is subjective global assessment of nutritional status? *J Paren Enter Nutr.* 1987;11:8–13.

3. Ireton-Jones CS, Hasse JM. Comprehensive nutritional assessment: the dietitian's contribution to the team effort. *Nutrition.* 1992;8:75–81.

4. Gray GE, Gray LK. Anthropometric measurements and their interpretation: principles, practices, and problems. *J Am Diet Assoc.* 1980;77:534–539.

5. Fischer JE. Plasma proteins as indicators of nutritional status. In: Levenson SM, ed. *Nutritional Assessment: Present Status, Future Directions and Prospects.* Columbus, Ohio: Ross Laboratories; 1982:25–26.

6. Rothchild MA, Oratz M, Schreiber SS. Albumin synthesis. *N Engl J Med.* 1972;286:748–757, 816–821.

7. Carpentier YA, Barthel J, Bruyns J. Plasma protein concentrations in nutritional assessment. *Proc Nutr Soc.* 1982;4:405–417.

8. Boles JM, Garre MA, Youinou PY, et al. Nutritional status in intensive care unit patients: evaluation in 84 unselected patients. *Crit Care Med.* 1983;11:87–90.

9. Winkler MF, Gerrior SA, Pomp A, Albina JE. Use of retinol-binding protein and prealbumin as indicators of the response to nutrition therapy. *J Am Diet Assoc.* 1989;5:684–687.

10. Tuten MB, Wogt S, Dasse F, Leider Z. Utilization of prealbumin as a nutritional parameter. *J Paren Enter Nutr.* 1985;9:709–711.

11. Vanlandingham S, Spiekerman AM, Newmark SR. Prealbumin: a parameter of visceral protein levels during albumin infusion. *J Paren Enter Nutr.* 1982;6:230–231.

12. Blackburn GL, Bistrian BR, Maini BS, et al. Nutritional and metabolic assessment of the hospitalized patient. *J Paren Enter Nutr.* 1977;1:11–22.

13. Pomp A, Bates M, Albina JE. Specialized nutritional support in surgical patients. *Prob Gen Surg.* 1988;5:271–295.

14. Moore EE, Moore FA. Immediate enteral nutrition following multisystem trauma. *J Am Coll Nutr.* 1991;10:633–648.

15. Alexander JW, MacMillan BG, Stinnett JD, et al. Beneficial effects of aggressive protein feeding in severely burned children. *Ann Surg.* 1980;192:505–517.

16. Mochizuki H, Trocki O, Dominioni L, et al. Mechanism of prevention of postburn hypermetabolism and catabolism by early enteral feeding. *Ann Surg.* 1984;200:297–310.

17. Harris JA, Benedict FG. *A Biometric Study of Basal Metabolism in Man.* Washington, DC: Carnegie Institute of Washington, Publication no. 279; 1919.

18. Long CL, Schaffel N, Geiger JW, et al. Metabolic response to injury and illness: estimation of energy and protein needs from indirect calorimetry. *J Paren Enter Nutr.* 1979;3:452–456.

19. Shanbhogue RLK, Chwals WJ, Weintraub M, et al. Parenteral nutrition in the surgical patient. *Br J Surg.* 1987;74:172–180.

20. Curreri PW, Richmond D, Marvin J, Baxter CR. Dietary requirements of patients with major burns. *J Am Diet Assoc.* 1974;65:415–417.

21. Hunter DC, Jaksic T, Lewis D, et al. Resting energy expenditure in the critically ill: estimation versus measurement. *Br J Surg.* 1988;75:875–878.

22. Ireton-Jones CS. Evaluation of energy expenditures in obese patients. *Nutr Clin Prac.* 1989;4:127–129.

23. Quebbeman EF, Ausman RK, Scheneider TC. A re-evaluation of energy expenditure during parenteral nutrition. *Ann Surg.* 1982;195:283–286.

24. Foster GD, Knox LS, Dempsey DT, Mullen JL. Caloric requirements in total parenteral nutrition. *J Am Coll Nutr.* 1987;6:231–253.

25. Dempsey DT, Guenter P, Mullen JL, et al. Energy expenditure in acute trauma to the head with and without barbiturate therapy. *Surg Gynecol Obstet.* 1985;160:128–134.

26. Weissman C, Kemper M, Damask MC, et al. Effect of routine intensive care interactions on metabolic rate. *Chest.* 1984;86:815–818.

27. Winkler MF, Pomp A, Caldwell MD, Albina JE. Energy expenditure in TPN patients. Presented at the American Dietetic Association; September, 1988; San Francisco, Calif.

28. Liggett SB, St. John RE, Lefrak SS. Determination of resting energy expenditure utilizing the thermodilution pulmonary artery catheter. *Chest.* 1987;91:562–566.

29. Bursztein S, Elwyn DH, Askanazi J, Kinney JM, eds. *Energy Metabolism, Indirect Calorimetry, and Nutrition.* Baltimore, Md: Williams & Wilkins; 1989.

30. Wolfe RR, Goodenough RD, Burke JF, Wolfe MH. Response of protein and urea kinetics in burn patients to different levels of protein intake. *Ann Surg.* 1983;197:163–172.

31. Greig PD, Elwyn DH, Askanazi J, Kinney JM. Parenteral nutrition in septic patients: effect of increasing nitrogen intake. *Am J Clin Nutr.* 1987;46:1040–1047.

32. Shaw JE, Wildbore M, Wolfe RR. Whole body protein kinetics in severely septic patients. *Ann Surg.* 1987;205:288–294.

33. Clifton GL, Robertson CS, Crossman RG. The metabolic response to severe head injury. *J Neurosurg.* 1984;60:687–696.

34. American Medical Association, Dept of Foods and Nutrition. Multivitamin preparations for parenteral use: a statement by the Nutrition Advisory Group. *J Paren Enter Nutr.* 1979;3:258–261.

35. American Medical Association, Dept of Foods and Nutrition. Guidelines for essential trace element preparations for parenteral use: a statement by an expert panel. *JAMA.* 1979;241:2051–2054.

36. Winkler MF, Albina JE. Vitamin status of TPN patients. *J Paren Enter Nutr.* 1990;14:16S.

37. Saito H, Trocki O, Alexander JW, et al. The effect of route of nutrient administration on the nutritional state, catabolic hormone secretion, and gut mucosal integrity after burn injury. *J Paren Enter Nutr.* 1987;11:1–7.

38. Alverdy JC, Chi HS, Sheldon GF. The effect of parenteral nutrition on gastrointestinal immunity. *Ann Surg.* 1985;202:681–684.

39. Lowry SF. The route of feeding influences injury responses. *J Trauma.* 1990;30:S10–S15.

40. Moore FA, Feliciano DV, Andrassy RJ, et al. Early enteral feeding compared with parenteral reduces postoperative septic complications. *Ann Surg.* 1992;216:172–183.

41. Wilmore DW, Smith RJ, O'Dwyer ST, et al. The gut: a central organ after surgical stress. *Surgery.* 1988;104:917–923.

42. Deitch EA, McIntyre Bridges R. Effect of stress and trauma on bacterial translocation from the gut. *J Surg Res.* 1987;42:536–542.

43. Alverdy JC, Aoys E, Moss GS. Total parenteral nutrition promotes bacterial translocation from the gut. *Surgery.* 1988;104:185–190.

44. Askanazi J, Rosenbaum S, Hyman AI, et al. Respiratory changes induced by the large glucose loads of TPN. *JAMA.* 1980;243:1444–1447.

45. Talpers SS, Romberger DJ, Bunce SB, Pingleton SK. Nutritionally associated increased carbon dioxide reduction: excess total calories versus high proportion of carbohydrate calories. *Chest.* 1992;102:551–555.

46. Weinsier R, Krumdieck CL. Death resulting from overzealous TPN: the refeeding syndrome revisited. *Am J Clin Nutr.* 1981;34:393–399.

47. Cerra FB, Cheung NK, Fischer JF, et al. Disease specific amino acid infusion (FO80) in hepatic encephalopathy: a prospective, randomized, double blind controlled trial. *J Paren Enter Nutr.* 1985;9:288–295.

48. Wahren J, Denis J, Desurmont P. Is intravenous administration of branched amino acids effective in the treatment of hepatic encephalopathy? A multicenter study. *Hepatology.* 1987;3:475–480.

49. Freund H, Dienstag J, Lehrich J, et al. Infusion of branched-chain enriched amino acid solution in patients with hepatic encephalopathy. *Ann Surg.* 1982;196:209–220.

50. Stehle P, Zander J, Mertes N, et al. Effect of parenteral glutamine peptide supplements on muscle glutamine loss and nitrogen balance after major surgery. *Lancet.* 1989;1:231–233.

51. Hammarqvist F, Wernerman J, Ali R, et al. Addition of glutamine to total parenteral nutrition after elective abdominal surgery spares free glutamine in muscle, counteracts the fall in muscle protein synthesis, and improves nitrogen balance. *Ann Surg.* 1989;209:455–461.

52. Ziegler TR, Young LS, Benfell K, et al. Clinical and metabolic efficacy of glutamine-supplemented parenteral nutrition after bone marrow transplant. *Ann Intern Med.* 1992;116:821–828.

53. Jeevanandam M, Ramias L, Shamos RF, Schiller WR. Decreased growth hormone levels in the catabolic phase of severe injury. *Surgery.* 1992;111:495–502.

54. Ziegler TR, Rombeau JL, Young LS, et al. Recombinant human growth hormone enhances the metabolic efficacy of parenteral nutrition: a double-blind, randomized controlled study. *J Clin Endocrinol Metab.* 1992;74:865–873.

55. Wilmore DW. Catabolic illness: strategies for enhancing recovery. *N Engl J Med.* 1991;325:695–702.

56. Standards of practice for nutrition support dietitians. *Nutr Clin Prac.* 1990;5:74–78.

57. Standards of practice: nutrition support nurse. *Nutr Clin Prac.* 1988;3:78–80.

58. Standards of practice: nutrition support pharmacist. *Nutr Clin Prac.* 1987;2:166–169.

59. Standards of practice: nutrition support physician. *Nutr Clin Prac.* 1988;3:154–156.

60. Mirtallo JM, Powell CR, Campbell SM, et al. Cost-effective nutrition support. *Nutr Clin Prac.* 1987;2:142–151.

61. Joint Commission on Accreditation of Healthcare Organizations. Characteristics of clinical indicators. *Quality Rev Bull.* 1989;15:330–339.

62. Skipper A. Collecting data for clinical indicators. *Nutr Clin Prac.* 1991;6:156–158.

Chapter 17

Geriatric Care

Charlette R. Gallagher-Allred

OVERVIEW

Good nutritional status contributes immeasurably to the quality of life of our nation's elderly population.[1] Conversely, poor nutritional status increases the number and severity of medical complications and contributes to early mortality, which not only detracts from quality of life but increases health care costs as well.[2] The role of the dietitian in caring for elderly persons involves assessing their nutritional well-being and implementing practices that can improve quality of life, minimize undesirable health consequences, and decrease health care costs caused by poor nutritional status. Three health care settings where dietitians frequently care for the elderly—long-term care facilities, home care programs, and palliative care (hospice) programs—will be discussed in this chapter.

LONG-TERM CARE

Issues in Long-Term Care

The growth and future of the long-term care industry in the United States are expected to be influenced by several factors. First is the aging of the U.S. population. As expected, the number of elderly living in long-term care facilities has risen over the past two decades[3] as the average age of the U.S. population has increased[4] and as the number of elderly, especially those over 85 years of age, has increased.[5] Second is the issue of health care costs. As cost constraints impinge on acute care facilities, incentives to limit length of stay are causing hospitals to discharge recuperating patients who still require skilled nursing care and advanced medical technologies to long-term care facilities that have skilled or subacute care units.[6] Indeed, Neu and Harrison[7] document that long-term care facilities are receiving more acutely ill patients than previously, and that the Medicare users are the sickest patients in each diagnosis-related group (DRG) category found within the skilled nursing facility. Third is the issue of increased regulation by governmental and insurance agencies and its impact on reimbursement. Regulations are rooted in the concept that quality of care must be high and payment for services must be reasonable and linked to care that is necessary.[8] In 1986 an Institute of Medicine (IOM) study documented concerns about the quality of care in U.S. nursing homes.[9] In 1987 the major changes suggested in the IOM study became Public Law 100-203, better known as Omnibus Reconciliation Act (OBRA) '87; amendments in 1989 and 1990, and issuance of the final regulations in 1991, further refined the original law. Today nursing homes are seeking to adhere to the guidelines for surveyors[10] that interpret the rules and regulations of OBRA and serve as standards by which nursing homes operate and receive reimbursement from federal and state Medicare and Medicaid programs. Fourth is the issue of quality of life and patient self-determination rights, or the advocated right to control one's personal health care decisions and to refuse medical treatment particularly through the use of advance directives.[11] This issue, among others, has contributed to the development of the home care industry in the United States.

The Role of the Dietitian in Long-Term Care

Just as the issues identified in the preceding paragraph are influencing the long-term care industry today, they influence the role of the dietitian in long-term care. There is a need for experienced dietitians with clinical expertise in providing cost-effective nutrition care for acutely and chronically ill elderly patients and with management expertise in initiating innovative, marketable dietary services to generate revenue.[12] Indeed, the diversified dietitian with expertise in quality food service and in achieving a dining experience that will maximize resident satisfaction can perform an invaluable marketing service, especially for facilities that wish to attract privately paying residents.[13]

The nutritional needs of long-term care residents today are highly demanding. Many patients present to nursing homes with malnutrition or develop malnutrition over time in long-term care facilities, and require medical nutrition therapy, including enteral and parenteral nutrition support, to optimize medical care. The number of tube-fed and parenterally fed residents, and the number of residents requiring specialized medical nutritional products as an adjunct to medical therapy, is high and rising. Therefore the long-term care dietitian must have up-to-date knowledge of the core science of nutrition and advances in nutrition support. With the plethora of prescribed and over-the-counter medications that elderly patients often take, nutrient–drug interactions are common and require examination by the dietitian and other health care professionals in order to minimize their potential negative outcomes. Additionally, the number of chronically ill residents who require assistance with activities of daily living, especially the post-stroke patient and the feeble patient who tires easily because of cardiopulmonary disease or cancer, has resulted in an increase in the number of residents who must be fed or assisted in eating. The dietitian's responsibilities therefore extend to developing a multidisciplinary feeding program and instructing nursing staff on feeding techniques. Also critical is the dietitian's expertise in quality of life issues and in helping residents and their families understand and make their wishes known concerning advance directives. Once sound food service and clinical nutrition programs are initiated, a system to monitor their success is needed, and dietitians are positioned to assume responsibilities for quality assurance and total quality management functions throughout the nursing home.[14]

Nutritional Screening and Assessment

OBRA '87[15] mandated that a long-term care facility that receives governmental monies must conduct, initially and periodically, a comprehensive, accurate, standardized, reproducible assessment of each resident's functional capacity. The assessment must include, among other components, the resident's nutritional and hydration status and requirements. OBRA directed the Health Care Financing Administration (HCFA) to define what would constitute an adequate assessment and to develop a process by which an interdisciplinary care plan would be developed from such an assessment. Subsequently, a resident assessment instrument was developed, which includes a Minimum Data Set (MDS). The broad-based MDS form includes information common to all nursing home patients, such as identification and background information, and data on cognitive patterns, communication/hearing patterns, vision patterns, physical functioning ability, continence, psychosocial well-being, mood and behavior patterns, activity pursuit patterns, disease diagnoses, health conditions, oral/nutritional status, dental status, skin condition, medication use, and special treatments and procedures. The MDS is a basic screening tool that identifies the resident's overall strengths, weaknesses, and risk factors associated with possible functional decline.

The federally developed MDS form (and subsequently several state-developed MDS-Plus forms) includes several questions about the resident's oral, nutritional, hydration, and skin status. Problems with chewing, swallowing, and mouth pain are elicited. Height, weight, and recent weight loss are recorded. Nutritional problems are noted, such as complaint about the taste of food, insufficient fluid and food consumption, and complaint of hunger. Presence of nutritional approaches, such as parenteral or enteral feeding tube, mechanically altered diet, therapeutic diet, need for special feeding equipment, and need for dietary supplements between meals, is also recorded. The MDS and MDS-Plus forms do not elicit all the information that is necessary to assess completely the resident's nutritional and hydration status or identify dietary needs. Therefore an additional nutritional assessment form is usually needed.[16]

Nutritional screens and assessments for today's long-term care residents need to be sophisticated because patient profiles are often highly complex. An initial nutrition screen performed by an admissions coordinator, nurse, dietary manager or technician, or food service supervisor at the time of the patient's admission to the facility may include information about the patient's height and weight; current diet order and previous dietary modifications; food intolerances, preferences, and religious, cultural, and ethnic requests; and ability to chew, swallow, and self-feed. Many long-term care facilities have found that the Determine Your Nutritional Health checklist (Exhibit 17–1) and the Level I Screen (Exhibit 17–2), developed by the Nutrition Screening Initiative, can effectively serve as a nutrition screen for long-term care residents upon admission. These tools can be especially helpful to the dietitian when they are completed by a discharge planner in an acute care facility prior to the resident's admission to the nursing facility or when they are completed by the resident, resident's family, or nursing staff upon admission to the nursing home.[17]

A more in-depth nutritional assessment, performed on admission and at least yearly thereafter, should include information about the resident's weight history; anthropometric, clinical, and laboratory indicators of nutriture; presence of conditions (such as pressure ulcers, dehydration, pulmonary disease, renal disease, cardiac disease, malabsorption, hypothyroidism, and multiple medication usage) that affect nutrient needs; a calculation of the resident's caloric expenditure, protein needs, and fluid requirements; and an evaluation of changes in the resident's nutritional condition since the last assessment. A nutritional assessment is incomplete until quality of life parameters (such as advance directives concerning syringe, tube, and parenteral feedings, and what, where, when, and with whom the resident desires to eat) are elicited from the resident and/or family. The comprehensive nutritional assessment form in Exhibit 17–3 includes questions that address quality of care, quality of life, and resident rights issues mandated by OBRA. Much of the information included on this form can be gathered by a dietary manager or dietetic technician from the medical record and interview with the resident and/or family with instruction from the dietitian; a dietitian or technician can complete the evaluation section of the form from the gathered information.

Exhibit 17–1 DETERMINE Your Nutritional Health Checklist

The Warning Signs of poor nutritional health are often overlooked. Use this checklist to find out if you or someone you know is at nutritional risk.

Read the statements below. Circle the number in the yes column for those that apply to you or someone you know. For each yes answer, score the number in the box. Total your nutritional score.

DETERMINE YOUR NUTRITIONAL HEALTH

	YES
I have an illness or condition that made me change the kind and/or amount of food I eat.	2
I eat fewer than 2 meals per day.	3
I eat few fruits or vegetables, or milk products.	2
I have 3 or more drinks of beer, liquor or wine almost every day.	2
I have tooth or mouth problems that make it hard for me to eat.	2
I don't always have enough money to buy the food I need.	4
I eat alone most of the time.	1
I take 3 or more different prescribed or over-the-counter drugs a day.	1
Without wanting to, I have lost or gained 10 pounds in the last 6 months.	2
I am not always physically able to shop, cook and/or feed myself.	2
TOTAL	

Total Your Nutritional Score. If it's—

0-2   **Good!** Recheck your nutritional score in 6 months.

3–5   **You are at moderate nutritional risk.** See what can be done to improve your eating habits and lifestyle. Your office on aging, senior nutrition program, senior citizens center or health department can help. Recheck your nutritional score in 3 months.

6 or more   **You are at high nutritional risk.** Bring this checklist the next time you see your doctor, dietitian or other qualified health or social service professional. Talk with them about any problems you may have. Ask for help to improve your nutritional health.

These materials developed and distributed by the Nutrition Screening Initiative, a project of:

 AMERICAN ACADEMY OF FAMILY PHYSICIANS

 THE AMERICAN DIETETIC ASSOCIATION

 NATIONAL COUNCIL ON THE AGING, INC.

Remember that warning signs suggest risk, but do not represent diagnosis of any condition. Turn the page to learn more about the Warning Signs of poor nutritional health.

continues

Exhibit 17–1 continued

> **The Nutrition Checklist is based on the Warning Signs described below. Use the word <u>DETERMINE</u> to remind you of the Warning Signs.**
>
> # Disease
> Any disease, illness or chronic condition that causes you to change the way you eat, or makes it hard for you to eat, puts your nutritional health at risk. Four out of five adults have chronic diseases that are affected by diet. Confusion or memory loss that keeps getting worse is estimated to affect one out of five or more older adults. This can make it hard to remember what, when or if you've eaten. Feeling sad or depressed, which happens to about one in eight older adults, can cause big changes in appetite, digestion, energy level, weight and well-being.
>
> # Eating poorly
> Eating too little and eating too much both lead to poor health. Eating the same foods day after day or not eating fruit, vegetables and milk products daily will also cause poor nutritional health. One in five adults skips meals daily. Only 13% of adults eat the minimum amount of fruits and vegetables needed. One in four older adults drinks too much alcohol. Many health problems become worse if you drink more than one or two alcoholic beverages per day.
>
> # Tooth loss/mouth pain
> A healthy mouth, teeth and gums are needed to eat. Missing, loose or rotten teeth or dentures which don't fit well or cause mouth sores make it hard to eat.
>
> # Economic hardship
> As many as 40% of older Americans have incomes of less than $6,000 per year. Having less—or choosing to spend less—than $25–$30 per week for food makes it very hard to get the foods you need to stay healthy.
>
> # Reduced social contact
> One-third of all older people live alone. Being with people daily has a positive effect on morale, well-being and eating.
>
> # Multiple medicines
> Many older Americans must take medicines for health problems. Almost half of older Americans take multiple medicines daily. Growing old may change the way we respond to drugs. The more medicines you take, the greater the chance for side effects such as increased or decreased appetite, change in taste, constipation, weakness, drowsiness, diarrhea, nausea, and others. Vitamins or minerals when taken in large doses act like drugs and can cause harm. Alert your doctor to everything you take.
>
> # Involuntary weight loss/gain
> Losing or gaining a lot of weight when you are not trying to do so is an important warning sign that must not be ignored. Being overweight or underweight also increases your chance of poor health.

continues

Exhibit 17–1 continued

NEEDS ASSISTANCE IN SELF CARE

Although most older people are able to eat, one of every five has trouble walking, shopping, buying and cooking food, especially as they get older.

ELDER YEARS ABOVE AGE 80

Most older people lead full and productive lives. But as age increases, risk of frailty and health problems increase. Checking your nutritional health regularly makes good sense.

 The Nutrition Screening Initiative, 1010 Wisconsin Avenue, NW, Suite 800, Washington, DC 20007
The Nutrition Screening Initiative is funded in part by a grant from Ross Laboratories, a division of Abbott Laboratories

Courtesy of The Nutrition Screening Initiative, Washington, DC.

A nutritional assessment is most accurate and useful when several disciplines are involved in its completion. For example, the nursing staff is often the best judge of the resident's eating ability and need for assisted feeding and devices. The physician evaluates both the presence of chronic or acute illnesses or conditions that affect the resident's nutritional status and the possible signs and symptoms of malnutrition; the physician and pharmacist perform a medication review that can identify possible food-nutrient-drug interactions. A dysphagia evaluation by the speech therapist/pathologist, an upper extremity evaluation and an evaluation of the need for assistive eating devices by the occupational therapist, and an oral and dental assessment by the dentist are invaluable services that can contribute to the development of a plan of care that will maximize the resident's nutritional status, quality of care, and quality of life.

Malnutrition and the Geriatric Patient

Protein-energy malnutrition (PEM) is prevalent in many long-term care institutions[18,19]; its risk factors are multifaceted (Exhibit 17–4). Characteristics common to elderly persons diagnosed with PEM are (1) age 70 years or older, (2) low to marginal income, (3) inadequate social support structure, and (4) a relatively recent change in mental status.[20] Because PEM resembles the signs and symptoms of the aging process, PEM may be overlooked without rigorous assessment.

A geriatric syndrome recently termed *failure to thrive*[21] is currently under study by the National Institute on Aging (NIA).[22] This syndrome is loosely

Exhibit 17–2 Nutrition Screening Initiative Level 1 Screen

Level 1 Screen

Body Weight

Measure height to the nearest inch and weight to the nearest pound. Record the values below and mark them on the Body Mass Index (BMI) scale to the right. Then use a straight edge (ruler) to connect the two points and circle the spot where this straight line crosses the center line (body mass index). Record the number below.

Healthy older adults should have a BMI between 24 and 27.

Height (in):_____
Weight (lbs):_____
Body Mass Index:_____
(number from center column)

Check any boxes that are true for the individual:

❑ Has lost or gained 10 pounds (or more) in the past 6 months.

❑ Body mass index <24

❑ Body mass index >27

For the remaining sections, please ask the individual which of the statements (if any) is true for him or her and place a check by each that applies.

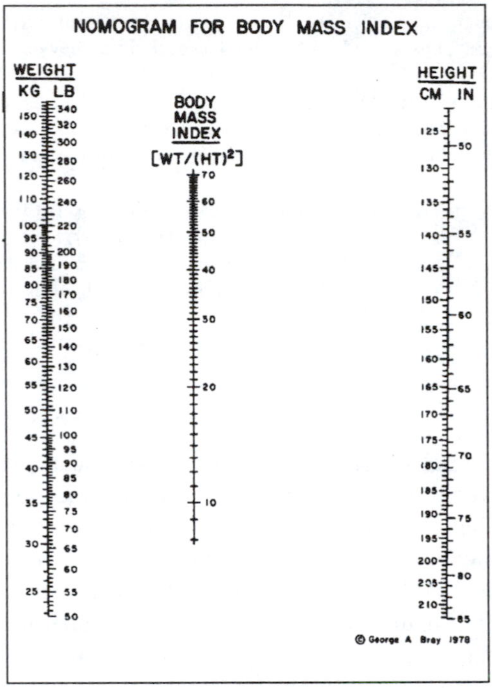

NOMOGRAM FOR BODY MASS INDEX

WEIGHT KG LB

HEIGHT CM IN

BODY MASS INDEX

$[WT/(HT)^2]$

© George A Bray 1978

Eating Habits

❑ Does not have enough food to eat each day

❑ Usually eats alone

❑ Does not eat anything on one or more days each month

❑ Has poor appetite

❑ Is on a special diet

❑ Eats vegetables two or fewer times daily

❑ Eats milk or milk products once or not at all daily

❑ Eats fruit or drinks fruit juice once or not at all daily

❑ Eats breads, cereals, pasta, rice, or other grains five or fewer times daily

❑ Has difficulty chewing or swallowing

❑ Has more than one alcoholic drink per day (if woman); more than two drinks per day (if man)

❑ Has pain in mouth, teeth, or gums

LEVEL I SCREEN   Name :   Date:

continues

Exhibit 17–2 continued

A physician should be contacted if the individual has gained or lost 10 pounds unexpectedly or without intending to during the past 6 months. A physician should also be notified if the individual's body mass index is above 27 or below 22.

Living Environment

☐ Lives on an income of less than $6000 per year (per individual in the household)

☐ Lives alone

☐ Is housebound

☐ Is concerned about home security

☐ Lives in a home with inadequate heating or cooling

☐ Does not have a stove and/or refrigerator

☐ Is unable or prefers not to spend money on food (<$25-30 per person spent on food each week)

Functional Status

Usually or always needs assistance with (check each that apply):

☐ Bathing

☐ Dressing

☐ Grooming

☐ Toileting

☐ Eating

☐ Walking or moving about

☐ Traveling (outside the home)

☐ Preparing food

☐ Shopping for food or other necessities

If you have checked one or more statements on this screen, the individual you have interviewed may be at risk for poor nutritional status. Please refer this individual to the appropriate health care or social service professional in your area. For example, a dietitian should be contacted for problems with selecting, preparing, or eating a healthy diet, or a dentist if the individual experiences pain or difficulty when chewing or swallowing. Those individuals whose income, lifestyle, or functional status may endanger their nutritional and overall health should be referred to available community services: home-delivered meals, congregate meal programs, transportation services, counseling services (alcohol abuse, depression, bereavement, etc.), home health care agencies, day care programs, etc.

Please repeat this screen at least once each year--sooner if the individual has a major change in his or her health, income, immediate family (e.g., spouse dies), or functional status.

These materials developed by the Nutrition Screening Initiative.

Courtesy of The Nutrition Screening Initiative, Washington, DC.

Exhibit 17–3 Comprehensive Nutritional Assessment Form

NUTRITIONAL ASSESSMENT

Diagnosis _____

Sex: _____ Age: _____ yrs   Admission Date: _____

Diet order (date): _____

    Perceived Rationale for Diet Order:_____

Route: Oral: ☐   Feeding tube: ☐   Parenteral/IV: ☐   Combinations: _____

    Oral supplementation: ☐   Describe: _____

Height: _____ Weight: _____ Ideal body weight: _____

Resident's desired body weight: _____ Interdisciplinary team goal weight: _____

Percent weight change since last assessment: Intentional change?   Yes ☐   No ☐

    New assessment: ☐   Yearly assessment: ☐   Explain change:_____

ABILITY TO PROVIDE FOOD PREFERENCE/OPINIONS ABOUT MEALS/MEALTIMES/DIET

Method of Communication:

    ☐ Oral   ☐ Writing

    ☐ Communication board   ☐ Signs/gestures/sounds

    ☐ Unable to communicate and make self understood

    ☐ Information from family/others   (Name): _____

Ability to understand others:	Adequate ☐	Inadequate ☐	Variable ☐
Visual ability to see tray food:	Adequate ☐	Inadequate ☐	Variable ☐
Visual ability to see written menu:	Adequate ☐	Inadequate ☐	Variable ☐

Food preferences: _____

Food allergies/sensitivities: _____

Food dislikes: _____

Likes diet order:	Yes ☐	No ☐	Unable to determine ☐
Understands reason for diet order:	Yes ☐	No ☐	Unable to determine ☐
Likes foods offered on menu:	Yes ☐	No ☐	Unable to determine ☐
Has difficulty choosing what to eat:	Yes ☐	No ☐	Unable to determine ☐
Likes foods received at snacks:	Yes ☐	No ☐	Unable to determine ☐
Receives food preferences:	Yes ☐	No ☐	Unable to determine ☐
Likes time of meals/snacks:	Yes ☐	No ☐	Unable to determine ☐
Chooses (or likes) meal partners:	Yes ☐	No ☐	Unable to determine ☐

Presence of advanced directives including feeding restrictions: Yes ☐   No ☐

    Signed by:_____   Date:_____

Change since last assessment: Yes ☐   No ☐   New assessment ☐

    Explain: _____

ABILITY TO SELF-FEED

Route of feeding: Self-feed ☐   Self-feed with assistance ☐   Unable to self-feed ☐

Feeding devices: _____

Able to use feeding devices:	Yes ☐	No ☐	Devices not needed ☐
Difference in feeding self in mornings and evenings:	Yes ☐	No ☐	Does not self-feed ☐

Physical functioning disabilities affecting ability to self-feed:

Bedfast all or most of the time:	Yes ☐	On dominant side ☐	No ☐
Hemiplegia/hemiparesis/quadriplegia:	Yes ☐	On dominant side ☐	No ☐
Arm: partial or total loss of voluntary movement:	Yes ☐	On dominant side ☐	No ☐
Hand: lack of dexterity or presence of contractures:	Yes ☐	On dominant side ☐	No ☐
Trunk: partial or total loss of ability to position:	Yes ☐	On dominant side ☐	No ☐

    Amputee (explain):_____

    Other: _____

Observation of ability to self-feed:_____

Resident desires to increase self-feeding: Yes ☐   No ☐   Unknown ☐   N/A ☐

Resident believes is capable of increased independence in self-feeding: Yes ☐   N/A ☐   No ☐

Direct care staff believe resident is capable of increased independence in self-feeding: Yes ☐ No ☐ N/A ☐

Change since last assessment: Yes ☐   No ☐   New assessment ☐

    Explain: _____

NAME _____ PHYSICIAN _____ ROOM NUMBER _____

    Last   First   Middle

Exhibit 17–3 continued

ABILITY TO EAT AS DESIRED
Forgets meals: Yes ☐ No ☐
Eats at desired place: Yes ☐ No ☐ Unable to determine desired place ☐ Usual place for meals _____
Eats away from facility on occasion: Yes ☐ No ☐ How often _____
Factors affecting ability to eat meals in desired place: None ☐
      ☐ Behavioral problems (eg, throws/steals food, verbally disruptive)
      ☐ Mobility limitations   ☐ Psychosocial problems (eg, fear)
      ☐ Facility limitations   ☐ Wanders
      ☐ Resident's safety   ☐ Other _____
Change since last assessment: Yes ☐ No ☐ New assessment ☐
    Explain: _____

USUAL FOOD AND FLUID INTAKE
Food intake prior to admission: Good ☐ Fair ☐ Poor ☐ Unknown ☐
Resists assistance with feeding: Yes ☐ No ☐ N/A ☐
Consumes adequate fluid to prevent dehydration: Yes ☐ No ☐
Order to force or limit fluids: Yes to force ☐ No ☐ Yes to limit ☐
Regularly complains of hunger: Yes ☐ No ☐ If yes, when _____
Complains about taste of many foods: Yes ☐ No ☐
Leaves 25+% food uneaten at most meals: Yes ☐ No ☐
Refuses meals/substitutes/supplements: Yes ☐ No ☐ How often _____
Consumes varied well-balanced diet daily: Yes ☐ No ☐
    _____ % time eats 4-6 oz meat/fish/poultry/meat substitute
    _____ % time eats/drinks 2 servings dairy products
    _____ % time eats 4 servings breads/cereals/grains
    _____ % time eats 2 vegetables (1 deep-yellow or leafy-green)
    _____ % time eats 2 fruits (1 citrus)
    _____ % time eats substitute if less than 75% of meal eaten; takes oral supplement as ordered
    _____ % time eats evening snack
Consumes foods other than at mealtimes: Yes ☐ No ☐ Sometimes ☐
    Eats or drinks at activities: Yes ☐ No ☐ Sometimes ☐
    Has food at bedside: Yes ☐ No ☐ Sometimes ☐
    Food brought in from outside facility: Yes ☐ No ☐ Sometimes ☐
    Uses vending machine: Yes ☐ No ☐ Sometimes ☐
Receives foods consistent with cultural/ethnic/religious background: Yes ☐ No ☐
Enjoys relationships with staff/family who feed: Yes ☐ No ☐ Unknown ☐ N/A ☐
Food becomes unpalatable or staff removes tray before resident has finished eating: Yes ☐ No ☐
Change since last assessment: Yes ☐ No ☐ New assessment ☐
    Explain: _____

DISEASES/CONDITIONS THAT DECREASE NUTRIENT AND FLUID INTAKE: None ☐
_____ Alzheimer's disease or other dementias   _____ Inadequate environment/staff at facility
_____ Anorexia   _____ Lethargy-tiredness
_____ Complaint about taste/variety of foods   _____ Nausea
_____ Depression/anxiety   _____ Pain
_____ Food preferences/idiosyncrasies   _____ Possible food-drug interaction
_____ Frequent refusal to eat   _____ Shortness of breath
_____ Impaired mentation   _____ Unrealistic fear of food or eating
Change since last assessment: Yes ☐ No ☐ New assessment ☐
    Explain: _____

DISEASES/CONDITIONS THAT INCREASE NUTRIENT AND FLUID REQUIREMENTS: None ☐
_____ Burns   _____ Motor agitation (pacing, wandering, tremors)
_____ Cancer   _____ Pneumonia
_____ Emphysema/asthma/COPD   _____ Pressure ulcers/stasis ulcers
_____ Fractures (date/location _____)   _____ Septicemia/infection/fever
_____ Hyperthyroidism   _____ Surgical wounds (date _____)
_____ Malabsorption/diarrhea/ostomy losses   _____ Vomiting
Increased requirements for which nutrients? _____
Change since last assessment: Yes ☐ No ☐ New assessment ☐
    Explain: _____

continues

Exhibit 17–3 continued

DISEASES/CONDITIONS THAT MAY SUGGEST NEED FOR THERAPEUTIC DIET OR FOOD TEXTURE MODIFICATION: None ☐

_____ Cardiovascular disease/stroke
_____ Chewing problems
    _____ facial paralysis
    _____ broken, loose, decayed or missing teeth
    _____ presence of ill-fitting dentures
    _____ refusal to chew
    _____ other _____
_____ Congestive heart failure
_____ Dehydration
_____ Diabetes mellitus/gastroparesis
_____ Edema/ascites
_____ Gastrointestinal surgery/food intolerances
(explain) _____
_____ Hypertension
_____ Immune disorders/immunosuppression/AIDS
_____ Liver failure/alcoholic liver disease
_____ Other _____

_____ Mouth problems
    _____ inability to suck through a straw
    _____ oral abscess
    _____ swollen or bleeding gums
    _____ toothache
    _____ other _____
_____ Renal failure
_____ Swallowing problems
    _____ fear of choking
    _____ history/potential for choking or aspiration
    _____ refusal to swallow
    _____ inability to or difficulty in swallowing
    _____ pain on swallowing
    _____ pockets food in cheeks
    _____ cannot swallow thick liquids
    _____ cannot swallow thin liquids

Change since last assessment: Yes ☐   No ☐   New assessment ☐
    Explain:_____

DISEASES/CONDITIONS THAT MAY SUGGEST NEED FOR SUPPLEMENTATION: None ☐

_____ Alcohol/drug abuse
_____ Anemia/internal bleeding
_____ Constipation/fecal impaction (chronic)
_____ Dehydration (ICD Code # _____)
_____ Erratic food consumption
_____ Fever
_____ Malabsorption/diarrhea (chronic)

_____ Malnutrition (ICD Code # _____)
_____ Osteoporosis/fractures
_____ Polypharmacy
_____ Pressure ulcers/stasis ulcers
    (number _____ stage _____)
_____ Urinary tract and other infections
_____ Other _____

Which nutrients may need to be supplemented? _____
Change since last assessment: Yes ☐   No ☐   New assessment ☐
    Explain:_____

MEDICATIONS AND TREATMENTS/PROCEDURES THAT AFFECT NUTRITIONAL STATUS OR DIET ORDER
(Identify name, dose, frequency)

Medications   None ☐

_____ Analgesics _____
_____ Antacids _____
_____ Antibiotics _____
_____ Anticoagulants _____
_____ Anticonvulsants _____
    _____
_____ Antihypertensives _____
    _____
_____ Anti-Parkinsonian _____
_____ Cardiac glycosides _____
_____ Diuretics _____
_____ Insulin/hypoglycemic agents _____
    _____
_____ Laxatives _____
_____ Lipid lowering _____
_____ Non-steroidals _____
_____ Psychotherapeutic drugs _____
    _____
_____ Steroids _____
_____ Vitamin/mineral supplements _____
    _____
_____ Other _____
_____ Possible food-drug interactions (identify) _____

Treatments/procedures   None ☐

_____ Catheter (indwelling urinary) _____
_____ Chemotherapy _____
_____ Dialysis _____
_____ Enema _____
_____ Isolation _____
_____ Ostomy (type) _____
_____ Oxygen _____
_____ Prosthesis (type) _____
_____ Radiation _____
_____ Speech therapy _____
_____ Suctioning (oral) _____
_____ Suctioning (gastric) _____
_____ Other _____

continues

Exhibit 17–3 continued

LABORATORY DATA INDICATIVE OF NUTRITIONAL STATUS   Date(s) _____

	High	Low	WNL			High	Low	WNL
Hgb (g/dL)					Serum Na+ (mEq/L)			
Hct (%)					Serum K+ (mEq/L)			
MCV/MCH (m³/μμg)					BUN (mg/dL)			
Total Lymph Count					Creatinine (mg/dL)			
Glucose (mg/dL)					Osmolality (mosm/kg)			
Albumin (g/dL)					Blood pressure			
Cholesterol (mg/dL)					Thyroid (T3/T4/FTI)			

Other: _____

Change since last assessment: Yes ☐   No ☐   New assessment ☐
          Explain:_____

SYMPTOMS POTENTIALLY INDICATIVE OF POOR NUTRITIONAL STATUS: None ☐
_____ Cachexia, loss of body fat/muscle   _____ Muscles, wasted, weak, calf pain
_____ Edema, bilateral, generalized   _____ Nails, clubbed, pale nailbeds
_____ Eyes, dull, pale, xerosis   _____ Pressure ulcers/open wounds
_____ Hair, dry, dull, thin, easily plucked   _____ Skin, poor turgor, pale, petechiae, dermatosis
_____ Irritability   _____ Tongue, swollen, dry, scarlet, magenta
_____ Lips/gums, dry, pale, angular fissures   _____ Dry mucous membranes
Change since last assessment: Yes ☐   No ☐   New assessment ☐
          Explain:_____

SUMMARY: LEVEL OF NUTRITIONAL CARE
_____ Basic: Weight within normal/desired/stable range. Lab data essentially within normal range. Medical
          condition stable. Food and fluid intake well-balanced and varied.
_____ Moderate: Weight fluctuates. Lab data consistent with potential for malnutrition. Medical condition
          unstable. Food and/or fluid intake fluctuates.
_____ Intensive: Excessive weight loss or gain. Lab data/diagnosis consistent with potential for or presence of
          malnutrition. Food and/or fluid intake poor. Resident receives tube feeding, has pressure
          ulcers, or is in critical medical condition.
Change since last assessment: Yes ☐   No ☐   New assessment ☐
Summary Rationale or Explanation of Change Since Last Assessment: _____
_____
_____

ESTIMATED DAILY NUTRIENT NEEDS
     REE: _____ kcal   Total energy: _____ kcal   Protein:_____ g   Fluid: _____ mL

GOALS: _____
_____
_____

SUMMARY OF RESIDENT AND FAMILY INPUT INTO NUTRITIONAL CARE: _____
_____
_____

DISCHARGE POTENTIAL   Good ☐   Fair ☐   Poor ☐

          Need for Nutrition Education for Home Care: Yes ☐   No ☐   Unknown ☐

PLAN OF CARE, consistent with assessment and goals, developed/revised on (date): _____

Signature: _____   Date: _____

Exhibit 17–4 Risk Factors for Malnutrition in Long-Term Care

1. Reduced Appetite
   - Reduced taste and smell due to aging or zinc deficiency
   - Anorectic effects of medications
   - Chronic and acute illnesses
   - Depression and dementia
   - Loss of control over meal timing
   - Loss of control over food choices
   - Non-conducive environment (agitated residents, noise, poor climate control, other distractions)
   - Poor food presentation (inadequate temperature, not visually attractive or appetizing)
   - Psychosocial factors (inattention to cultural, ethnic, religious or personal preferences of pre-institutionalization habits)
2. Decreased Nutrient Utilization
   - Increased nutrient need due to acute or chronic disease (cancer, infection, etc.)
   - Decreased calorie intake with attendant decrease of intake of other nutrients (inactivity, decreased body mass/weight, treatment for obesity)
   - Drug/nutrient interaction (decreased food absorption/metabolism)
   - Medical illness (infections, renal failure, COPD, CHF, gastrointestinal disease, malabsorption)
   - Iatrogenic—dietary restriction by physician (calorie restriction, low sodium or cholesterol)
3. Decreased Caloric Need
   - Low body weight
   - Reduced muscle mass
4. Feeding Problems
   - Hand and upper extremity disability (weakness and paralysis, tremor, contractures, arthritis and pain)
   - Dementia and depression
   - Agitation or wandering during meals
   - Delirium or depressed consciousness
   - Weakness of chewing
   - Gum or oral cavity disorder or pain
   - Poor dentition/edentulousness
   - Poorly fitting and lost dentures
   - Dysphagia

Source: Reprinted with permission from Dimant, J, The Psychosocial and Environmental Approach to Nutritional Management in Long Term Care. *Journal of Medical Directors*, Vol. 2, No. 2, p. 53, with permission of the American Medical Directors Association, © 1992.

described by the NIA as consisting of weight loss, decreased appetite, and inactivity, often accompanied by dehydration, depressive symptoms, impaired immune function, and low serum cholesterol. The syndrome is probably multi-factorial in origin, perhaps associated with specific chronic disease processes and acute conditions, micronutrient deficiencies, alterations in endocrine factors affecting metabolism, inflammatory mediators, and depressive changes in mentation. The end result is impaired functional status, morbidity from infection, pressure ulcers, and increased mortality. Research currently is underway to describe the progression of failure to thrive in various specific groups of older persons with different chronic diseases and disabilities, and to elucidate potential differences and commonalities in pathophysiologic mechanisms and clinical course. The effectiveness of nutritional support intervention on the clinical outcome of failure to thrive and loss of appetite has not been rigorously tested.[22] Long-term care dietitians will want to keep abreast of developments in the area of adult failure to thrive.

Laboratory Tests

The nutritional status of elderly residents can be assessed and monitored by biochemical tests (see Chapter 11), anthropometric data (see Chapter 8), dietary intake information (see Chapter 10), and clinical and physical signs and symptoms of nutritional well-being (see Chapter 6).

Protein studies generally include serum albumin, transferrin, and prealbumin. Albumin is assumed to be useful as an indicator of nutrition status because (1) a serum albumin value of less than 2.8 g/dL is related to the development of generalized edema in kwashiorkor,[23] (2) a low serum albumin concentration is assumed to correlate with visceral protein impairment,[24] and (3) a low serum albumin is correlated with poor clinical outcome.[25,26] Additionally, a serum albumin value of less than 3.5 g/dL is a screening criteria for visceral protein depletion and is used to define ICD-9-CM codes for Medicare and Medicaid populations.[27] However, serum albumin as an indicator of visceral protein losses has not been well correlated with reference methods for body composition analysis[28] or functionally significant changes, and albumin is unreliable in identifying clinically significant malnutrition at serum concentrations between 3.1 and 3.5 g/dL.[29] Additionally, with its 17- to 21-day half-life, albumin is not a useful indicator of the effectiveness of nutritional support. Further, and of significance in long-term care, it has long been known that albumin decreases with the aging process.[30–33] Multiple factors also common in long-term care, such as congestive heart failure, trauma, hypoxia, sepsis, renal failure, bedrest, fluid and electrolyte imbalance, hepatic failure, and major surgery, can modify serum albumin levels.

Serum transferrin, with its half-life of eight to ten days, responds more quickly than albumin to nutritional deficiency and repletion with aggressive nutritional support, but it too is unsuitable for use in assessing a rapid response to nutrition support. Like albumin, transferrin decreases with age.[34] It is increased in iron deficiency, but it is reduced in anemia of chronic disease, in inflammation, and in chronic infection, conditions that often affect the elderly nursing home resident.

Prealbumin, also called transthyretin and thyroxine-binding prealbumin, is a transport protein synthesized by the liver, which is transported in the blood complexed with retinol-binding protein and vitamin A. Prealbumin is a sensitive indicator of protein deficiency and repletion because of its rapid two-day turnover rate.[35,36] Despite its superiority as a sensitive and cost-effective marker in identifying nutrition status and monitoring the adequacy of a nutrition support plan,[37] it is more expensive than serum albumin on a multichemistry panel (about $3.00 versus $0.25 per patient).[29] Prealbumin may be elevated in patients who are treated with corticosteroids, which is an important consideration for many patients in long-term care facilities.

A hematological assessment, including a complete blood count with mean corpuscular indices, should be a routine part of assessing a patient's nutritional well-being. Common problems in nursing home residents that limit the ability to assess the severity of anemia include dehydration and polycythemia, caused by chronic obstructive lung disease. Nutritional anemias in the elderly include iron deficiency,[38] folate deficiency, and vitamin B_{12} deficiency.[39] Impaired cognitive function and neuropsychiatric disorders treatable with cobalamin therapy may occur in elderly patients even in the absence of anemia and signs of frank vitamin B_{12} deficiency.[40] When a hemoglobin and hematocrit are low and an elevation in mean corpuscular volume and mean corpuscular hemoglobin is present (indicating a macrocytosis anemia and a potential folate or vitamin B_{12} deficiency), then serum and red blood cell folate tests and a serum vitamin B_{12} test should be evaluated in addition to a dietary intake assessment for folate and vitamin B_{12}. Folate deficiency in the elderly is most commonly caused by low intake of dietary folacin, but it may also be caused by a malabsorption syndrome or drugs, including trimethoprim, diphenylhydantin, barbiturates, cholestyramine, aspirin, and alcohol.[41] The common causes of vitamin B_{12} deficiency in the elderly are pernicious anemia and late effects of gastrectomy or ileal resection, which lead to a severe reduction in vitamin B_{12} absorption.[39]

A hypochromic anemia with low hemoglobin, hematocrit, mean corpuscular volume, and mean corpuscular hemoglobin values indicates the necessity of further studies for iron deficiency, such as serum iron, ferritin, and transferrin. In the elderly, chronic iron deficiency is most often caused by blood loss resulting from drug intake (such as aspirin, nonsteroidal anti-inflammatory drugs, and anticoagulants), hemorrhage from a peptic ulcer, or carcinoma of the colon. Roe admonishes health professionals that "no time should be wasted in assessing the iron intake of an elderly person with evidence of iron deficiency anemia until these and other causes related to blood loss have been excluded."[42(p137)]

A normocytic, normochromic anemia of chronic disease generally is not associated with iron, folate, or vitamin B_{12} deficiencies but probably is associated with chronic illness, including chronic renal or hepatic insufficiency, chronic infection, and bone marrow dyscrasias.[43] Treatment is not nutritional but is directed at the underlying disorder.[44]

A low serum cholesterol level (below 160 mg/dL) has been suggested to be an indicator of poor nutritional status.[45,46] Similarly, tests of the immune system, including total lymphocyte count, have been suggested to be indicators of nutritional status, but they are influenced by a variety of factors that occur with aging and are therefore rarely of definitive assistance in diagnosing malnutrition in the elderly.[42]

Functional Tests and Nutrition Implications

The goal of geriatric care is to keep residents active, independent, and psychologically stable.[47] Therefore a geriatric assessment should focus on the resident's functional and cognitive abilities. The Activities of Daily Living (ADL) Index[48] covers most basic activities required of adults to be independent: maintaining continence, arising, toileting, bathing, dressing, and eating. The ADL Index is most suitable for the aging individual who may be moving from independence to dependence, e.g. from home care to nursing home care. It helps clinicians understand the impact of disease on function and prepares the clinician to assist in making decisions about therapy and support. An Instrumental Activities of Daily Living (IADL) Scale evaluates more sophisticated functions than the ADL Index. It is best used with active individuals living in the community who may require only home care services. It provides information about how well a patient functions in telephoning, shopping, preparing food, housekeeping, handling laundry, using transportation, taking medications, and managing finances.[47]

Normal physiological changes that occur with aging can affect the elderly resident's functional capacity and thereby affect nutritional status. For example, aging is associated with a decline in the cardiac and respiratory output following exercise, which may result in decreased blood and oxygen flow to the gastrointestinal tract and thereby cause satiety rather than hunger following physical activity.[49] Many elderly residents will benefit from relaxation prior to meals.

Anatomic and functional changes of the oral and gastrointestinal tract significantly affect food ingestion and nutrient utilization. Over half of the U.S. elderly population is completely edentulous.[50,51] Mouth pain associated with improperly fitting dentures or poor oral health causes many elderly to consume a limited variety of liquid or soft foods.[52] In addition, a decrease in gustatory and olfactory sensitivity occurs with aging, which is explained by a loss of papillae on the tongue and a loss of taste buds on the papillae.[53,54] A loss of the ability to taste sweet and salt flavors is of significance and results in many elderly patients' complaints that food has no flavor or tastes bitter or sour.[55–57] The implications for nutrition care are not to overly restrict sweet and salty foods unless restriction is both medically necessary and proven effective; indeed, a low-simple-sugar diet for diabetes and glucose intolerance,[58,59] and a no-added-salt diet for salt-sensitive hypertension,[60,61] have been shown to be adequate dietary modifications for these conditions.

The processes of esophageal motility and peristalsis change with age, which can cause dysphagia (difficulty in swallowing). Swallowing normally initiates a peristaltic wave in the esophagus that helps move food toward the stomach, which normally is followed by a relaxation wave that causes the esophageal sphincter to open and food to pass into the stomach. Peristaltic waves decrease with aging, which can allow the esophagus to collect food in its lower portion, resulting in pain and regurgitation.[61] The *Dining Skills*[62] handbook, developed by the Consultant Dietitians in Health Care Facilities (a dietetic practice group of the American Dietetic Association), is an excellent resource in caring for dysphagic residents.

Aging also appears to cause bowel muscle atrophy, which, when accompanied by inactivity, may predispose the elderly patient to constipation.[63] Increasing physical activity and responding at the time of urging to defecate are often the best ways to prevent constipation.[64] A high-fiber diet, accompanied by a high fluid intake, may eliminate the need for expensive laxatives, but may be contraindicated in residents who have muscle atrophy or atonic colon, which is sometimes associated with long-term diabetes mellitus.[65]

Changes in hepatic function with aging include decreased rates of protein synthesis, reduced capacity for gluconeogenesis, and decreased ability to metabolize toxic substances, including alcohol and drugs. Reduced renal function also may occur with age because of a loss of kidney nephrons, changes in tubular function, and decreased blood flow.[66] Creatinine clearance, commonly thought to be representative of renal function, is quite variable among the elderly. Thus a patient should be followed longitudinally to determine how test results change and how significant they may be. Concomitantly, a reduced daily urine flow, increased blood urea concentrations, and diminished excretory and reabsorptive capacity of the renal tubules result in a decreased glomerular filtration rate, which may have implications for fluid and protein intake.[67]

Reduced fluid intake, which can result in dehydration, often occurs in the elderly because of a decreased thirst sensation associated with aging.[68,69] Dehydration can also occur quickly in the elderly patient who has limited total body water reserves because of limited lean body mass. On the other hand, water intoxication can occur with disease states, such as congestive heart failure, renal dysfunction, and cirrhosis.

A loss of total body protein occurs with aging, largely because of decreased skeletal muscle mass, which can be considerably improved by exercise.[70] The reduction in total body protein, skeletal muscle mass, and renal and kidney function may have implications for dietary intake of protein. Since muscle mass often decreases with age, protein requirements might be expected to decrease commensurately. And because renal and kidney functions also decrease with age, it might be expected that decreased protein intake should be recommended. Several nitrogen balance studies, however, have addressed the protein requirements of the elderly, and results are inconsistent.[71] Most studies suggest that the protein needs of healthy elderly adults are met by the Recommended Dietary Allowance (RDA) of 0.8 g protein/kg body weight, but chronic diseases may alter this level to maintain nitrogen balance.[72] Immobile, nonambulatory patients are often in negative nitrogen balance because of inactivity, and extra dietary protein does not reverse this process. The RDA for protein coupled with exercise or physical therapy may, however, help preserve muscle mass and decrease the rate of body protein loss in the elderly. A high-protein diet with greater than 15 percent of total calories as protein does not appear to precipitate problems in elderly patients without preexisting renal disease.[73]

The presence of osteoporosis can make it difficult to obtain accurate height and weight measurements in the elderly. Evaluation of height and weight measurements, and of indices of body composition derived from these values, is complicated by the loss of stature and changes in body composition associated with aging. Therefore accuracy in interpreting the collected data is compromised, and, with a lack of appropriate standards, interpretation is highly subjective. However, it is highly recommended that weight be measured and hydration status and edema be noted at least monthly for all nursing home residents. Weight loss is significant when there is a 1 to 2 percent loss in one week, 5 percent in one month, 7.5 percent in three months, or 10 percent in six months; greater losses than these are considered severe.[10] Measurement of a resident's height can be estimated from recumbent length, arm span, total arm length, and knee height when direct measurement is not possible because of a bedridden condition or the presence of contracted extremities, spinal curvature, or amputation.[74]

Nursing Home Medications and Drug–Nutrition Interactions

In nursing homes, 45 percent of residents take five or more medications, and virtually all take at least one; the average number of medications received daily by residents in skilled nursing homes is eight.[75] Digoxin is the most commonly prescribed drug for residents over age 65, followed by a furosemide diuretic.[76]

Chronic use of medications has the potential to significantly alter nutritional status by affecting nutrient absorption, distribution, metabolism, or elimination.[42] Drugs that cause protein-energy malnutrition are usually those that induce nausea and vomiting, such as cancer chemotherapeutic drugs and digoxin, or those that induce other adverse reactions to food, such as those that cause malabsorption. Vitamin deficiencies may be caused by antacids, hypocholesterolemic agents, H_2 receptor antagonists, laxatives, antibiotics, and specific antagonists to folic acid, vitamin B_6, and vitamin K. Mineral depletion can be induced by diuretics, laxatives, glucocorticoids, chelating agents, antacids, and non-narcotic analgesics.

Undernourishment can affect the transport, metabolism, and elimination of drugs. For example, protein malnutrition with hypoalbuminemia results in reduction in protein binding of drugs, which allows more of a drug to diffuse out of the vascular compartment and across interstitial spaces and tissues to reach drug receptor sites. Protein malnutrition also impairs drug metabolism in the liver. Additionally, renal excretion of drugs is diminished by the presence of edema, which may be associated with both protein malnutrition and congestive heart failure.[42]

Drugs that enhance the development of obesity include psychotropic drugs (phenothiazine and benzodiazepine tranquilizers) and antidepressant drugs (monoamine oxidase inhibitors, tricyclics, and lithium carbonate), presumably due to changes in appetite when relief from anxiety, depression, and phobias occur. On the other hand, phenothiazine or benzodiazepine tranquilizers may cause underweight, bedridden patients to eat less if tranquilizing and sedative effects detract from interest in food or cause patients to sleep through mealtimes.

Chapter 9 and many references[77–80] are available to enlighten the dietitian on the nutrition-related side effects of medications commonly used by the elderly. Medications of special importance to the dietitian in nursing homes include antipsychotics and sedatives, narcotic and non-narcotic analgesics (including morphine, aspirin, nonsteroidal anti-inflammatory drugs, and acetaminophen), digoxin, laxatives, corticosteroids, anticonvulsants, H_2 receptor blockers, antacids, hypocholesterolemic agents, antituberculosis agents, antihypertensive agents, antiparkinsonian drugs, anticoagulants, beta-blockers, and diuretics.

HOME CARE

"For every elderly person admitted to a nursing home in the U.S., there are two to three equally dependent elderly individuals remaining in the community."[18(p178)]

These individuals constitute the 15 percent of the community elderly (or about 3.75 million people) who require some assistance in their activities of daily living[81] because of the common conditions that they exhibit, including dementia, status post hip fracture, advanced arthritis, status post stroke, Parkinson's disease, and cardiovascular-pulmonary diseases.[82]

Evidence from national nutritional monitoring of the U.S. population does not indicate that protein energy malnutrition in the free-living elderly is widespread, but sociodemographic and economic conditions make sampling of frail, sick, poor, elderly difficult, and these are the very persons most likely to have problems in obtaining adequate food. Smaller-scale surveys suggest relatively high prevalence rates among dependent home-bound elderly and subgroups such as the demented or chronically ill with multiple comorbidities.[83] Posner et al.[84] reported that many intakes fail to meet the RDAs for nine essential nutrients in 40 to 80 percent of the Boston home-bound elders studied. The risk for poor nutritional status of home care patients can be identified through use of the Nutrition Screening Initiative screens (Exhibits 17–1 and 17–2), which identify common risk factors and indicators for malnutrition.

Judging an older patient's mental and emotional competence is just as critical as assessing physical function. Many screening instruments have been devised to use in the home care and nursing home settings. A familiar neuropsychologic instrument in geriatric medicine is the Mini-Mental State Examination (MMSE).[85] It assesses attention, memory, and language; a low score indicates delirium, dementia, or depression.

A number of depression screening instruments are available: the Yeasavage Geriatric Depression Scale, the Hamilton Depression Rating Scale, and the Beck Depression Inventory. It is important to remember that depression can be as functionally disabling as medical conditions. And in most elderly patients, depression can be relieved with judicious use of medication. Medical, financial, and family problems weigh heavily on the aged, especially because they may have a great deal of time on their hands, and improving circumstances may enhance their quality of life substantially.[47]

In non-nursing-home settings, 27 percent of older persons take at least one medication and 23 percent take at least five; most of the rest take between two and five medications.[76] The National Ambulatory Care Survey showed that of the top ten drugs prescribed for those aged 65 and older, three were antibiotics (Amoxil, amoxicillin, ampicillin), two each were diuretics—antihypertensives (Lasix or furosemide, Dyazide) and nonsteroidal anti-inflammatory agents (Motrin, Naprosyn), and one each were a cardiotonic (Lanoxin) and antiarrhythmic (Inderal) and a steroid (prednisone).[86] As with nursing home residents, drug profiles of home care elderly patients are extremely important to monitor closely. In addition to prescription medications, many older people take numerous over-the-counter medications. They are frequently reluctant to offer information about their medications, and often must be specifically asked about medications that they might consider routine or trivial.[87]

Many older persons in the United States take vitamin/mineral supplements, and usage is highest by those with higher family income and education level and by those who perceive themselves to be in "good health" compared to those with less resources and those who think themselves to be "less healthy."[55] Consumption is increasing by older users, particularly for vitamin E, vitamin C, calcium, and zinc.[88] Older persons are susceptible to fraudulent health practices, including nutrition and supplement abuse, and they spend billions of dollars yearly on practices that can result in significant harm, needless expenditure, and delay in seeking appropriate medical intervention for perceived or real health problems.[89,90]

Because of the trend to decrease length of hospital stay, home care programs are receiving more acutely ill patients with more nutrition-related diagnoses than in previous years.[91] Home care providers also are pressured to discharge patients sooner, due to limits imposed on the number of home care visits that may be reimbursed, which leads to limited opportunities to provide appropriate nutrition care to patients with nutritional problems. Even though home care administrators are anxious to provide efficient and effective nutrition care, Medicare/Medicaid and many insurance companies do not reimburse directly for the services of a dietitian, which means that home care agencies that employ dietitians often absorb costs for nutrition services in administrative or overhead cost centers. Until such time as nutrition services provided by dietitians are routinely reimbursed by both private and public third-party payers, dietitians can serve as consultants to a home care program.[92,93]

The home care consultant dietitian can devise nutrition information forms (such as the forms in Exhibits 17–1 and 17–2) and referral systems that enable efficient, thorough collection of nutrition data from which the level of the patient's nutritional needs can be determined and prioritized. The consultant dietitian can also plan and implement a nutrition teaching program for nursing staff [94] to help the nurse provide appropriate nutrition care and assure referral of appropriate patients to the dietitian when necessary. Following an analysis of the patient population serviced, referral to the dietitian might be based on levels of acuity and diagnosis.[92]

The current trend for increased demand for home health services is expected to continue in the future.[95] Likewise, research is expected to continue to validate the increasingly important prophylactic, therapeutic, and palliative roles of nutrition in the management of home care patients.[96] Several resources have been published to assist the dietitian in planning nutrition interventions for home care patients.[97–99]

PALLIATIVE (HOSPICE) CARE

Palliative or hospice care advocates that when the length of a patient's life can no longer be extended by aggressive medical care, the quality of that life should be maximized.[100] Eating, mealtimes, and nutrition are major contributors to a patient's quality of life. Therefore, when eating is an enjoyable experience, its practice should be maximized; if it is not, its practice should not be overemphasized. The goals of the provision of nutritional care to terminally ill patients and their families include the following[101]:

- relief of troublesome symptoms (diet can be an effective adjunct to medical and nursing interventions)
- enhancement of pleasurable experiences of living
- prevention or treatment of malnutrition, which could be the unavoidable cause of death, if death by starvation or dehydration is unacceptable to the patient, family, and/or health care team

The dietitian is an important member of hospice care programs,[102] and can achieve these goals by performing several functions, including the following[101]:

- assessing the patient's physical and psychological condition for the role that curative and palliative treatments, food, and mealtimes have on causing symptoms; ascertaining if dietary modifications can alleviate these symptoms and improve well-being
- identifying the patient's and family's nutritional concerns and dietary questions
- establishing goals of treatment and integrate dietary intervention as appropriate into the overall plan of care
- counseling the patient and family on specific and practical dietary modifications that can enhance well-being
- reevaluating nutritional goals and intervention periodically, and implementing changes when appropriate

A nutritional assessment of terminally ill patients may be significantly different than an assessment of acutely ill patients. Exhibit 17–5 is an assessment instrument that includes important nutrition-related questions that the palliative care dietitian or nurse might ask the patient and family. Identification of specific questions, issues, and concerns that patients and their families have is also of utmost importance.

Exhibit 17–5 Nutrition Assessment Instrument for Hospice Setting

---

1. Does the patient experience any of the following problems?
   - nausea and/or vomiting   Yes ☐   No ☐
     if so, is it associated with:
     —taste of specific foods   Yes ☐   No ☐
     —sight or smell of particular foods   Yes ☐   No ☐
     —temperature of foods   Yes ☐   No ☐
   - diarrhea   Yes ☐   No ☐
   - constipation or gastrointestinal obstruction   Yes ☐   No ☐
   - mouth sores   Yes ☐   No ☐
   - difficulty chewing   Yes ☐   No ☐
   - difficulty swallowing   Yes ☐   No ☐
   - dry mouth   Yes ☐   No ☐
   - poor appetite   Yes ☐   No ☐
     if so, is it caused by:
     —pain or other symptoms   Yes ☐   No ☐
     —depression or anxiety   Yes ☐   No ☐
     —early satiety, fatigue, or weakness   Yes ☐   No ☐
   - pressure sores   Yes ☐   No ☐

2. Does the patient take any vitamin, mineral, or other food supplements?   Yes ☐   No ☐

3. Does the patient have a gastrointestinal or intravenous feeding tube in place?   Yes ☐   No ☐

4. Does the patient or family express significant remorse about weight change or food intake?   Yes ☐   No ☐
   - If the patient has lost a lot of weight, does the weight change make the patient more dependent on others?   Yes ☐   No ☐
   - Does the patient or family want to try to reverse the weight loss with enteral or parenteral nutritional support?   Yes ☐   No ☐

5. Does the family exhibit any of the following behaviors?
   - inappropriate use of food as a crutch for emotional problems   Yes ☐   No ☐
   - belief that disease is caused by what the patient did or did not eat   Yes ☐   No ☐
   - fear that if the patient doesn't eat, he or she will feel hunger pains   Yes ☐   No ☐
   - fear that if the patient becomes dehydrated, he or she will suffer   Yes ☐   No ☐
   - fear that if the patient quits eating, he or she will die soon   Yes ☐   No ☐
   - belief in unorthodox nutritional therapies such as vitamin C, laetrile, the macrobiotic diet, enzymes   Yes ☐   No ☐

Source: Reprinted with permission from Gallagher-Allred C.R., Nutritional Care of the Terminally Ill Patient and Family, in *Palliative Care for People with Cancer,* J. Penson and R. Fisher, eds., p. 94, with permission of Edward Arnold, © 1991.

Assessment instruments for terminally ill patients rarely include biochemical laboratory tests. Tests may be performed, however, if the results will potentially alter the patient's management, and if their invasiveness does not cause more discomfort than is warranted by the information to be gained.[103] Often, what an "eyeball" test does not tell probably does not need to be known. In contrast, dietary assessment and the assessment of possible nutrient and drug interactions are often important. Appropriate dietary assessment questions may include the following[100]:

• Do you enjoy eating?
• What are your favorite foods?
• Are there any foods that you can think of that you would like to eat and that anyone can get for you?
• Do you want to change how much you eat? Where you eat? When you eat? How can we help you to do so?
• Is there any assistance such as Meals on Wheels, food stamps, or food supplements that we can try to obtain for you?

Identifying the many medications that a terminally ill patient may be taking and identifying their effect on food intake is important. For example, many hospice patients receive narcotic analgesics that cause nausea, vomiting, and constipation.[104] Dietary alterations are an important adjunct to medical and nursing treatment of these conditions. Additionally, diarrhea can be medication, disease, or treatment induced, and dietary modification can be of therapeutic value.[100]

Asking about weight is probably appropriate only when the patient or family expresses sadness or concern about weight loss (or weight gain that occurs with some medications). An appropriate assessment question includes the patient's and family's views of aggressive nutritional support. Upon accepting a palliative care program, a patient and patient's family generally will sign an informed consent document indicating that they do not want extraordinary treatments to be instituted to keep the patient alive. This consent document often includes a statement about aggressive nutritional support. When conducting the nutritional assessment, the palliative care dietitian should ascertain whether the patient and/ or the patient's family are comfortable with their acceptance of the policy of no aggressive nutritional support. Many patients and/or individual family members may want to discuss tube and parenteral feedings with the dietitian. Many resources are available to assist the clinician in managing issues associated with nutrition support of terminally ill patients.[105–107]

CONCLUSION

Assessment is the component upon which appropriate and individualized nutritional care for elderly patients is based. Indeed, a nutritional care plan can only be as good as the completeness and accuracy of the assessment upon which it is based. The roles and expectations of dietitians will continually change as more is learned about the nutritional needs of elderly patients and as environmental and economic factors affect health care in general and geriatric care in particular. By serving as a patient advocate, the dietitian, in collaboration with other health care providers, can assure that quality of care and quality of life are maximized for our nation's elderly in long-term care, home care, and palliative (hospice) care settings.

REFERENCES

1. Leaf A, ed. Aging: nutrition and the quality of life. *Am J Clin Nutr.* 1992;55:1191S–1273S.

2. Reilly JJ, Hull SF, Albert N, et al. Economic impact of malnutrition: a model system for hospitalized patients. *J Paren Enter Nutr.* 1988;12(4):371–376.

3. US Senate Special Committee on Aging and the American Association of Retired Persons. *Aging America: Trends and Projections.* Washington, DC: American Association of Retired Persons; 1984.

4. National Center for Health Statistics. *Health, United States, 1987.* Washington, DC: US Government Printing Office; 1988. DHHS publication No. (PHS) 88–1232.

5. Spencer G. Projections of the population of the United States by age, sex and race: 1983–2000. *Current Population Reports.* 1987;25:952.

6. US Dept of Health and Human Services. *Secretary's Commission on Nursing Support Studies and Background Information.* Washington, DC: Government Printing Office; 1988:II-7.

7. Neu CR, Harrison S. *Post Hospital Care before and after the Medicare Prospective Payment System.* Santa Monica, Calif: Rand/UCLA Center for Health Care Financing Policy Research; 1988.

8. US Dept of Health and Human Services, Health Care Financing Administration. Medicare and Medicaid programs: survey, certification and enforcement of skilled nursing facilities and nursing facilities. *Federal Register.* 1992;57(168):39278–39315.

9. Institute of Medicine, Committee on Nursing Home Regulation. *Improving the Quality of Care in Nursing Homes.* Washington, DC: National Academy Press; 1986.

10. US Dept of Health and Human Services, Health Care Financing Administration. *Part II. Guidance to Surveyors for Long Term Care Facilities.* Washington, DC: US Government Printing Office; 1992.

11. American Bar Association Commission on Legal Problems of the Elderly. *Patient Self-Determination Act State Law Guide.* Washington, DC: American Bar Association; 1991.

12. Ross Products Division. *Positioning Clinical Nutrition for Leadership in Long-Term Care: Report of the First Ross Forum on Long-Term Care for Clinical Nutrition Services.* Columbus, Ohio: Ross Products Division; 1994.

13. Breeding C, Smith Edge M. Consultant dietitians: the opportunity is now. *J Long-Term Care Admin.* 1992;20(3):25–27.

14. Puckett R. JCAHO's agenda for change. *J Am Diet Assoc.* 1991;91:1225–1226.

15. US Dept of Health and Human Services, Health Care Financing Administration. Medicare and Medicaid programs: requirements for long term care facilities. *Federal Register.* 1989;54(21): 5316–5373.

16. Dimant J. The psychosocial and environmental approach to nutritional management in long term care. *J Med Dir.* 1992;2(2):52–58.

17. Gallagher-Allred CR. *Implementing Nutrition Screening and Intervention Strategies.* Washington, DC: Nutrition Screening Initiative; 1993.

18. Rudman D, Feller AG. Protein calorie undernutrition in the nursing home. *J Amer Geriatr Soc.* 1989;37:173–183.

19. Pinchofsky-Devin GD, Kaminski MV. Incidence of protein calorie malnutrition in the nursing home population. *J Am Coll Nutr.* 1987;7:109–112.

20. Lipschitz DA, Mitchell CO. Nutritional assessment of the elderly: special considerations. In: Wright RA, Heymsfield S, McManus III CB, eds. *Nutritional Assessment.* Boston, Mass: Blackwell Scientific Publications Inc.; 1984:131–139.

21. Institute of Medicine. *Extending Life, Enhancing Life: A National Research Agenda on Aging.* Washington, DC: National Academy Press; 1991.

22. Request for Proposal (RFP). Failure to thrive syndrome among older persons. *NIH Guide for Grants and Contracts.* 1992;21(42):12–15.

23. Whitehead RG, Coward WA, Lunn PG. Serum albumin concentration and the onset of kwashiorkor. *Lancet.* 1973;1:63.

24. Jeejeebhoy KN. The functional basis of assessment. In: Kenney JM, Jeejeebhoy KN, Hill GL, Owen OE, eds. *Nutrition and Metabolism in Patient Care.* Philadelphia, Pa: WB Saunders Co; 1988:739–751.

25. Agarwal N, Acevedo F, Leighton LS, Cayten CG, Pitchumoni CS. Predictive ability of various nutritional variables for mortality in elderly people. *Am J Clin Nutr.* 1988;48:1173–1178.

26. Reinhardt GF, Myscofski JW, Wilkens DB, et al. Incidence and mortality of hypoalbuminemic patients in hospitalized veterans. *J Paren Enter Nutr.* 1980;4:357.

27. *International Classification of Diseases—Clinical Modifications.* 9th rev, 4th ed. New York, NY: McGraw-Hill; 1994.

28. Shizgal HM. Nutritional assessment. In: Winters RW, Greene HL, eds. *Nutritional Support of the Seriously Ill Patient.* New York, NY: Academic Press; 1983:267–278.

29. Bernstein LH. Monitoring quality of nutrition support: a chemical marker. *Diet Curr.* 1992;19(2):5–8.

30. Greenblatt DJ. Reduced serum albumin concentration in the elderly: a report from the Boston collaborative drug surveillance program. *J Am Geriatr Soc.* 1979;27(1):20–22.

31. Miller AK, Adir J, Vestal RE. Tolbutamide binding to plasma proteins of old and young human subjects. *J Pharm Sci.* 1978;67:1192–1193.

32. Gersovitz M, Bier D, Matthews D, et al. Dynamic aspects of whole body glycine metabolism: influence of protein intake in young adult and elderly males. *Metabolism.* 1980;29:1087–1094.

33. Gersovitz M, Munro HN, Udall J, Young VR. Albumin synthesis in young and elderly subjects using a new stable isotope methodology: response to level of protein intake. *Metabolism.* 1980;29(11):1075–1086.

34. Henderson CT. Nutrition. In: Cassell CK et al., eds. *Geriatric Medicine.* 2nd ed. New York, NY: Springer-Verlag; 1990.

35. Winkler MF, Gerrior SA, Pomp A, Albina JE. Use of retinol-binding protein and prealbumin as indicators of the response to nutritional therapy. *J Am Diet Assoc.* 1980;89:684.

36. Bernstein LH, Leukhardt-Fairfield CJ, Pleban W, Rudolph RA. Usefulness of data on albumin and prealbumin concentrations in determining effectiveness of nutritional support. *Clin Chem.* 1989;35:271.

37. Mears E. Prealbumin and nutrition assessment. *Diet Curr.* 1994;21(1):1–4.

38. Kalchthaler, Rigor Tan ME. Anemia in institutionalized elderly patients. *J Am Geriatr Soc.* 1980;28:108–113.

39. Chanarin I. *The Megaloblastic Anemias.* Oxford, UK: Blackwell Scientific Publications, Ltd; 1969;457–474.

40. Lindenbaum J, Healton EN, Savage DG, et al. Neuropsychiatric disorders caused by cobalamin deficiency in the absence of anemia or macrocytosis. *N Engl J Med.* 1988;318:1720–1728.

41. Blumberg JB. Changing nutrient requirements in older adults. *Nutr Today.* 1992;27:15–20.

42. Roe DA. *Geriatric Nutrition.* 3rd ed. Englewood Cliffs, NJ: Prentice Hall Inc; 1992.

43. Lipschitz DA. Nutrition and the aging haemopoietic system. In: Hutchinson M, Munro HN, eds. *Nutrition and Aging.* New York, NY: Academic Press; 1986:251–262.

44. Hobbs J, Guthrie TH, Brubaker LH, Bilodeau PA. Hematology. In Rakel RE, ed. *Textbook of Family Practice.* 4th ed. Philadelphia, Pa: WB Saunders Co; 1990:1336.

45. Rudman D, Mattson DE, Nagraj HS, et al. Prognostic significance of serum cholesterol in nursing home men. *J Paren Enter Nutr.* 1988;12(2):155–158.

46. Verdery RB, Goldberg AP. Hypocholesterolemia as a predictor of death: a prospective study of 224 nursing home residents. *J Gerontol Med Sci.* 1991;47:M84.

47. Beck JC, Freedman ML, Warshaw GA. Geriatric assessment: focus on function. *Patient Care.* February 28, 1994:10–28.

48. Katz S, Ford A, Moskowitz R, et al. Studies of illness in the aged: the index of ADL—a standardized measure of biological and psychosocial function. *JAMA.* 1963;185:914–919.

49. Shephard RJ. Nutrition and the physiology of aging. In: Young EA, ed. *Nutrition, Aging, and Health.* New York, NY: Alan R. Liss Inc.; 1986:1–23.

50. Rozovski SJ. Nutrition for older Americans. *Age Aging.* 1984;344:49.

51. US Dept of Health and Human Services. The national nursing home survey: 1977 summary for the United States. Hyattsville, Md: National Center for Health Statistics; 1979. PHS 79-1794 (Vital and Health Statistics, Series 13, #43).

52. Jernigan AK. *Nutrition in Long Term Care Facilities: A Handbook for Dietitians.* Chicago, Ill: American Dietetic Association; 1987.

53. Bartoshuk LM. Taste: robust across the age span? *Ann NY Acad Sci.* 1989;561:65–75.

54. Schiffman SS, Covey E. Changes in taste and smell with age: nutritional aspects. In: Ordy JM, Harman D, Alfin-Slater RB, eds. *Nutrition in Gerontology.* New York, NY: Raven Press; 1984: 43–64.

55. Nutrition Screening Initiative. *Report of Nutrition Screening I: Toward a Common View.* Washington, DC: The Nutrition Screening Initiative; 1992.

56. Schiffman SS, Moss J, Ericksonn RP. Thresholds of food odors in the elderly. *Exp Aging Res.* 1976;2:389–398.

57. Schiffman SS. Food recognition by the elderly. *J Gerontol.* 1977;32:586–592.

58. Coulston AM, Mandelbaum D, Reaven GM. Dietary management of nursing home residents with non-insulin-dependent diabetes mellitus. *Am J Clin Nutr.* 1990;51:67–71.

59. Rosen WK. The diabetic diet reconsidered: a medical care evaluation study. *Ann Med Dir.* 1991;1(1):44–47.

60. Zemel MB, Sowers JR. Salt sensitivity and systemic hypertension in the elderly. *Am J Cardiol.* 1988;61(16):7H–12H.

61. Hollis JB, Castell DO. Esophageal function in elderly men: a new look at "presbyesophagus." *Ann Intern Med.* 1974;80:371–374.

62. *Dining Skills: Practical Interventions for the Caregivers of the Eating-Disabled Older Adult.* Pensacola, Fla: Consultant Dietitians in Health Care Facilities; 1992.

63. Young EA, Urban E. Aging, the aged, and the gastrointestinal tract. In: Young EA, ed. *Nutrition, Aging, and Health.* New York, NY: Alan R. Liss Inc.; 1986:91–131.

64. Alessi CA, Henderson CT. Constipation and fecal impaction in the long-term care patient. *Clin Geriatr Med.* 1988;4(3):571–588.

65. Thompson MP, Tollison JW. Caring for the elderly. In: Rakel RE, ed. *Textbook of Family Practice.* 4th ed. Philadelphia, Pa: WB Saunders Co; 1990:162–163.

66. Lindeman RD. Age changes in renal function. In: Goldman R, Rockstein M, eds. *The Physiology and Pathology of Human Aging.* New York, NY: Academic Press Inc; 1975:19–38.

67. Epstein M. Effects of aging on the kidney. *Fed Proc.* 1979;38:168–172.

68. Rolls BJ, Phillips PA. Aging and disturbance of thirst and fluid balance. *Nutr Rev.* 1990;48: 137–144.

69. Silver AJ. Aging and risks for dehydration. *Clev Clin J Med.* 1990;57:341–344.

70. Zehng JJ, Rosenberg IH. What is the nutritional status of the elderly? *Geriatrics.* 1989;44: 57–64.

71. Chernoff R, Lipschitz DA. Nutrition and aging. In: Shils ME, Young VR, eds. *Modern Nutrition in Health and Disease.* 7th ed. Philadelphia, Pa: Lea & Febiger; 1988:982–1000.

72. Munro HN, Suter PM, Russell RM. Nutritional requirements of the elderly. *Ann Rev Nutr.* 1987;7:23–49.

73. Tobin J, Spector D. Dietary protein has no effect on future creatinine clearance. *Gerontologist.* 1986;26:59A.

74. Chumlea WC, Roche AF, Mukherjee D. *Nutritional Assessment of the Elderly Through Anthropometry.* Columbus, Ohio: Ross Laboratories; 1987.

75. Beers MH, Ouslander JG, Rollingher I, Reuben DB, Brooks J, Beck JC. Explicit criteria for determining inappropriate medication use in nursing home residents. *Arch Intern Med.* 1991;151:1825–1832.

76. Lamy PP, Michocki RJ. Medication management. *Clin Geriatr Med.* 1988;4:623–638.

77. Kerstetter JE, Holthausen BA, Fitz PA. Malnutrition in the institutionalized older adult. *J Am Diet Assoc.* 1992;92:1109–1116.

78. Roe DA. *Handbook on Drug and Nutrient Interactions: A Problem-Oriented Reference Guide.* 5th ed. Chicago, Ill: The American Dietetic Association; 1992.

79. Murray JJ, Healy MD. Drug-mineral interactions: a new responsibility for the hospital dietitian. *J Am Diet Assoc.* 1991;91:66–70.

80. Smith CH. Drug-food/food-drug interactions. In: Morley JE, Glick Z, Rubenstein LZ, eds. *Geriatric Nutrition.* New York, NY: Raven Press; 1990:371–396.

81. Dawson D, Hendershot G, Fulton J. Aging in the eighties: functional limitations of individuals age 65 years and over. Advance data from *Vital and Health Statisics of the National Center for Health Statistics.* No. 133, June 10, 1987. Rockville, Md: US Dept of Health and Human Services, Public Health Service.

82. Kovar MG. Health of the elderly and use of health services. *Pub Health Rep.* 1977;92:9–19.

83. Dwyer JT. *Screening Older Americans' Nutritional Health: Current Practices and Future Possibilities.* Washington, DC: Nutrition Screening Initiative; 1991.

84. Posner BM, Smigelski CG, Krachenfels MM. Dietary characteristics and nutrient intake in an urban home-bound population. *J Am Diet Assoc.* 1987;87:452–456.

85. Folstein MF, Folstein SE, McHugh PR. "Mini-Mental State:" a practical method for grading the cognitive state of patients for the clinician. *J Psychiatr Res.* 1975;12:189–198.

86. Koch H, Knapp DA. Highlights of drug utilization in office practice: national ambulatory medical care survey, 1985. Advance data from *Vital and Health Statistics of the National Center for Health Statistics,* No. 134, May 19, 1987. Rockville, Md: US Dept of Health and Human Services, Public Health Service.

87. Chernoff R. Physiologic aging and nutritional status. *Nutr Clin Prac.* 1990;5(1):8–13.

88. Hale WE, May FE, Marks RG, Stewart RB. Drug use in an ambulatory elderly population: a 5 year update. *Drug Intell Clin Pharm.* 1987;21:530–535.

89. Lamy PP. Nonprescription drugs and the elderly. *Am Fam Phys.* 1989;39(6):175–179.

90. Subcommittee on Health and Long-Term Care of the Select Committee on Aging, House of Representatives, 98th Cong, 2nd ses. Comm. Pub. No. 98-435. *Quackery: A $10 Billion Scandal.* Washington, DC: US Government Printing Office; 1984.

91. Posner BM, Krachenfells MM. Nutrition services in the continuum of health care. *Clin Geriatr Med.* 1987;3(2):261–274.

92. Rebovich EJ, Mahovich P, Blair KS. Nutrition services in home care. *Caring.* 1990;9:8–14.

93. Ross Products Division. *Clinical Nutrition Services: An Integral Component of Home Care: Report of the First Ross Forum on Home Care for Clinical Nutrition Services.* Columbus, Ohio: Ross Products Division; 1994.

94. Foundation for Hospice and Homecare, and Ross Laboratories. *Nutrition: A Partner in Home Care.* Columbus, Ohio: Ross Laboratories; 1990.

95. Sounding Board: Home Care—Who Cares? *New Engl J Med.* 1986;314(14):917–920.

96. *The Surgeon General's Report on Nutrition and Health: Aging.* Washington, DC: US Government Printing Office; 1988. US Dept of Health and Human Services (DHHS) publication PHS 88-50210.

97. Finn SC, ed. Nutrition and home care. *Caring.* 1990;9(10):1–82.

98. Nutrition Screening Initiative. *Nutrition Interventions Manual for Professionals Caring for Older Americans.* Washington, DC: Nutrition Screening Initiative; 1992.

99. Dantone JJ. *Bridging the Gap: Procedure and Instructional Manual for Dietary and Nursing Interventions.* Grenada, Miss: Nutrition Education Resources; 1993.

100. Gallagher-Allred CR. *Nutritional Care of the Terminally Ill.* Gaithersburg, Md: Aspen Publishers, Inc; 1989:27.

101. Gallagher-Allred CR. Nutritional care of the terminally ill patient and family. In: Penson J, Fisher R, eds. *Palliative Care for People with Cancer.* Dunton Green, Kent, UK: Edward Arnold; 1991:91–104.

102. Gallagher-Allred C. Dietitians are necessary in hospice programs. *Am J Hospice Care.* 1985;2(6):11–12.

103. Cassileth PA. Common medical problems. In: Cassileth BR, Cassileth PA, eds. *Clinical Care of the Terminal Cancer Patient.* Philadelphia, Pa: Lea & Febiger; 1982:16–17.

104. Cassileth BR, Cassileth PA. *Clinical Care of the Terminal Cancer Patient.* Philadelphia, Pa: Lea & Febiger; 1982.

105. Position paper of the American Dietetic Association: Issues in feeding the terminally ill adult. *J Am Diet Assoc.* 1992;92(8):996–1005.

106. Gallagher-Allred CR. Managing ethical issues in nutrition support of terminally ill patients. *Nutr Clin Prac.* 1991;6:113–116.

107. Gallagher-Allred CR, Amenta MO. Nutritional care of the terminally ill. *Hospice J.* In press.

Part IV

Nutrition Monitoring, Evaluation, and Productivity

Chapter 18

Nutrition Monitoring in the United States

Catherine E. Woteki

OVERVIEW

Monitoring is a process done for both observing individual changes of patients or clients or as part of large-scale surveillance systems. Additionally, subsets of patients in institutions or agencies can be compared with national statistics or to monitor changes that occur in the nutritional or health status of a group. This chapter focuses on a national monitoring system.

Nutrition monitoring makes use of two sources of information to help policy makers plan and evaluate policy decisions and food programs designed to improve the health and well-being of the population. The sources of information are administrative records and surveys. Examples of administrative records include birth and death certificates, program participation records, and food export and import records. Surveys use statistical sampling methods to select representative samples of a population and then interview or examine the elements of the sample. Populations could consist of institutions (such as hospitals or schools), households, or individuals.

Government agencies at federal, state, and local levels collect and analyze nutrition-monitoring data to provide a basis for designing policies and programs, for regulatory decisions about food safety, and for evaluating decisions. Because the data are made available to researchers, the records and surveys are useful for epidemiologic research. In addition food companies frequently use the data for product development and marketing purposes.

HISTORICAL PERSPECTIVE

In the United States, *nutrition monitoring* is defined as "watching over nutrition, in order to make decisions which will lead to improvements in nutrition in populations."[1] This term is identical to the term *nutrition surveillance*, which is widely used in other countries and by the World Health Organization. Probably because of the association of *surveillance* with the covert activities of intelligence agencies, the term *nutrition surveillance* is rarely used in the United States.

At the federal level, a dozen different agencies in six departments conduct and analyze nutrition-monitoring activities. The agencies with the greatest responsibilities are the Human Nutrition Information Service of the U.S. Department of Agriculture (USDA) and the Centers for Disease Control (CDC) of the U.S. Department of Health and Human Services (DHHS). Both the USDA and the DHHS conduct large, multipurpose population surveys and maintain and analyze record-based systems. The Departments of Defense, Labor, Commerce, and State conduct more targeted activities to meet their needs for information on topics relevant to their missions or related to the needs of the special population groups that they serve. The activities of all six departments are collectively referred to as the National Nutrition Monitoring and Related Research Program, which was codified by the passage of the Nutrition Monitoring and Related Research Act of 1990.[2]

Nutrition-monitoring data are analyzed in six different ways:

1. to determine the adequacy of the food supply at the national, household, and individual levels
2. to estimate the prevalence of health and nutritional characteristics of the population and of subgroups in the population
3. to produce normative values of nutrition and health status indicators in population groups
4. to evaluate interrelationships among health, sociodemographic, economic, and nutrition variables
5. to monitor changes over time
6. to study the etiology and natural history of nutrition-related diseases through longitudinal studies of survey participants

COMPONENTS OF NUTRITION MONITORING

Record-Based Systems

The availability of administrative records and the large numbers of cases contained in them make them a desirable source of data for nutrition-monitoring purposes. But administrative records sometimes pose special problems in data analysis and interpretation because of the cursory and incomplete nature of some types of records; changing or different eligibility criteria for programs; errors in reporting, recording, or transcribing the information; and lack of standardization in obtaining the data. Despite these limitations, administrative records provide valuable information for nutrition monitoring.

Two of the record-based systems were established early in the 20th century and provide historical trend data. These are the food supply data and the vital statistics program. More recently, the CDC has begun using food assistance programs as the basis for surveillance programs. Three examples of the most frequently used record-based systems are described below.

Food Supply Data

The USDA has made annual estimates of the per capita availability of food and nutrients since 1909. The estimates are analogous to a food balance sheet. Quantities of food disappearing into the wholesale or retail systems are estimated by summing the amounts of food produced, imported, and in inventory at the beginning of the year and then by subtracting exports, year-end inventories, and nonfood uses. The result is an estimate of the pounds available for consumption of approximately 350 different food items. For reporting purposes, these estimates are divided by the number of people in the U.S. population that year, multiplied by the nutrient composition of the edible portion per pound of food, summed across all food categories, and divided by 365 days per year to yield estimates of nutrients available per capita per day.

Food supply data are used to assess the potential of the U.S. food supply to meet the nutritional needs of the population, to monitor trends in per capita food and nutrient availability over time, to estimate complete demand systems that measure price and income elasticities of demand in a consistent way, and to study relationships between diet and disease over time. For example, the amount of iron in the food supply is approximately 17 mg per capita per day,[3] an amount that exceeds the Recommended Dietary Allowances[4] for all sex/age groups except pregnant women. The amount of iron in the food supply increased in response to the introduction of iron-enriched flour in the 1940s and iron-fortified cereals in more recent years.

Vital Statistics

The vital statistics program was initiated in 1915, and data have been collected continually and published annually since then. Registering births, deaths, fetal deaths, and induced terminations of pregnancy is the responsibility of the individual states. The National Center for Health Statistics of the DHHS administers the decentralized, cooperative system that collates and makes data available on the national, state, and local levels. Uniformity in the data collection is achieved by the use of standard certificates for recording information and through periodic issuing of recommended standards. In developing countries, there are frequently problems with underreporting of births and deaths and with a lack of coverage of some regions. In developed countries such as the United States, reporting is considered to be nearly universal.

A number of descriptive and outcome variables are recorded for births and deaths. Descriptive variables for births include age, education, race, and Hispanic origin of mother and father; marital status and nativity of mother; and sex, birth order, and plurality of the infant. Currently, the outcome variables recorded for births include the infant's birth weight, gestational age, and Apgar score. The mother's weight gain during pregnancy; her alcohol and tobacco use; and other medical risk factors of pregnancy such as anemia, diabetes, and hypertension are included as well.[5] For deaths, the descriptive variables include sex, age, education, marital status, race, and Hispanic origin of the decedent, type and place of death, geographic place of death, occupation and industry of the decedent, residence, and whether an autopsy was performed. The outcome variables recorded on death certificates include the underlying and multiple causes of death.[5]

Mortality rates, particularly infant and child mortality rates, are frequently used as indicators of the overall health and nutritional status of a population. Discrepancies between the rates of groups with different incomes, education levels, or racial/ethnic backgrounds or from different geographic regions may signal an underlying nutritional problem that warrants further investigation. Any precipitous change in rates also warrants a closer look. For example, infant mortality rates and life expectancy at birth by race are tracked as part of the overall monitoring of health status in the United States.[6] The leading causes of death also are monitored because of the etiologic role that diet plays in many diseases. In the United States five of the ten leading causes of death are diet related—heart disease, cancer, stroke, diabetes mellitus, and atherosclerosis—and three—chronic liver disease and cirrhosis, accidents, and suicides—often result from excessive ingestion of alcoholic beverages. Taken together, these eight causes of death account for nearly 70 percent of all deaths in the United States each year.[7] As part of the National Nutrition Monitoring and Related Research Program, the causes of death are monitored.[3]

Because most countries collect both mortality and food supply data in a similar manner, mortality data have been analyzed together with food supply data to generate hypotheses on the relationship between diet and disease. For example, several international studies have shown direct correlations between the per capita availability of fat and breast cancer mortality.[8] This type of observation provides the basis for further epidemiological studies in human populations and laboratory studies to attempt to determine the mechanism by which dietary fat may cause or modify the course of breast cancer.

CDC Surveillance Systems

The CDC has developed record-based surveillance systems for children and pregnant women who participate in federally funded food assistance, nutrition, and health programs. Started in 1974, the Pediatric Nutrition Surveillance System (PedNSS) continually monitors selected indicators of nutritional status among low-income infants and children younger than 18 years of age. Since 1979, a similar program, called the Pregnancy Nutrition Surveillance System (PNSS), was started for pregnant women. Simple indicators of nutritional status such as short stature, underweight, overweight, anemia, and low birth weight are obtained from the routine clinical measurements that public health clinics record. The CDC collates and analyzes the data provided by participating states and provides the information back to the states for their use in program planning and evaluation.[8]

Data can be analyzed by clinic, county, and state, permitting policy makers to identify high-risk areas for targeted interventions. For example, the PNSS data are used to describe the prevalence of anemia among pregnant, low-income women seeking prenatal care in public health clinics. The prevalence of anemia increases during the second and third trimesters and is higher among black women than for any other ethnic/racial group. The PNSS data also show that early enrollment in the Special Supplemental Food Program for Women, Infants, and Children (WIC) program is associated with a lower prevalence of anemia.[8] As another example, the PedNSS has been used to track trends in the prevalence of anemia among low-income children in the United States. Based on data from six states, a steady decline in anemia prevalence was found from 1975 to 1985,[8] suggesting that distribution of iron-fortified infant formula and cereals through the WIC program had a beneficial effect.

The CDC surveillance system data have proven to be useful to state policy makers, but the data have limitations that need to be kept in mind when generalizing to the national level. The surveillance populations are those who seek care in public health settings and who meet the program eligibility criteria, which may vary from state to state. The clinics participating in the system use different equipment and methods for conducting the routine measurements and tests that are reported, and quality control and standardization among clinics and states are difficult.

Surveys

Surveys take advantage of well-developed statistical methods to provide information that can be generalized to an inference population. Most of the federal nutrition surveys have large sample sizes and use a technique called multistage area probability sampling to identify households or individuals who are interviewed and/or who undergo physical examinations to yield data on dietary and nutritional status that can be generalized to regional and national levels.

Surveys provide information on three areas of importance to nutrition monitoring—food and nutrient consumption at the household and individual levels; nutrition and related health measurements; and knowledge, attitudes, and behavior assessments. The most frequently cited federal nutrition surveys—the Nationwide Food Consumption Survey (NFCS) conducted by the USDA and the National Health and Nutrition Examination Survey (NHANES) conducted by the CDC—will be described in more detail.

Food and Nutrient Consumption

The USDA has conducted the NFCS, a national survey of household food consumption, about every ten years since 1936. The sample of households is drawn from the 48 coterminous states, and recent surveys have consisted of a basic sample of all households and a sample of low-income households with incomes at or below 130 percent of the poverty threshold. The person most knowledgeable about food purchased and prepared by the household (called the "household food manager") is interviewed about the amounts and prices of food used by the household during a seven-day period. Since 1965, individual household members have been interviewed about what they ate on the previous day and then asked to keep a diary of foods eaten that day and the following day.

The descriptive variables obtained on participating households include income, family size, education of male and female heads, cash assets, region, urbanization, tenancy, and participation in the Food Stamp and WIC programs. Individuals report their sex, age, race, ethnicity, employment status, height, and weight, and whether they are pregnant or lactating. Outcome variables for households are the quantity in pounds of food used, its monetary value, and its nutrient content. For individuals, the outcome variables include intakes of food and nutrients.[5]

To provide more continual coverage of the population in the years between large decennial surveys, the USDA began a smaller survey in 1985 called the Continuing Survey of Food Intakes by Individuals. Like the decennial survey, this one consists of a basic sample and a low-income sample drawn from 48 states. However, different age groups and methods of obtaining dietary intake data have been used. In 1985–1986, the ages surveyed were restricted to men and women 19 to 50 years of age and children ages 1 to 5. Six 24-hour recalls of dietary intake were obtained through in-person interviews of participants initially, and telephone interviews subsequently. For data collected in

1989–1991, the same method was used as in the decennial survey (all ages, and 24-hour recall plus two-day diary).

Data from the household and individual intake surveys are used to assess the adequacy of food available at the household level, the adequacy of nutrient intakes of individuals, and the size and nature of populations that may be at risk due to inadequate or excessive intake of nutrients. As shown in Exhibit 18–1, a wide range of other uses are made of the data.

Nutrition and Related Health Measurements

The White House Conference on Food, Nutrition, and Health held in 1969 recognized the importance of a reliable assessment of the nutritional status of Americans, particularly the extent of malnutrition and hunger. Consequently the first NHANES was undertaken in 1971. Three national surveys have been conducted in 1971–1974, 1976–1980, and 1988–1994, and a special survey of Mexican Americans, Puerto Ricans, and Cubans residing in the continental United States was conducted in 1982–1984.

Each survey has used multistage probability sampling to select a representative sample of the civilian noninstitutionalized population. Nutritional and health status are evaluated from data generated through interviews conducted in the home and physical examinations conducted in mobile examination centers. The interviews include 24-hour dietary recalls; a food frequency questionnaire; questions related to eating habits, lifestyle, and other nutrition-related practices; and medical history. Physical examinations include body measurements, hematological and biochemical assessments, and medical and dental examinations. The results of these surveys have multiple uses that include determining the prevalence of health and nutritional characteristics of the population and subgroups in the population; producing normative values for nutrition and health status indicators; evaluating interrelationships among health, nutrition, and sociodemographic variables; and monitoring changes over time. Examples of these data uses are listed in Exhibit 18–1. Mortality follow-up studies are being conducted on the cohorts for all the NHANES, and these studies will permit epidemiologic studies of the etiology and natural history of disease in the United States.

Knowledge, Attitudes, and Behavior

With the recognition of the important role that diet plays in chronic disease etiology, agencies have undertaken a number of surveys to obtain information on people's food and nutrition knowledge, attitudes, and behaviors. These surveys tend to have smaller sample sizes (generally in the range of 1,500 to 2,500 respondents), have more targeted samples, and use computer-assisted

Exhibit 18–1 Uses of Survey Data

Assessment of Dietary Intake	*Economics of Food Consumption*
Provide detailed benchmark data on the food and nutrient intake of a population.	Provide detailed benchmark data on domestic consumption—quantities of foods, food costs and nutrients available—for foods used by U.S. households.
Monitor nutritional quality of diets.	Assess demands for agricultural production, marketing facilities, and services.
Determine size and nature of populations at risk because of inadequate or excessive intake of nutrients.	Study effects of socioeconomic factors (income, size, composition of households) on total food consumption and expenditures and on food consumption-expenditure patterns for various food commodities.
Identify appropriate interventions (food assistance, fortification, or education) for at risk populations.	Analyze relationships between socioeconomic characteristics of and nutrient availability for selected population groups.
Obtain better understanding of variation in intake of nutrients among individuals and of intake of individuals over time.	Determine importance of home food production and of foods received as gifts or pay in food consumption of households.
Explain relationships of food and nutrient intake to nutritional and health status of a population.	Determine importance of food bought and eaten away from home on food consumption of households and individual household members.
Show dietary change required to meet proposed guidelines for improved health and well-being.	Determine importance of use of "convenience" foods on food consumption of households.
Identify socioeconomic factors associated with diets that meet and fail to meet nutritional criteria.	Determine differences in kinds and amounts of food that households report as used and individual household members report as eaten.
Identify food intake patterns and eating patterns (how often, when, where, and with whom) associated with diets that meet and fail to meet nutritional criteria.	Determine extent of seasonal variability in food and nutrient consumption among households.
Provide a basis for identification of foods on which composition data are needed.	
Predict need and market for new products and characteristics of likely consumers.	
Determine nutritional significance of food enrichment and fortification.	

continues

Exhibit 18–1 continued

Food Programs and Food Guidance

Determine factors affecting participation
in food programs and effect of
participation on food expenditures, diet
quality, nutritional status, and health
status, to predict change in participation
and effects that would result from
modification in the program.

Assess dietary national and health status
changes associated with food program
participation.

Analyze effect of food programs on the
market for commodities.

Identify populations at nutritional risk for
possible intervention with food
assistance, fortifications, and education
programs.

Identify changes in food and nutrient
consumption that might be expected to
reduce risk.

Develop for administrative and educational purposes food guides and food
plans that reflect food consumption
practices and meet nutritional and cost
criteria.

Determine reasonable amounts of foods
and surplus to distribute to families.

Nutrition and Health Status Assessment

Relate food consumption patterns and
nutrient intakes of subpopulations to
physical and physiological indicators of
health status.

Examine interactions of nutrition-related
variables with health conditions
determined through health histories and
clinical examinations.

Describe general nutritional health status
of the population and determine
subgroups at risk.

Monitor trends in nutritional status to
determine whether observed problems
are changing.

Historical and Secular Trends

Appraise history of food consumption,
dietary, and nutritional status relative to
economic, technologic, and other
factors.

Predict changes in food consumption,
dietary, and nutritional status as they
may be influenced by economic,
technologic, and other developments.

Attempt to correlate food consumption,
dietary, and nutritional status with
prevalence of diseases over time.

Food Safety Considerations*

Determine intake of incidental
contaminants, food additives, and
naturally occurring toxic substances.

Identify patterns of use of foods and food
components in the diets of a population.

Identify extreme and unusual patterns of
intake of foods or food ingredients,
including food additives.

continues

Exhibit 18–1 continued

Historical and Secular Trends	*Food Safety Considerations**
Assess reasonableness of dietary standards relative to food intake of healthy populations over time.	Identify size and nature of at risk populations from use of particular foods and food products.
Attempt to follow food consumption and nutritional status through the life cycle.	Determine number of food items in which a food additive may be permitted and in what amounts.
	Determine need to modify regulations in response to changes in food consumption.

*These include determining human exposure to food additives, pesticides, animal drugs, feed additives, GRAS substances, environmental contaminants, and naturally occurring toxic substances.

Source: Adapted with permission from Food and Nutrition Board, Coordinating Committee on Evaluation of Food Consumption Surveys, *National Survey Data on Food Consumption: Uses and Recommendations.* Washington, DC: National Academy Press; 1984.

telephone interviewing more frequently than the large multipurpose surveys described earlier. Examples of these surveys include the Behavioral Risk Factor Survey, conducted since 1984 by the CDC; the Nationwide Survey of Nurses' and Dietitians' Knowledge, Attitudes, and Behavior Regarding Cardiovascular Risk Factors, conducted by the National Institutes of Health; the Point of Purchase Labeling Studies, conducted in 1981–1986 by the FDA; and the Diet and Health Knowledge Survey, conducted in 1989–1991 by the USDA.[5]

Food Composition

Data on the composition of food and on the bioavailability of nutrients in food are critical elements of nutrition monitoring. Survey leaders use the food composition data to estimate the population's nutrient intake, and the food supply data based on food composition data are used to estimate the nutrients available per capita.

A number of national and international tables of food composition are in existence, each designed to meet the needs of their developers. In the United States, the USDA is responsible for maintaining the national food composition database. Nutrient composition data are obtained from scientific publications, university and government laboratories, and food processors and trade groups, and through contracts for generating needed food composition data. Most values released are supported by laboratory analyses. Values not available from laboratory analyses are imputed from data for other forms of the food or from data for similar foods. In addition, the federal government supports other databases that include levels of naturally occurring toxicants, contaminants, and allergenic compounds.

IMPROVEMENTS NEEDED

America's nutrition-monitoring system is widely recognized as the most comprehensive in the world, but many areas still need improvement. These include increased coverage of populations thought to be at greatest nutritional risk, more small-area data, improved timeliness of data release, and better policy analysis.

Population Coverage

The population surveys of the National Nutrition Monitoring System are incomplete in their coverage of the American population both over time and in the inclusion of groups suspected to be at higher risk of malnutrition. The record-based systems are more complete, although the food supply data are limited to the civilian population.

Survey timing has at times been well planned and at other times been haphazard. For example, during the 1970s, coverage was very good, with NHANES-I and -II in continual operation from 1971 to 1975 and 1976 to 1980, the NFCS collecting data in 1979–1980, and the low-income NFCS conducted in 1979–1980. No national surveys were conducted in the early 1980s, when dramatic changes were occurring in poverty rates among children and elderly persons in the United States. Since 1985, a national survey has been planned and conducted every year to collect information, at a minimum, on food and nutrient intakes of selected age/sex groups, and NHANES-III will cover a six-year time span from 1988 to 1994.

Coverage of populations at nutritional risk poses problems of different types. The national surveys are designed to be representative of the civilian, noninstitutionalized population in the United States. This definition and the method of sampling either eliminate or limit the sizes of some subgroups in the survey samples. Groups in the population that are frequently not covered adequately include racial/ethnic minority groups, pregnant or lactating women, homeless persons, Native Americans living on reservations, and institutionalized persons. Because oversampling to boost the numbers of these persons in surveys is prohibitively costly, about the only way to remedy the information deficits is to conduct special studies in these groups.

Small-Area Data

States, counties, and cities need information specific to their own populations, but the national surveys frequently can only be analyzed at the national or regional level. The CDC surveillance systems arose in part to help fill the states' information needs. Other, innovative ways need to be explored to help smaller areas meet their needs for information about the nutritional status and health of their residents.

Timeliness

The time required to plan, collect, and analyze data for the national surveys can extend up to ten years, but the need for information on which to base policy decisions is immediate. For large population surveys, two years of planning and one year of pilot testing before beginning data collection are not unusual, and at least one year of data cleanup and processing are needed before survey files are ready for analysis. The introduction of computer-assisted interviewing is helping to reduce the data processing time following collection of interviews, but it also tends to increase the planning time.

Policy Analysis

The primary reason for conducting nutrition monitoring is to provide information for policy decisions, and federal agencies perform much of the policy-relevant analyses. However, the survey data are rarely analyzed as completely as desirable, and many important policy issues can be at least partially addressed through analysis of existing monitoring data. At times, this occurs because the agencies responsible for nutrition programs may not be aware of the existing data. The agencies that conduct the surveys and maintain the record-based systems make the data available to researchers on public-release data tapes, and the analysis of these data is a fruitful endeavor for researchers.

REFERENCES

1. Mason JB, Habicht JP, Tabatabai H, Valverde V. *Nutritional Surveillance*. Geneva: World Health Organization; 1984:14.
2. Pub. L. No. 101-445. National Nutrition Monitoring and Related Research Act of 1990.

3. Life Sciences Research Office, Federation of American Societies for Experimental Biology. *Nutrition Monitoring in the United States: An Update Report on Nutrition Monitoring.* Washington, DC: US Government Printing Office; 1989:64, 77.

4. Food and Nutrition Board, Subcommittee on the Tenth Edition of the RDAs. *Recommended Dietary Allowances.* 10th ed. Washington, DC: National Academy Press; 1989:205–213.

5. Interagency Board for Nutrition Monitoring and Related Research. J Wright (ed.). *Nutrition Monitoring in the United States: The Directory of Federal and State Nutrition Monitoring Activities.* Hyattsville, Md: Public Health Service; 1992:25, 39.

6. National Center for Health Statistics. *Health, United States, 1990.* Hyattsville, Md: Public Health Service; 1991:1, 11–12, 22.

7. Public Health Service. *The Surgeon General's Report on Nutrition and Health.* Washington, DC: US Government Printing Office; 1988:22.

8. Food and Nutrition Board, Committee on Diet, Nutrition, and Cancer. *Diet, Nutrition, and Cancer.* Washington, DC: National Academy Press; 1982:73, 205–206, 215–216.

Chapter 19

Evaluating Nutrition Services To Achieve Quality

Julie O'Sullivan Maillet and Linda Jahn Toohey

OVERVIEW

The goal of any nutrition service in the 1990s is to improve quality of service in a cost-effective manner. Any and all systems can improve, and continual improvement is fundamental to the process of good service. The current wording is *total quality management (*TQM*)*, or *continuous quality improvement (*CQI*)*; however, the precise wording is not the issue. The titles and processes have evolved and will continue to evolve. For 20 years, the health care system, including dietetics, has been focusing on various systems to enhance quality of care. The Joint Commission on Accreditation of Healthcare Organizations (Joint Commission) has developed an institution-wide assessment, implementation, and evaluation process to assist in quality control. These standards place emphasis on the role of all leaders in the hospitals and the interaction across departments to assess and to enhance patient care through flexible quality management and improved processes.[1]

DEFINING QUALITY ASSURANCE PROGRAMS

Early quality assurance focused on problem identification, analysis, and correction, whereas current quality review focuses on improving services that may not have major problems. Terminology has included *quality assurance* (QA*)*, *quality control* (QC), *quality improvement* (QI), and *continuous process* *improvement* (CPI). Distinct from the original terminology and intent, TQM or CQI "is a management philosophy that is customer focused and quality driven to improve care by examining the systems and processes to which care is provided. These processes require each member of the care delivery team to build quality into every step of service development and delivery."[2] Quality is integrated into all points of service and takes a primary prevention position.

The TQM method is based on principles established by W. Edwards Deming.[3] As a statistician, he was interested in measuring the degree of difference between the goal of the service and the actual service based on the user's rather than the provider's expectations.[4] "Success is determined by the extent to which the product or service is valued by the user, not by the absence of deficiencies as defined by the producer."[4(p1126)]

The goal of quality assessment is to improve health care by making decisions based on scientific data or standards of care so that the outcome of the decision is more predictable. The measurement of quality has changed from an externally driven to an internally driven force, with the focus on client outcomes rather than on organizational structure. The successful departments have every member of the staff view himself or herself as a partner in a team achievement. The goal is to empower the staff so that problem solving occurs at the most basic level. Whereas quality assurance was targeted at "assuring" a more perfect system, quality improvement is aimed at continually "improving" the process and producing measurable outcomes. The current strategies emphasize efficiency of services as well as effectiveness.

The design to achieve quality within a nutrition service depends on a planned, systematic method for evaluating quality and appropriateness of services. Quality assurance includes measurement of professional standards of practice and establishment of criteria for practice; the transition to TQM/CQI shifts the focus toward client-centered care. For example, quality assurance focuses on measurable objectives provided by the practitioner—did the patient receive the nutrition assessment within the given time frame?—rather than client-focused care—did the nutrition assessment result in a measurable change in patient outcome? A nutrition assessment accurately and neatly written affects nothing if it is tucked away in the medical chart. The dietitian has accomplished no measurable intervention unless he or she actively participates in the overall client care plan. TQM examines the process of care to change the outcome of care.

The emphasis is to make quality management a day-to-day part of work, where the information collected for quality evaluation is integrated into the overall organization, and collected and evaluated across disciplines. The input from staff, the respect for each individual's role, the importance of employees' pride in their contribution, and the philosophy of continuous improvement are essential aspects of TQM. The concept of teams to evaluate issues is also fundamental: a few managers should not determine changes needed and quality standards; rather a diverse group of individuals need to work as a team. The team concept should include all levels of employees, from clerical to chief administrators. This involvement or empowerment of the staff may also reduce turnover of staff and improve employee satisfaction.

The definition of quality includes meeting clients' ("customers' ") requirements. The department's structural needs take second place to client needs and may require reconfiguration to meet those needs. The use of cross-functional (cross-departmental) teams assists the organization in structural evaluation. The TQM agenda considers every employee a shareholder in the success and effectiveness of the total operation. Quality nutrition goes beyond the traditional benchmark of timely screening and assessment duties; it expands to the entire operation. Achieving nutritional needs depends on all food service units (purchasing, production, service) and is critical to a client's nutritional status and satisfaction. Quality patient care depends on communication across disciplines and departments to coordinate food intake with diagnostic and therapeutic services, to ready the client for meals, and to monitor response to therapy.

PUTTING THE CLIENT AS CUSTOMER FIRST

Nutrition professionals need to put the client first, devising systems that accommodate the client as customer, whether they are in a private office, ambulatory-based clinic, or food service department. Examples of food service systems-driven procedures rather than customer-responsive care are numerous. Consider the patient menu selection system in a hospital. Often, a majority of patients may not select their menus. An examination of the system might show that menu selection is traditionally conducted through a menu that is delivered in the morning at breakfast, collected by lunch, and served the next day. This may meet the schedule of the department of food and nutrition service; however, for the patient, a menu delivered at dinner might allow the families and friends to help in selection and would be closer to actual selection time. This might improve client intake. Or consider when dietetic technicians conduct pediatric nutrition screening: often it is during nonvisiting hours rather than when the family is available. Some of the customary systems need to be reconsidered, putting the client as customer first and the current system second. Examine the system of nutrition screening: it takes the dietetic technician 24 to 48 hours to conduct a screening that often contains duplicative information collected by other professionals upon assessment. Referral connections from the other disciplines, such as nursing, might expedite the screening and therefore expedite the needed interventions.

IMPLEMENTATION OF A PROCESS IMPROVEMENT STRATEGY

Institutional or departmental policies that commit the department to a systematic means of providing quality service and care are essential. A variety of implementation strategies may be used. An 11-step process is described below. There is no absolute process to follow: it needs to be tailored to the particular service.

1. Define the responsibilities and mission of the department/unit. This mission-vision directs all future activities.
2. Establish a mechanism to organize priorities based on client perceptions of quality, critical indicators, client risk, volume of service, or problem areas.
3. Identify the project or process to improve. Determine who has the authority to change the process.
4. Name the initiative or project team(s).
5. Have the teams assess the situation from all angles and all perspectives. Consider the policies, procedures, equipment, and people involved.
6. Analyze the reasons for the situations and processes and how to improve them.
7. Develop potential solutions to improve the process. Select the best alternative for a quality solution.
8. Implement the proposed system. Refine and evaluate as needed.
9. Institutionalize the improvement and continue to maximize the improvement opportunities. The goal is preventative maintenance of systems.
10. Train staff appropriately. Excellent service depends on well-trained staff.
11. Set up key objectives for the following year or designated time period and start the process again.

When defining the responsibilities and mission of the department/unit, the service/product provided must be determined. This encourages looking at the big picture of what the department or service does. Determining the future vision for the department or service focuses priorities. The mission identifies the responsibilities of the department or service, such as "to provide nutritionally appropriate and satisfying meals to clients." To accomplish this, the essentials are timely nutrition screening, assessment, and care; a safe and sanitary food service environment; staff training and education; and monitoring and evaluation. Ambulatory care units might expand their mission and add educational goals for clients. Discharge planning may be part of the mission. An outpatient obstetrics department's mission might be to provide nutrition evaluation and treatment to optimize the outcome of pregnancy and to promote quality nutrition practices for newborns.

Departmental or service visions must not exist in a vacuum. They are developed through examining the vision and strategies for the entire organization. All annual goals or objectives and tasks to accomplish the vision are aligned to achieve quality. Consumers' expectations of what and how your organization meets their needs help to determine how to accomplish your vision.

Establish a triage mechanism to organize priorities. The priorities arise from the mission and are based on criteria such as the effect on customer satisfaction, effect on large numbers of clients (high volume) or on high-risk clients (high risk), important functions established by external agencies, perceptions by the clients, input from staff, problem-prone activities, or resource reduction or cost containment. Provide an analysis of the reasons for the problems in the processes and develop potential solutions. When the process has many steps, each individual who works within the system should be considered the client of the preceding employee. For example, the dietetic technician should consider the client as the principal customer, but the dietitian, diet office, and possibly nursing service as additional customers of the service provided. Clear quality requirements are then defined in measurable terms for each client. Aim for small successes first—outcome improvements that can be seen in two to four months.

The priorities for improvement are determined by the collective group of top management after input from many individuals. A key factor is the determination of who has responsibility for the process, so as to include them in the analysis. Name the initiative or project team(s), and set objectives for the team(s). Have the team refine and further define the area to improve. Include a diversity of members, including cross-department representation on the team. Quality management meeting times vary. Schechter and Boss[5] cite a range from 1 to 12 hours a week for meetings, with 4 to 6 hours typical.

The teams assess the situation from all angles: client needs and perceptions, perceptions of direct care/service providers, input from audiences indirectly involved, such as administrators or staff, and analysis of the hard data available. The method needs to be clear, comprehensive, and a true measure of the situation to assess actual client requirements and desires. Numerous measurement tools are available and useful. Schematic pictures of the situation help team members to visualize the situation. Using flowcharts, check sheets, line graphs, Pareto charts, control charts, and cause-and-effect diagrams will help crystallize the process.[6]

The team should provide an analysis of the reasons for the quality problems and design parameters to measure quality service and develop potential solutions. Brainstorming, delphi techniques, and nominal group activities assist in ensuring that all members of the team participate. The best solution to improve the process and the standard to measure quality are proposed and implementation planned. Implementation will cause refinement of the process. A feedback loop connecting the system and the needs of the clients should be established.

Finally, set the standard in the institution for growth improvement. TQM is based on making the improvement a day-to-day part of service, with the enhanced expectation now the "norm." Continue to maximize the improvement opportunities identified by the process through monitoring. This must include training the staff appropriately. The best service is only as good as the weakest employee. Orientation to new systems and training systems for new employees need to be established to continue to achieve quality. CQI is achieved only when continuous improvement of employees is achieved.

Limit the initiatives in Year 1 to system refinement and then expand in reasonable increments to major system evaluation. Set up key objectives for the continuation of the process. Remember that other organizational units may identify processes or projects where you are a provider or customer; time for staff involvement in these projects is essential.

QUALITY NUTRITIONAL CARE

Dietetic reimbursement for services continues to be a professional goal. Dietetic practitioners need to define the value of their services provided, determine quality standards, and measure the results. Dietetic services have to be consistently provided, at the appropriate level, and without adverse outcome to the client; unnecessary procedures and collection of information that do not affect care and cost must be reduced.

Three indicators of quality are patient satisfaction, patient outcome, and variations in practice. Philip Caper[7] proposes three components of medical quality: efficacy of the diagnostic or treatment procedure to accomplish the goal; appropriateness of the procedure based on individual cost and benefit; and caring, the interpersonal aspects of the caregiver-patient relationship. These same criteria appear useful in dietetics. Although hard scientific data may not be available for many diagnostic procedures or treatments, it is time to establish this body of knowledge and to conduct comparisons of alternate ways of treating various conditions to establish nutritional standards. The appropriateness of care may be compared to consensus papers on treatment and monitoring protocols when scientific data are not available. These protocols may be used with professional judgment in our diagnostic or treatment procedures. Besides net effectiveness of care, cost-effectiveness of diagnosis and care must be considered. A sample guideline for care developed by the Dietitians in Nutrition Support, the dietetic practice group of the American Dietetic Association, appears in Exhibit 19–1. Other formats may include written guidelines or parameters, such as when enteral or parenteral nutrition is provided or the use of critical indicators such as "Nutrition education will be provided when blood glucose is greater than 140 mg/dl on three or more occasions in one month or when hemoglobin A1C is greater than 8 on last visit." Teams within the institution are needed to establish practice guidelines for the institution. A systematic procedure to assimilate new knowledge into the guidelines is essential.

The art of caring is intertwined with patient services. Clients of nutritional services can best assess this aspect of quality. A multifaceted approach to client satisfaction of nutritional services needs to be established; is the client satisfied with the food, with the written material provided, with the counseling sessions? This sensitivity to the customer's needs is essential. TQM is results-driven. Distinctions to be made include separating "customers' evaluations of current products and services from what they'd like to have in the future."[5(p110)] In addition, the relative value of the services as opposed to the overall satisfaction with the service needs to be separated. Food service departments, clinics, and universities can ask their clients to identify or rank factors in order of their importance to service satisfaction. Distinctions among expected, requested, and exciting expectations of services are helpful, as well as how services are below expectations.

Hunt[8] identifies eight dimensions of quality: performance, features, reliability, responsiveness, credibility, tangibles, courtesy, and security. She recommends that the customer's requirements be defined according to these dimensions and that a customer worksheet be developed to determine if the requirement is met and the importance of the requirement to the customer. Hunt also recommends use of flow diagrams to define services. Figure 19–1 illustrates a flowchart of patient services. A flowchart crystallizes the process and illustrates areas for potential improvement.[9]

PLANNING AND CHANGE

Progress is desired change. TQM and many management principles encourage strategic planning and being a visionary. Although the purpose of dietetic and nutrition services remains relatively constant, the techniques have advanced. Paradigms have shifted to meet different needs of the clients and incorporate new technologies and automated systems. Part of achieving quality is keeping abreast of changes and incorporating them into a successful service, a service valued by

Exhibit 19–1 Guidelines for Initial Nutrition Screening

Marion Feizelson Winkler and Lucinda K. Lysen

The degree of nutrition care required by a patient varies depending on past history and present condition. Nutrition screening should be completed on all patients in the hospital, in home care, or in an extended-care facility. Screening should identify the patient's degree of nutritional risk and the subsequent steps needed for a comprehensive nutrition consultation and diagnostic nutrition assessment. This process should be ongoing to alert the clinician to changes in the patient's condition that affect nutritional status.

Objective

To identify parameters that provide an objective and reliable indication of an adult patient's nutrition risk.

I. Initial consultation with patient and/or caregiver regarding:
   A. Physical ability to ingest food
   B. Food tolerance
   C. Previous diet modifications
   D. Weight history
   E. Alcohol and/or drug abuse

II. Review of medical management and evaluation of diagnostic tests and procedures
   A. Diagnosis and/or problem list. Injury, disease, or treatment that may affect the patient's nutritional status by:
      1. Altering metabolism and requirements for specific nutrients
      2. Interfering with the ability to ingest or digest food, absorb nutrients, or excrete fibrous waste
   B. Clinical evidence of nutritional status
      1. Weight history
         a) Weight on admission
         b) Height
         c) Usual body weight
         d) Percentage weight change
      2. Laboratory data
         a) Serum albumin level
         b) Hemoglobin and hematocrit
         c) Other tests specific to disease state
      3. General physical appearance
         a) Edema
         b) Cachexia
         c) Obesity
         d) Open or draining wound
         e) Pressure sore
         f) Skin turgor and appearance
   C. Treatment that may affect nutritional status
      1. Dialysis
      2. Chemotherapy, radiation
      3. Surgery
      4. Medication with known drug-nutrient interaction and/or effect on appetite or metabolism

continues

Exhibit 19–1 continued

    D. Gastrointestinal function
    E. Diet prescription
       1. Diet order
       2. Number of days NPO (taking nothing by mouth) or on clear liquid diet without supplements
       3. Oral supplements
       4. Enteral nutrition support
       5. Total parenteral nutrition

III. Assessment of degree of nutritional risk is based on conclusions drawn from initial consultation with patient and review of medical management.
    A. A patient *may* require specialized nutrition support in the following situations:
       1. Poor intake—inability to meet nutrient and fluid requirements for more than 5 days
       2. Weight loss
          a) Unintentional weight loss of >10% of usual weight in 6 months
          b) Involuntary loss of >5 lb in 1 month
       3. Admission serum albumin level <3.5 g/dL
       4. Diagnosis or treatment interferes with intake of food or utilization of nutrients
    B. Documentation of assessment and need for nutrition intervention
       1. Patients identified at nutritional risk receive comprehensive nutrition consultation and diagnostic assessment
       2. Patients not at nutritional risk are periodically reevaluated

Bibliography

Hannaman KN, Penner SF. A nutrition assessment tool that includes diagnosis. *J Am Diet Assoc.* 1985;85:607–609.

Hedberg AM, Garcia N, Weinmann-Winkler S, Gabriel ML, Lutz AL. Nutritional risk screening: development of a standardized protocol using dietetic technicians. *J Am Diet Assoc.* 1988;88:1553–1556.

Hunt DR, Maslovitz A, Rowlands BJ, Brooks B. A simple nutrition screening procedure for hospital patients. *J Am Diet Assoc.* 1985;85:332–335.

Ireton-Jones CS, Hasse JM. Comprehensive nutritional assessment: the dietitian's contribution to the team effort. *Nutrition.* 1992;8:75–81.

Kamath SK, Lawler M, Smith AE, Kalat T, Olson R. Hospital malnutrition: a 33-hospital screening study. *J Am Diet Assoc.* 1986;86:203–206.

Noel MB, Wojnaroski SM. Nutrition screening for long-term care residents. *J Am Diet Assoc.* 1987;87:1557–1558.

Potosnak L, Chudnow LP, Simko MD. A simple tool for identifying patients at nutritional risk. *QRB Qual Rev Bull.* 1983;9:81–83.

Seltzer MH, Bastidas JA, Cooper DM, Engler P, Slocum B, Fletcher HS. Instant nutritional assessment. *JPEN J Parenter Enteral Nutr.* 1979;3:157–159.

Thompson JS, Burrough CA, Green JL, Brown GL. Nutritional screening in surgical patients. *J Am Diet Assoc.* 1984;84:337–338.

Tramposch TS, Blue LS. A nutrition screening and assessment system for use with the elderly in extended care. *J Am Diet Assoc.* 1987;87:1207–1210.

Screening: Reviewers

Alison Arkin, Linda M. Bayer, Leah M. Bennett, Peter J. Fabri, Linda S. Horace, Linda Kocinski, Julie O'Sullivan Maillet, Denise B. Schwartz, Ezra Steiger, 1991–92 Dietitians in Nutrition Support Executive Committee.

Source: Reprinted from Winkler, M.F. and Lysen, L.K., Suggested Guidelines for Nutrition and Metabolic Management of Adult Patients Receiving Nutrition Support. 2d ed. 1993; Sect. 1, 2–5.

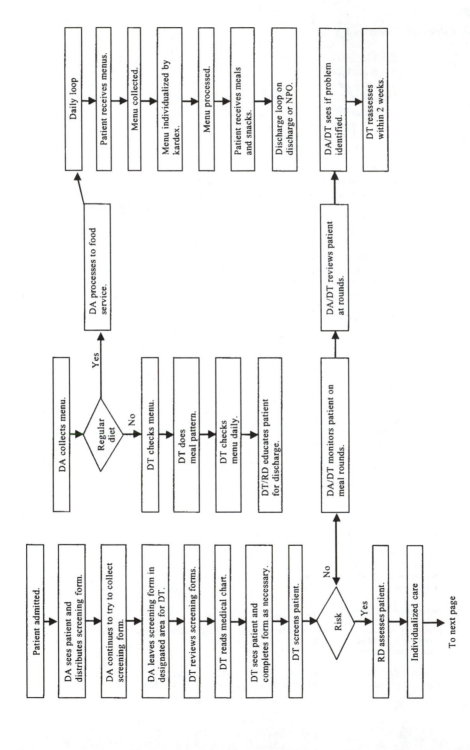

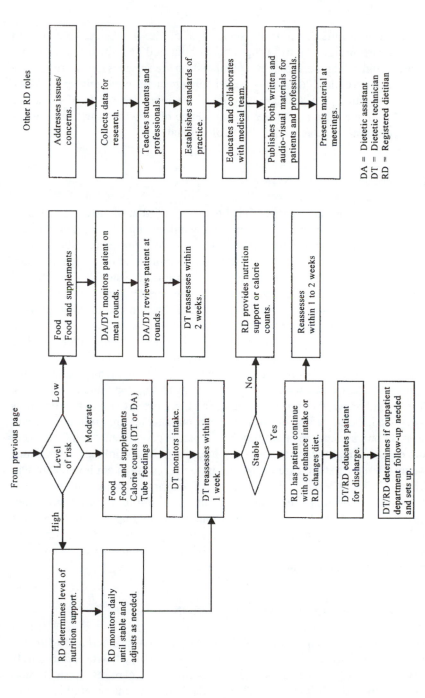

Figure 19–1 Flowchart of the Process of Patient Nutritional Care. *Source:* Reprinted from *Handbook for Clinical Nutrition Services Management* by M.R. Schiller, J.A. Gilbride, J. O'Sullivan Maillet, pp. 72–73, Aspen Publishers, Inc., © 1991.

the client. Long waits for nutrition services in clinics, nonselective menus in long-term care, weight control programs without body composition data, and laborious hand calculations of menu composition are services that were acceptable during most of the 20th century but will change in the next century. As Mary Abbott Hess said, "We are experts only if we meet the needs of those we serve."[3(p1127)] Each of us must meet the challenge of viewing nutrition services from the customer side as well as the professional side.

THE PROCESS OF CHANGE

Change of systems is complex. Kurt Lewin,[10] the father of the classic change theory, defined a three-phase process involving unfreezing, moving, and refreezing to obtain the desired change. During the *unfreezing* phase, the clinical manager has to raise the question to the Food Service and other departments: "Are we satisfied with the current quality monitoring system?" The clinical manager can shift the paradigm of producing single-discipline reports to integrating the CQI concepts into everyday care through communicating with other departments. To reduce the collection of parallel data tracks, the clinical manager should discuss care issues with other departments, identify data collection methods, and determine how to streamline the data collected.

The second phase, *moving*, brings the clinical nutrition manager toward the new goal—collaboration with other departments to develop mutual indicators. In this second phase, the forces for change and the forces to maintain the status quo may be in conflict. The clinical manager must foster integration of patient care issues across departmental lines. The separate department "solo" period in health care and quality management is gone, and multidisciplinary teams must move up from the patient care environment to the management level. Duplication of services will be reduced to lower costs. For example, think of the resources that are utilized to admit one client—each discipline doing its initial screening/ assessment. The clinical manager must communicate, campaign, and lobby the benefits of the new systems while understanding the resistance to the new systems. Each individual deserves the right to discuss the new systems and participate in the refinement of the system.

DATA BUT VERY LITTLE INFORMATION

Traditionally, a person could walk into a Department of Food and Nutrition and locate easily the neatly bound Quality Assurance Manual, with each monthly report precisely filed. The hard question that the health care revolution targets is, What is the value of the content? Have the bound data generated improved outcomes in care? Are the indicators limited to the "usual" indicators (diet accuracy, diet transmission, discharge notification), or should the clinical managers examine broader multidisciplinary issues?

EXAMPLES:

Traditional QA	CQI Today
Notification of 24-hour discharge diet instruction	Patient education, learner readiness, and appropriate environment for teaching
Nutrition screening completed within 24 hours of admission	Nutrition screening prior to elective admissions Incorporating nutrition screening into one multidisciplinary database
Meals delivered on time	Peak times for patient food consumption

One almost universal goal in a Food and Nutrition Department's operational system is to adequately nourish the patient. The traditional nutrition assessment within 72 hours of admission and three meals a day may not achieve this goal with sicker patients and shorter hospital stays.

The clinical dietitian's part of patient care begins with the nutritional assessment. Quality implementation depends on the liaisons between the clinical and operational units of the department. The prescription for nutritional care is diagnosed by the dietitian and filled in the purchasing, production, and assembly unit of the Food and Nutrition Department.

Traditionally, the clinical nutrition manager defines the service provided as inpatient care. Thus labor spent in "menu modification," whether by the pencil-and-paper method or computerized, is done without patient input and education. The clinical nutrition manager must consider what this menu correction activity accomplishes for the client. For a diabetic the hospital has artificially controlled blood glucose through the staff's guarding of activities, yet the client/patient has not been empowered regarding his or her food choices. When the client is discharged to the community, it is no surprise that his or her blood glucose curve takes a different direction.

CQI means taking a hard look at long-term "activities": What is their worth? What is the level of resource consumption to outcome levels? Can we do it a different way? Asking questions is critical to improving service in the 21st century health care system.

Successful change is not an overnight phenomenon. Persons involved in the change must participate in the planning phase. Persons affected by the change must be kept informed. This is where cross-disciplinary teamwork and consensus building occurs. CQI techniques point out the benefits of the collaborative approach, reducing costly and labor-intensive data collection with improved results. Simply, everyone "owns" the process and indicator.

EXAMPLES:

The Clinical Manager, acting alone:	The Clinical Manager, cooperating with the team:
Tracks drug-and-diet interaction notification via the clinical RD reviewing charts to evaluate if the unit is meeting the standard care. Results show less than 50% adherence. Then the clinical manager talks to the Pharmacy Director.	"Talks first" to the pharmacists and nurse to ascertain commonly ordered drugs, then shares the Food and Nutrition Department's Standard of Care Related to Drug and Nutrient Interaction Counseling and invites all providers to develop mutual indicators in the interest of productive patient care.
Tracks first	Talks first
Talks second	Tracks second
Result: resistance to change	Result: opportunities for improvement

CONCLUSION

The revised 1994 Joint Commission standards have shifted from a department set of services, such as dietetic services, to services provided, such as assessment and intervention. Nutrition and food service are essential to quality client care—it is the time to seize the opportunity these changes have created.

The final phase of Lewin's theory involves *refreezing*, characterized by consolidation and adoption of new ideas. The public, institutions, and the government are ready for new ideas—to deliver improved health care, more efficiently, with better results. CQI is the model by which these goals can be actualized. The process of CQI is continuous: it is a systematic way of working each and every day. The keys are to have a vision, establish baseline data as to how you are doing from the customer's perspective, improve the processes within your service, and continue to check and improve the service.

REFERENCES

1. American Hospital Association Staff. Standards for the Joint Commission for the Accreditation of Healthcare Organizations; Chicago, Ill: AHA; 1994.
2. Wiseman L. *Making the Transition from Quality Assurance to Continuous Quality Improvement.* Fayetteville, NC: Continuing Education Resources; 1992.
3. Walton M. *The Deming Management Method.* New York, NY: Perigee Books; 1986.
4. Hess MA. President's Page: minding your TQMs. *J Am Diet Assoc.* 1991;91(9):1126–1128.

5. Schechter M, Boss D. Putting quality management to work. *Food Management*. November 1992:102–113.

6. Ridway D. Introduction to Total Quality Management seminar. December 3, 10, 16, 17, 1993; Newark, NJ.

7. Caper P. Defining quality in medical care. *Health Affairs*. Spring 1988:49–61.

8. Hunt A. Total quality management in dietetics. Presented at American Dietetic Association Annual Meeting; October 21, 1992; Washington, DC.

9. Schiller R, Gilbride J, Maillet JO. *Handbook of Clinical Nutrition Management*. Gaithersburg, Md: Aspen Publishers, Inc; 1991.

10. Lewin K. *Field Theory in Social Science*. New York, NY: Harper & Row; 1951.

Chapter 20

Productivity and Cost-Effectiveness in Nutrition Services

Martha T. Conklin

OVERVIEW

Productivity is the relationship between outcomes and the resources used to create those outcomes. In the nutrition literature, outcomes have been typically defined as the volume of nutrition care tasks generated by professional labor. For example, the productivity of clinical dietitians has been described as the ratio of patient contacts versus the number of scheduled work hours for dietitians.[1] When productivity is defined in this manner, outcomes are phrased in terms of treatments applied to patients or services rendered to clients. Counting the number of nutritional assessments or the number of counseling sessions given per dietitian hour certainly is one way to look at productivity, but it tends to limit the scope of the analysis to the process of treating rather than curing, to teaching rather than learning.

Another paradigm for productivity is to define outcome in terms of changes that occur to the patient or client. A different productivity equation is used that defines inputs as the treatments or services given by professionals that achieve positive health outcomes in the target population. For example, instead of counting the number of nutritional care plans written as an indicator of productivity, this new equation determines the reduction in length of hospital stay for patients who received nutritional support that enhanced their nutritional status and thereby led to a quicker recovery. This type of productivity equation is harder to construct because so many factors associated with the health of patients/clients are not under the control of a dietitian, but viewing productivity in this manner places the focus on effectiveness in achieving positive health outcomes, and that is where the emphasis should be.

The current economic climate requires that government fund only those projects whose benefits to society outweigh the costs. In this era of health care financing reform, the focus on productivity is not on delivery of service but on health outcomes resulting from the delivery of service. This is forcing the dietetic profession to document its effectiveness or risk the shift of support from government and social agencies to other competing services. Resources are not unlimited, and choices must be made. When decisions are reached regarding the continuation or expansion of programs, the preferred alternative will be the one that produces the greatest impact on the most targets for the same expenditure, or that produces the same impact for the least expenditure. If nutrition services and therapies are to be included as a standard benefit in health care reform, evidence needs to be compiled that links the work of dietitians to health outcomes.

Studies using standard, evaluative research methodologies can be used to demonstrate the contribution a dietitian can make to improved patient care. The results of these studies can also supply the data to document the effectiveness of nutrition services that are needed to make legislative and administrative decisions regarding program funding, reimbursement formulas, and staffing requirements.

The objectives of this chapter are (1) to explain why documentation of program effectiveness is the first issue to be addressed in program evaluation; (2) to explain how questions of economic efficiency fit into overall program evaluation; (3) to define two techniques, cost-benefit and cost-effectiveness analyses, for evaluating the allocation of program resources; and (4) to suggest methods practitioners can use to collect data for analyzing program efficiency.

PROGRAM EVALUATION

According to Knickman, there are two separate components of program evaluation.[2] The first phase of evaluating a program is concerned with measuring what the program does. Research in this stage of evaluation involves determining whether the program intervention or treatment is carried out as planned, is providing services to the target population, and is resulting in changes or modifications consistent with the intended outcomes. In other words, did a program make a significant difference, and what was the probability of success attached to the outcome?[2,3]

Practitioners need information to plan nutrition intervention programs that are structured to obtain valid, objective data formulated in terms of outcome criteria. A program is effective, and therefore the professionals working in that program are productive, if positive health outcomes occur in the target population. If a program fails to demonstrate achievement of its goals, it may be decided that the program should be abandoned or changed. No further expenditure of resources is justifiable if a program is not successful. In this sense, professionals also should not be judged productive, even though treatment was rendered as planned, if their labor did not result in positive health outcomes.

Only after effectiveness is substantiated should an analyst determine whether program funds have been used efficiently in terms of alternative uses of the same resources. This is the second phase of program evaluation. Cost-benefit analysis and cost-effectiveness analysis are both used in this second phase. Whereas the question of a program's effectiveness is answered by impact studies, the calculation of the value of these effects and the efficiency with which resources are allocated is specific to the cost-benefit framework of economic analysis.[2,3]

Cost containment is not a procedure pertinent to economic analysis, although it is a fiscal reality in making budgetary decisions for existing health care programs. Cost containment implies the setting of explicit expenditure goals or "caps" and then altering budgets and expenditures so that these goals are met by the end of a specific fiscal period.[4] Cost-benefit analysis is used in deciding whether a program should be initiated or continued; cost containment, on the other hand, is related to operational expenditures in an existing program or facility. The former is an analytical tool; the latter is an operational constraint placed upon a department or organization by administration or government funding formulas.

COST-BENEFIT ANALYSIS

Cost-benefit analysis is a strategy for determining how to allocate finite resources. Using this analytical method, policy makers and program planners attempt to decide which alternative use of resources will best improve the well-being of individuals, given existing institutional structures, public programs, and distribution of private funds.[3]

Cost-benefit analysis provides decision makers with information designed to facilitate their ability to make rational decisions. The methodology is based on the reasonable assumption that any objective fact brought into a decision-making process is better than none. However, cost-benefit analysis is not intended to be the sole decision-making criterion. Its economic information must be balanced with social, political, humanitarian, and other information in order to reach a just decision.[5] Nor is it meant to alter the practitioner-client relationship. As pointed out by Klarman, clinicians caring for their patients are not expected to assume an economic posture, and they should not. They must continue to act as if human life and health are invaluable. It is society's role to introduce cost-benefit constraints into the decision-making process.[6]

Computing Costs and Benefits

A comprehensive cost-benefit analysis requires estimates of all the benefits and costs of a program. The first question to be addressed is, "Benefits and costs to whom?" Factors vary depending upon the perspective used in the analysis. Before benefits and costs are calculated, the accounting perspective must be declared to be either that of the individual receiving the program, an agency delivering the service, or society. This perspective will dictate relevant costs and benefits.[7]

Once determined from a specific perspective, the benefits and costs are translated into dollars. The benefits and costs can then be compared by computing either a benefit-to-cost ratio (B/C) or net benefits (B-C). A project is economically efficient if the benefits are greater than the costs: that is, if the ratio is greater than one and the net benefits are greater than zero.

When one is determining the benefits of a program, it is essential to identify all end results. This means all direct and indirect effects of the program, including the rate of success or the probability of outcome attached to each result. Resources that are saved because of the program are also considered to be benefits.

The cost-benefit methodology requires that the benefits have an economic value to individuals in order to be included in the analysis. Economic value is defined as the money people would be willing to pay to ensure that a project is undertaken. The value is placed on a direct benefit by finding its market price in the private sector or by determining the price of an equivalent substitute in the market.[2] The benefits of saved resources are calculated by summing the costs that were averted as a result of the program being in effect . For example, in a health care context this includes the cost of personnel, materials, and expenses that would be incurred to treat people if they were to remain ill.[8] Indirect benefits may be harder to ascertain and require much more judgment in their calculation, but they are nonetheless pertinent. Indirect benefits of an alcoholism rehabilitation program, for example, could be how successful participants of the program avoid the social costs of absenteeism and reduced productivity.

The costs used in cost-benefit analysis include both direct and indirect resources required to conduct the program. Direct costs are items from a budget—personnel, facilities, materials, equipment, financing, and so forth. Indirect costs include "opportunity costs," that is, the value of foregone opportunities because resources were used in a given project when they could have been used in an alternative manner. For example, the potential loss of income because a patient is enrolled in a time-consuming treatment program is an indirect cost.[3] Other indirect costs are losses of labor resources due to mortality and morbidity.[9]

Discounting and Sensitivity Analysis

Both costs and benefits are calculated to extend into the future—for example, to extend throughout a lifetime. In calculating these values, economists use a technique called discounting. Discounting is predicated on the theory that a dollar earned in the future is never worth a full dollar.[10] The reason is that a dollar not spent now can be invested productively to yield a larger number of real dollars in the future; also, the recipients of the dollar might not be alive in the future to collect what is owed them. In other words, a dollar in 1994 is worth more to a consumer than it will be in 2004 because of the immediate gratification associated with spending in the present or the delayed gratification of accrued investment. Discounting, the inverse of compound interest, weights future dollars by a discount factor to make them equivalent to present dollars. The level of the discount rate is a controversial issue among economists because the higher it is, the lower the benefit or cost will be valued.[3,11,12]

In order to test the sensitivity of the results of a cost-benefit study to various assumptions that were made by the analyst, well-conceived studies also engage in a process called sensitivity analysis. In this process various assumptions such as the level of the discount rate are changed and the benefit-cost ratio is recalculated. If the project or program still yields net benefits with changed analytical assumptions, the analysis is considered even more cogent.[3] For a review of the terms used in this discussion, see the definitions listed in Exhibit 20–1.

Limitations

By converting all factors into monetary terms, cost-benefit analysis allows a comparison of the economic efficiency of program alternatives, even when the interventions are not aimed at common goals. Using this technique, one can ascertain the worth or merit of a single project, and also compare which of two or more projects in different areas produces better returns.[3] The program that yields the greatest net benefit would logically be the one supported.

Cost-benefit analysis does have limitations, however, as a decision-making tool. The requirement that costs and benefits be measured in monetary terms is both an advantage and a disadvantage. Using this method, costs and benefits could be compared and a decision could be made to undertake only those projects with benefits exceeding costs. However, the measurement of benefits in dollar

Exhibit 20–1 Definitions of Terms in Economic Analysis

Perspective: Accounting view taken by the analyst. Examples include the patient, the dietetic department, the agency, or society.

Discounting: Process of computing the present value of future outcomes or resources.

Sensitivity Analysis: Test of the stability of the analysis by changing the assumptions, estimates, or judgments used by the analyst.

Direct Benefits: Outcomes associated with the program or intervention that can be directly related to savings or averted expenditures. In a health care context, this might be savings associated with not treating a person who has been cured of an illness, with a decrease in hospital days, with reduction in or elimination of drugs required by a patient, or with the extended life of a patient who then remains a productive member of society.

Indirect Benefits: Outcomes that result from the program, but for which the measurement of value involves a less direct calculation that may involve making several assumptions; nonetheless, a value in monetary terms can be placed on the benefit. For example, the social costs of absenteeism, lost productivity, and other morbidity factors related to a person having a chronic disease that are averted as a result of the intervention.

Direct Costs: Costs directly related to the program or intervention. These costs may come from the budget or be factored from budgetary expenditures. They may also include the direct use of resources that are not "paid for" by the organization, depending on the perspective from which the analysis is approached. Direct costs are personnel, equipment, materials, supplies, and overhead.

Indirect Costs: Costs associated with the program in a less direct fashion. Opportunity costs, the value of foregone opportunities because resources were used in a given project when they could have been used in an alternative manner, are calculated under indirect costs. Indirect costs could be cost of travel to receive treatment, cost of waiting time to receive treatment, and loss of income due to treatment. The accounting perspective will determine which indirect costs are pertinent.

---

terms biases cost-benefit analysis in favor of those programs that preserve the most "productive" people in terms of earnings, namely male workers and younger individuals.[8] The criterion used in cost-benefit analysis requires only that the sum of benefits across all individuals be greater than the sum of costs across all individuals. Thus the cost-benefit ratio justifies the existence of some programs that cause people in society to be worse off than they would be in the absence of those programs. It ignores the question of which person benefits and focuses exclusively on determining the aggregate quantity of benefits.[2]

COST-EFFECTIVENESS ANALYSIS

As we have seen, the major disadvantage of cost-benefit analysis is the requirement that human lives, quality of life, and other social benefits be valued in dollars.[11] The ethical and judgmental problems encountered in attempting to monetize the benefits of social programs or health service projects are precisely the reason that many researchers use cost-effectiveness analysis instead of cost-benefit analysis to evaluate resource allocation. Cost-effectiveness analysis does not make judgments regarding the relative desirability of project objectives; rather it compares the costs of alternative strategies for achieving a given goal. Cost-effectiveness requires the calculation of program costs and benefits, but the benefits do not have to be converted into dollars; only the costs must be. The benefits are expressed as the documented results of the program.

This type of analysis is particularly useful to managers in assessing the efficacy of a program. The cost-effectiveness approach can be used by a department whose goals have already been established by administration; the central focus of attention can then be concentrated on determining which combination of resources is the most efficient, or least costly, in meeting those goals.[2,3] It is important to emphasize that no program can, by itself, be judged as cost-effective. By definition, the nature of the analysis is comparative. A new program can be compared with the old way of accomplishing the same objectives, or two or more effective programs with the same objectives can be compared to determine which is the most efficient.

The criterion for cost-effectiveness used with most health care programs is the ratio of the net increase of health care costs to net effectiveness expressed in outcome criteria, usually enhanced life expectancy and quality-adjusted life years.[10,13] "The lower the value of this ratio, the higher the priority in terms of maximizing benefits derived from a given health expenditure."[10(p1954)]

The computation of the numerator (cost) and the denominator (effectiveness) employs a rationale very similar to that used in cost-benefit analysis. Costs include only the resources drawn from the health care budget. The formula used to calculate costs derives the net changes in the total number of dollars spent on health care as a result of the program or practice under consideration.

The denominator of the equation, net health effectiveness, includes life and other health benefits conferred. These are usually measured in lives, life years, or quality-adjusted life years,[10] but they could also be expressed in terms of a specific outcome. As in cost-benefit analysis, discounting is applied to future costs or outcomes.[8,10]

In summary, both cost-benefit and cost-effectiveness studies in health care should be evaluated by the following criteria: effectiveness or impact determined by use of an experimental or quasiexperimental design with random assignment of subjects,[14] calculation of all immediate costs of the program, costs of subsequent workup and/or treatments, costs of evaluating and treating complications with the program, future costs averted due to the program's effectiveness, and increased health care costs during prolonged life. If the study takes a societal or patient perspective, measurement of quantity and quality of life should be addressed. Future dollar costs and benefits should be discounted and sensitivity analyses performed on the discount rate and other key variables.[13]

COST-BENEFIT AND COST-EFFECTIVENESS ANALYSIS APPLIED TO NUTRITION PROGRAMS

Well-designed and -executed cost-benefit or cost-effectiveness studies on nutrition services are not easily found in the literature. The difficulty in conducting economic research on nutrition programs is in separating the impact of nutrition intervention from the entire spectrum of prevention and treatment outcomes. This is precisely the problem identified by the Ambulatory Nutrition Care Research Study Committee of the American Dietetic Association (ADA). The chairperson of this committee wrote that the committee began in 1977 with the assumption that the relative costs and benefits of nutritional counseling were unknown. After extensive literature review, that assumption was judged correct.[15,16]

The committee developed a model for testing the cost benefits of nutritional counseling (see Figure 20–1). The first linkage in the model was found to be the least well documented because of the variation in clinical practice and inconsistent documentation. As one follows the model to the right, there is more proof in the literature concerning altered risk factors affecting health outcomes, leading to economic benefits.[15] It is important to note that the first step in the model is where dietitians contribute their unique knowledge and skills in translating treatment or prevention objectives into realistic meal patterns for patients or clients.

Since this time, research on the cost-effectiveness of nutrition services has continued to be an area of vital interest to the dietetic profession. Dietitians have been challenged to reexamine process-oriented standards of care and productivity and to measure the effectiveness of nutrition services in terms of patient or client outcomes.[16] Studies that focus on establishing the effectiveness of services rendered by dietitians have continued to be underscored as the first requirement in building a body of evidence associated with the cost benefit or cost-effectiveness of nutrition care.[17,18]

In May of 1990, ADA funded a project to provide members of the profession with realistic recommendations regarding the current status of information and the need for future studies on costs and benefits of nutrition care services. The

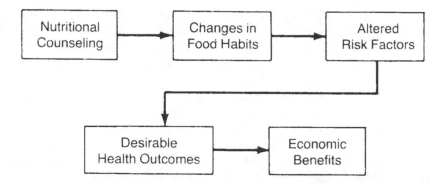

Figure 20–1 American Dietetic Association Model for Testing Cost Benefits of Nutrition Counseling. *Source:* Reprinted from Mason, M, et al., Requisites of Advocacy, Philosophy, Research, Documentation: Phase II of the Costs and Benefits of Nutrition Care, *Journal of the American Dietetic Association*, Vol. 80, p. 213, with permission of the American Dietetic Association, © 1982.

---

subsequent report indicated that the biggest problem in the literature was not the number of studies on effectiveness, cost, and cost-effectiveness of nutrition care, but the *quality* of the studies. The studies "suffered from poor design, arbitrarily selected samples, unaccounted for concomitant or confounding factors, and inappropriate statistical analyses."[19] (pS-10) Incidently, very few of these studies were conducted by dietitians. This led the project director to suggest that dietitians become more active in the planning, implementing, and reporting of cost-effectiveness studies.

Despite the problems of quality, results of this literature review indicated that it was possible to link nutrition care to important clinical outcomes in four areas: acute illness such as burns and surgery, prenatal care, obesity, and diabetes.[19] Results from several studies confirmed direct benefits for patients and the hospital due to fewer medical complications and reduced length of stay when nutrition intervention was administered to patients in hypermetabolic stress associated with burns and surgery.[20] Even stronger evidence had been accumulated on the cost benefits associated with nutrition intervention in prenatal care. Nutrition intervention had been linked to improved pregnancy outcomes, which translated into healthier infants and cost savings to the health care system.[21] A recent study found that participation in the Special Supplemental Food Program for Women, Infants, and Children (WIC) improved birth outcome to the extent that it could be estimated that for each $1.00 spent funding WIC, Medicaid would save $2.91 in costs for newborn medical care.[22] Studies that demonstrated short-term weight loss after nutrition intervention were common, but more investigators needed to follow the participants for more than 12 months. The costs of weight control programs had been measured in cost per pound lost, cost per participant, and cost per 1 percent decrease in percentage overweight.[23] The success of nutrition intervention in promoting normal levels of blood sugar and lipids had been well documented; however, more studies were needed to investigate the long-term effect of diabetes education on program participants.[24]

Two strong recommendations came from the report. The first was that practice guidelines for nutrition care be developed, validated, and studied to ascertain the impact of the delivery of nutrition care according to practice guidelines on patient health outcomes and cost-effectiveness. The second recommendation was that the American Dietetic Association fund studies to develop a strong database of scientific research on nutrition care. The Nutrition Services Payment Systems (NSPS) Committee of ADA identified non-insulin-dependent diabetes mellitus (NIDDM) as the first area for study.

In 1991, ADA awarded a contract to develop, field test, and evaluate nutrition care practice guidelines for NIDDM written by an interdisciplinary consensus panel and field tested through a randomized clinical trial.[25] The actual study will take several years to complete, but the process of developing and validating practice protocols has already created significant dialogue in the professional community about appropriate outcomes to use in determining effectiveness. The study design can also serve as a model for the study of cost-effectiveness in nutrition care for other diseases and conditions.[26]

The profession of dietetics through the American Dietetic Association has continued to emphasize the importance of cost-benefit and cost-effectiveness studies in documenting the contribution of nutrition care to the health of patients and clients. Most recently these efforts have made it possible for leaders in the association to put forth a legislative platform entitled *Economic Benefits of Nutrition Services.* This document specifically addressed the cost-effectiveness of nutrition services and therapies and the scientific expertise of the registered dietitian. It was sent to all policy makers, legislators, and their staff to explain the value of nutrition services in promoting the health of individuals.[27,28]

PRIMER FOR THE PRACTITIONER

Conducting efficiency analyses correctly is not an easy enterprise. Should the average dietetic practitioner be involved in this type of activity? The answer is a qualified "yes!" It is qualified by the fact that ADA is making considerable strides in developing efficacious protocols for determining the cost-effectiveness of nutrition services.[26] As individuals we do not have the talent or resources to duplicate these efforts. Dietitians should, however, understand enough about the methodology to support the process and promote the results once they are generated.

The process of building a body of evidence that links nutrition services and therapies to health outcomes is long and tedious, and it does not exist in a vacuum. Practitioners help the profession in this process in several ways. First, they help by being aware of the factors involved in documenting cost benefit and cost-effectiveness. If they understand the methodology and begin to think in terms of client outcomes, they can be alert to case studies that will establish a relationship between nutrition services and cost savings in health care. The Massachusetts Dietetic Association members responded to a call from their state's senators for data documenting the positive benefits of nutrition services by collecting case study data.[29] One case may not be sufficient evidence within itself to establish the effects of nutrition services, but combined with other cases, a body of anecdotal evidence begins to build, and this may lead to funding of a full-fledged research project designed to establish this relationship more objectively. For example, case studies from several states were used as the foundation for the ADA legislative platform. These studies showed "that nutrition care saves health care dollars by reducing the need for long-term drug therapies, reducing treatment needs, and reducing hospitalization."[28(p1043)] It is apparent that evidence to support the cost-effectiveness of nutrition intervention does exist.

Secondly, practitioners can help by conducting small studies in their own work environment that document the cost benefit or cost-effectiveness of their practice. When one is designing a study of this type, the most logical accounting perspective to assume is that of the department or agency that funds the program or intervention. Using this perspective, the analysis most closely resembles what is termed a *private profitability analysis*. The program sponsor accounting perspective is most appropriate when the sponsor must make choices between alternative programs in the face of a fixed budget,[3] and this is the situation most practitioners find themselves in today.

Documenting Benefits of Nutrition Intervention

In order to conduct research within a cost-benefit or cost-effectiveness framework, the impact of a specific program has to be determined. Whether the benefits are then valued in monetary terms depends on which methodology is used. Sound program evaluation research focusing on effectiveness must be the foundation of conclusions regarding any benefits claimed. Remember that economic analysis is used to decide how to allocate money between competing, effective services. If a service or intervention does not achieve its intended objectives—if it does not affect positive health outcomes—there is no need to proceed any further. Funds should be withdrawn from this endeavor.

Direct Benefits

A direct benefit is any outcome directly attributable to the nutrition project under consideration. An example of a direct benefit is a change in diet or food habits as a result of nutrition counseling. From this change, an increase or decrease in the intake of specific nutrients could be documented. Another direct benefit is the change in the functioning of the body due to altered food intake. This could be identified by fluctuations in weight; changes in gastrointestinal functioning, such as reduced constipation; adequate weight gain during pregnancy; altered biochemical and clinical conditions associated with the amelioration of nutrient deficiencies; reduction of hypertension or the severity of diabetes due solely to weight loss; or any other factor that is a documented outcome of a program.

Placing a value on such benefits is most easily done by determining the cost of the treatment alternatives necessitated by the absence of improved food habits. In economic terms, these are called *market substitutes* and *saved resources*. For example, the value of reduced constipation is the cost of laxatives; for a geriatric population, it is the cost of treating fecal impactions multiplied by the probability of occurrence. In a similar calculation reported in the literature, it was determined that $44,000 was saved per year in the cost of laxatives by the initiation of a dietary fiber supplementation program.[30] Davidson et al. used this methodology in calculating the benefits of a nutrition counseling program for diabetics.[31]

Indirect Benefits

An indirect benefit of a nutrition program would be the saving of physicians' time and other organizational resources due to the prevention or reduction in severity of a disease. This could be documented by decreases in admissions into acute care or long-term care facilities and/or decreases in the length of stay. An example would be the Nutrition Program for the Elderly, which could help maintain an individual in the community and potentially contribute to the avoidance or delay of institutionalization. The ultimate indirect benefit from a nutrition program would be saved or extended lives. Cost-benefit procedures require that a value be placed on human life, and there is a body of literature dedicated to making this value judgment.[9,10,12] The potential savings generated by a change in the cost of food required to meet a specific regimen as compared to the traditional food consumed can also be considered an indirect benefit of nutrition intervention. Such a calculation has been done for a nutrition education program designed to teach the principles and applications of a sodium-restricted diet, including methods for preparing low-sodium foods at home. The results showed that the cost of preparing a 500 mg sodium diet at home did not differ from that of a regular diet, whereas low-sodium convenience food items specifically formulated for home consumption caused a significant increase in cost as compared to the cost of a regular diet.[32] This calculation alone showed the potential economic impact of education provided by a registered dietitian. The direction of the change in cost that is associated with a change in food habits would dictate whether it should be considered an indirect benefit, an indirect cost, or a neutral consideration.

Cost-Effectiveness Format

The complexities in determining all the benefits of nutrition intervention and then placing a value on those benefits are innumerable and involve many assumptions. The simpler approach, one that is defensible in terms of current knowledge, is the use of a cost-effectiveness format. With this method, a dietitian documents program effectiveness in terms of observable outcomes without converting them into dollars. The efficiency in resource allocation is then evaluated by comparing the costs of the alternatives associated with delivering the service. The formula for the cost-effectiveness calculation is:

Average cost per client/average outcome per client

For example, in a cholesterol reduction program, the formula might be average cost per patient to deliver the program divided by the average percent decrease in LDL cholesterol resulting from the program. The analysis would yield the cost for each 1 percent decrease in LDL cholesterol. The treatment protocol that achieved the least cost per 1 percent decrease in LDL cholesterol would be considered cost-effective. As with cost-benefit analysis, there are no set guidelines for the cost-effectiveness approach other than the application of common sense, documented program effectiveness, current costs tallied from a consistent perspective, and professional judgment.

Documenting Costs of Nutrition Intervention

Once program effectiveness is documented and the rate of success is known, ascertaining program costs becomes the next issue in calculating either cost benefits or cost-effectiveness. The accounting perspective must be declared first, because costs are specific to the viewpoint of the analysis. Both direct and indirect costs need to be determined. Direct costs are the resources consumed by the program. These should be calculated as the real costs or those reflected in an operating statement as opposed to an anticipated budget. The salaries of the dietitians, nurses, physicians, dietetic technicians, and others working on the project would be direct costs. For example, the salaries of the registered dietitian and a dietary clerk assigned to a dialysis unit would be pertinent to the cost of a program delivering nutritional services to renal patients.

Documenting Time

When the nature of a dietitian's job involves a variety of functions, as in a public health setting or community hospital, it may be necessary to determine the percentage of time spent in various categories of activity such as screening, assessing, planning direct delivery of services to the client, making arrangements for delivery of services through others, and other activities defined by the particular job description. Data from this type of activity sampling can also be collected in terms of diagnoses. A log of time spent in various professional activities related to levels of nutrition intervention or diagnoses should be maintained systematically. The percentage of time spent in each activity category along with the estimate of the number of patients to be treated or counseled within a given time can lead to a cost figure for dietitian time per diagnosis, professional activity, or specific program. Similar information can be used to anticipate or justify staffing patterns for services. This methodology is outlined by the staffing study sponsored by the American Dietetic Association.[33]

Documenting Direct Costs

Other direct costs of nutrition programs are the equipment, supplies, rent, maintenance, administration, and other overhead expenses that are derived from financial statements. Even in an interdisciplinary program, these costs can be apportioned by using accounting techniques, such as allocating costs for rent and maintenance by applying a factor related to the percentage of square footage occupied by the nutrition service component, or assigning costs by a factor related to the patients the dietitian counsels as a percentage of the whole patient population.

Documenting Indirect Costs

Indirect costs focus on "opportunity cost." What could the department or agency have been doing if it were not engaged in the project under study? If a department decides to forego a revenue-producing community project in weight control in order to focus attention on screening and delivering more intensive nutrition services to inpatients, the indirect cost of that decision is the revenue that could have been generated by the weight control project.

If a client accounting perspective is used, the value of the participants' inputs and time spent in the program should be calculated as an indirect cost. An indication of average earnings or worth is necessary to determine this figure, and the time spent in traveling and waiting should be considered as well as the actual treatment time.[3] The extra cost of food and vitamin supplements consumed while in the program would also be a participant input.

An indirect cost that is difficult to determine, but of importance if the societal accounting perspective is used, is the cost to society of the death and disability related to the untreated people who could have benefited from nutrition intervention but did not have access to it. Health statistics could supply some of this information, but the dietitian could begin by considering the total demand for nutrition services. In other words, how many people needed the services of dietitians but did not get them? Parenthetically, this same information is needed by an administrator or program director when making plans for the future. Exhibit 20–2 summarizes some of the potential costs of nutrition intervention. It illustrates how an analyst might display costs in order to make sure that all costs have been considered while only those costs pertinent to the chosen accounting

Exhibit 20–2 Worksheet for Determining Costs

	Accounting Perspective		
Costs	*Agency*	*Client*	*Society*
Salaries			
Dietitian's time	X		X
Time of other health professionals	X		X
Time of nonprofessionals	X		X
Time of administrators	X[a]		X
Time of patients/clients		X	X
Facilities			
Office space	X		X
Equipment	X		X
Supplies	X		X
Maintenance	X		X
Overhead	X		X
Transportation	X[b]	X	X
Treatment			
Charges to patient/client		X	
Extra food		X[c]	
Nutrient supplements		X[c]	
Loss to society from lack of treatment			X

TOTAL COSTS

[a]Only if administrative time is in budget.
[b]Only if home visits are part of treatment regimen.
[c]Only if change in habits represents additional costs.

perspective are included. The "Xs" illustrate costs that would typically be included in analyses from the various accounting perspectives.

MODEL OF A COST-EFFECTIVENESS STUDY

In this section, a model cost-effectiveness study is presented that could be used to evaluate alternative weight control programs. It does not represent a comprehensive model because issues of discounting and sensitivity analysis are not addressed. It is also a study designed from the agency or operational perspective. It was written to give a broad-based example of some of the considerations and calculations that would be required in a study of this type. Other models exist in the literature. A hospital model associated with inpatient nutrition care was published as a result of a consensus panel in the medical and dietetic profession.[34] An additional model of a cost-effectiveness study on a community-based lipid screening project has been published.[35] Both of these examples are resources where dietitians can find answers to questions about designing a cost-effectiveness study in their own practice setting.

Parameters

Let us assume that the Ramar Corporation was considering sponsoring a weight control program for its senior executives and middle managers. The entire cost of the program would be paid by the company as a health benefit to the employees. The Ramar Corporation's personnel department, with the aid of a company economist and a consulting dietitian, found three alternative programs for achieving this objective:

1. a medical model, using appetite-suppressant drug therapy and vitamins prescribed by a physician
2. a psychosocial model, using peer counseling, psychosocial incentives, and a low-calorie diet, high in protein and low in carbohydrate, that was unilaterally prescribed to all participants
3. an interdisciplinary model, using nutrition counseling concentrating on an individualized, reduced-calorie meal plan, behavioral modification, and an exercise program, all of which were tailored to the lifestyles of the participants.

Whereas the professional expertise of the registered dietitian (RD) was used in all three models, the RD was involved only as a consultant for the participants who had nutritional complications in Models 1 and 2. In the interdisciplinary team Model 3, the dietitian was the team leader and the primary professional involved in the planning and implementation of the program.

The study team from the personnel department collected information concerning costs and effectiveness from ongoing programs in order to calculate the cost-effectiveness of each program alternative. The Ramar Corporation was prepared to fund the most cost-effective method of ensuring weight control for its executives.

Methodology

A cost-effectiveness study was conducted on the costs of each alternative program in relation to the outcome criteria. The criteria used in evaluating program impact were the average number of pounds lost by the participants and the percentage of participants who maintained that weight loss for at least one year. Information on costs and program impact was accumulated from a record review of existing programs that were treating population groups similar to the employees of the proposed program (see Table 20–1). Based on this information, the cost-effectiveness calculation was as follows:

Program	Program Cost	Outcome Calculation	Cost-Effectiveness Ratio
1	$48,600	$(325 \times 21\# \times .03 = 205\#)$	$237: 1# wt. loss
2	$53,803	$(460 \times 18\# \times .05 = 414\#)$	$130: 1# wt. loss
3	$76,460	$(300 \times 23\# \times .10 = 690\#)$	$111: 1# wt. loss

The interdisciplinary team model would be the most cost-effective program, based on the established outcome criteria and the data available. This program had a cost-effectiveness ratio of $111 per pound of weight lost and maintained for at least one year, as opposed to $237 and $130 for Model Programs 1 and 2, respectively. According to this study, the Ramar Corporation would be using company resources most efficiently if it developed and funded an interdisciplinary weight control program administered by a registered dietitian.

Model Program 3 had the highest cost, and the study team might well have rejected this alternative if they had just compared program costs. A more informed decision was made only after comparing the costs to the outcome. When effectiveness was brought into the equation, the program that initially appeared to be the most costly became the most cost-effective because of a higher degree of performance on the outcome criterion. This shows the strength of economic analysis as a decision-making tool.

Table 20–1 Cost-Effectiveness Data on Three Weight Control Programs

Program Model	Annual Expense Categories	Percent of Time	Annual Cost	No. Pts.	Aver. Wt. Loss (lbs.)	One-Year Maintenance (Percent)
1. Medical model	*Staffing required*			325	21	3
	Physician	20	$20,000			
	Registered nurse	25	7,500			
	Registered dietitian	5	1,400			
	Clerk	25	4,160			
	Pharmaceutical supplies, rent, utilities, maintenance, miscellaneous expenses		15,540			
	Total cost		$48,600			
2. Psychosocial model	*Staffing required*			460	18	5
	Clinical psychologist	50	31,500			
	Registered dietitian	5	1,400			
	Clerk	50	8,320			
	Materials and supplies		550			
	Rent, utilities, maintenance, telephone answering service, miscellaneous expenses		12,033			
	Total cost		$53,803			
3. Interdisciplinary team model	*Staffing required*			300	23	10
	Registered dietitian	100	28,000			
	Physician	5	5,000			
	Fitness trainer	25	7,000			
	Clerk	50	8,320			
	Materials and supplies		1,890			
	Rent (including exercise facilities), utilities, maintenance, miscellaneous expenses		26,250			
	Total cost		$76,460			

Note: All data are hypothetical.

CONCLUSION

The calculation of costs and benefits is only one way to evaluate the "worth" of nutritional services, but it is a method that has persuasive power in legislative and administrative arenas. Although it is not a panacea for all the problems in the profession, the discipline imposed by trying to conduct this type of analysis, or even becoming involved in the collection of its raw data, can help with daily managerial decisions and have a potentially positive effect on the practice of dietetics. Knowledge of effectiveness can also help dietitians market their skills with other members of the health care team. Ultimately, it falls to dietetic professionals, not economists, to document the net benefit of their services and to use the resources at their disposal efficiently. Each dietitian bears the responsibility to become involved in the process, not only to document one's own worth but to establish how the profession contributes to the prevention and treatment of disease and disability.

REFERENCES

1. Leyshock PJ, Tracy DL. Using a computerized system to monitor clinical dietetic productivity. *Top Clin Nutr.* 1992;7:69–77.

2. Knickman J. Conceptual and technical considerations in cost-benefit analysis. In: Sutherland J, ed. *Management Handbook for Public Administrators.* New York, NY: Van Nostrand Rheinhold; 1978:663–668.

3. Rossi PH, Freeman HE. *Evaluation—A Systematic Approach.* 5th ed. Newbury Park, Calif: Sage Publications; 1993.

4. Richards G. Cost containment: the heat is on, and up. *Hospitals.* 1982;56:82.

5. Swint M, Nelson WB. The application of economic analysis to evaluation of alcoholism rehabilitation programs. *Inquiry.* 1977;14:63.

6. Klarman HE. Present status of cost-benefit analysis in the health field. *Am J Pub Health.* 1967;57:1948–1953.

7. Hellinger FJ. Cost-benefit analysis of health care: past applications and future prospects. *Inquiry.* 1980;17:204–215.

8. Tolpin, HG. Economics of health care. *J Am Diet Assoc.* 1980;76:217–221.

9. Cooper BS, Rice DP. The economic cost of illness revisited. *Soc Security Bull.* 1976;39:21.

10. Rice DP, Cooper BS. The economic value of human life. *Am J Pub Health.* 1967;57:1954–1966.

11. Weinstein MC, Stason WB. Foundations of cost-effectiveness analysis for health and medical practices. *N Engl J Med.* 1977;296:716.

12. Landefeld JS, Soskin EP. The economic value of life: linking theory to practice. *Am J Pub Health.* 1982;72:555–565.

13. Ganiats TG, Wong AF. Evaluation of cost-effectiveness research: a survey of recent publications. *Fam Med.* 1991;23:457–462.

14. Yates BT. Cost-effectiveness analysis and cost-benefit analysis: an introduction. In Cordray DS, Lipsey MW, eds. *Evaluation Studies: Review Annual, Vol 11.* Newbury Park, Calif: Sage Publications; 1987:315–342.

15. Mason M, Hallahan IA, Monsen E, et al. Requisites of advocacy, philosophy, research, documentation: Phase II of the cost and benefits of nutritional care. *J Am Diet Assoc.* 1982;80: 213–214.

16. Disbrow DD. The costs and benefits of nutrition services: a literature review. *J Am Diet Assoc.* 1989;89(suppl 89):S6–S55.

17. Simko MD, Conklin, MT. Focusing on the effectiveness side of the cost-effectiveness equation. *J Am Diet Assoc.* 1989;89:485–487.

18. Splett, PL. Assessing effectiveness of nutrition care: prerequisite for cost-effectiveness analysis. *Top Clin Nutr.* 1990;5:26–33.

19. Splett PL. Phase I: Status report of existing data on the effectiveness, cost, and cost effectiveness of nutrition care services. *J Am Diet Assoc.* 1991;91(suppl 91):S9–14.

20. Paulsen LM, Splett PL. Summary document of nutrition intervention in acute illness: burns and surgery. *J Am Diet Assoc.* 1991;91(suppl 91):S15–17.

21. Trouba PH, Okereke N, Splett PL. Summary document of nutrition intervention in prenatal care. *J Am Diet Assoc.* 1991;91(suppl 91):S21–26.

22. Buescher PA, Larson LC, Helson MD, Lenihan AJ. Prenatal WIC participation can reduce low birth weight and newborn medical costs: a cost-benefit analysis of WIC participation in North Carolina. *J Am Diet Assoc.* 1993;93:163–166.

23. Geppert J, Splett PL. Summary document of nutrition intervention in obesity. *J Am Diet Assoc.* 1991;91(suppl 91):S31–35.

24. Geppert J, Splett PL. Summary document of nutrition intervention in diabetes. *J Am Diet Assoc.* 1991;91(suppl 91):S27–30.

25. Franz MJ. Practice guidelines: road maps for nutrition care. *J Am Diet Assoc.* 1992;92:1136.

26. Mazze RS, Franz MJ, Monk A, et al. Methodologies for field-testing and cost-effectiveness analysis. *J Am Diet Assoc.* 1992;92:1139–1142.

27. American Dietetic Association. *Economic Benefits of Nutrition Services: Legislative Platform of The American Dietetic Association.* Unpublished technical paper; 1992.

28. Finn SC, Gallagher A. President's Page: Health care reform—where ADA stands. *J Am Diet Assoc.* 1993;93:1043–1044.

29. Johnson EQ, Folkman JW, Lunch M, et al. Nutrition services improve health and save money: evidence from Massachusetts. *J Am Diet Assoc.* 1993;93:A–50. Abstract.

30. Hull C, Greco RS, Brooks, DL. Alleviation of constipation in the elderly by dietary fiber supplementation. *J Am Geriatr Soc.* 1980;28:410.

31. Davidson JK, Delcher HK, Englund A. Spin-off cost/benefits of expanded nutritional care. *J Am Diet Assoc.* 1979;75:250–257.

32. Kris-Etherton PM, Kisloff L, Kossouf RA, Rogers C. Teaching principles and cost of sodium-restricted diets. *J Am Diet Assoc.* 1982;80:55–58.

33. Dietetic Staffing Study Committee. Identification of clinical dietetic practitioners' time use for the provision of nutrition care. *J Am Diet Assoc.* 1981;79:708–715.

34. Doing a cost-benefit analysis of nutrition services. In: *Benefits of Nutrition Services: A Costing and Marketing Approach. Report of the Seventh Ross Roundtable on Medical Issues.* Columbus, Ohio: Ross Laboratories; 1987:23–29.

35. Disbrow DD, Dowling RA. Cost-effectiveness and cost-benefit analyses: Research to support practice. In: Monsen ER, ed. *Research: Successful Approaches.* Chicago, Ill: The American Dietetic Association; 1992:272–294.

Chapter 21

Strategies and Practical Approaches—Case Models on Nutrition Assessment

Catherine Cowell, Judith A. Gilbride, and Margaret D. Simko

OVERVIEW

In this chapter two cases are included that illustrate how the information and examples presented in this book can be integrated into practice. One model describes application in a community health agency; the second simulates systems planning in a 500-bed medical center in a large metropolitan area. It is hoped that these models will assist readers in adapting relevant material in this volume to develop their own individualized programs for nutrition intervention.

MODEL I—COMMUNITY PROFILE

The Setting

The setting for this model is a county where the majority of people live in urban communities or in some scattered rural areas. Their community reflects the impact of growing poverty and unemployment due to the loss of major industries and a continuing downturn in the economy. Planning is underway for an additional WIC site (Supplemental Food Program for Women, Infants, and Children) to be located in the county health department. The health care team for this program consists of a nutritionist, three nutrition aides, one public health nurse, a social worker, and a receptionist/clerk and other support team members.

The nutritionist has drawn upon maternal and child health data to document the need for an additional WIC site to be located in the county using the systems model and to expand the interpretation of nutrition into the delivery of prenatal care services (see Figure 1–1).

Step 1—Identification

First, the team determines if services are needed by answering the following questions raised by the system model:

- What does the population look like?
- What is the need for expanding the WIC nutrition intervention program?
- What part of the population is at nutritional risk based on available maternal and child health data?

To describe the population and the community in the light of these questions, the nutrition profile of Exhibit 5–1 is utilized. The completed profile using sources suggested in Exhibit 5–1 for the selected population is shown in Exhibit 21–1. The pertinent information covers the following areas:

1. *Boundaries*—The population area is a county (800 square miles). The population to be served by the health care agency or catchment area will be drawn from eligible people who reside within the geographical boundary lines of the county. The participants must be determined eligible on the basis of the state WIC income guideline and nutritional risk criteria.
2. *Population*—The total population of the county was 175,000 as of January 1994. To calculate the percentage in each age group, the number in each age group is divided by the total population. It is estimated that there are 4,700 children under one year of age. Thus that age group is calculated as being 2.7 percent of the total population (4,700/175,000). Percentages for the other age groups are calculated the same way.
3. *Socioeconomic Status*—Socioeconomic information on the population as of June 1993 is obtained from the county employment office. Sometimes it is not possible to find immediately all of the information noted on the profile; however, additional data may be added as they become available. In some instances, all of the information is not needed for a particular health care agency. For example, in working with young children and adolescents, it may not be important to collect information about other age groups like the elderly, especially if the nutrition intervention is age designated.
4. *Housing*—The number of individual households, 39,043, is determined from the county's housing office. The average size family is calculated by

Exhibit 21–1 The Nutrition Profile—Model I Community

I. POPULATION DESCRIPTION *(Describe the Characteristics of the Population Served)*

SUNRISE COUNTY—800 SQ. MILES   URBAN AND RURAL

Total Population in Area Served	Gender		As of (Date)
	Male	Female	JANUARY 1993

Age Distribution	Number	Percent	Ethnic Racial Composition	Number	Percent
Under 1 Year	4,700	2.7	American Indian .	2,220	1.3
1–14 Years	33,800	19.3	Asian/Pacific		
15–24 Years	45,500	26.0	Islander	1,980	1.1
25–44 Years	43,750	25.0	Black	41,700	23.8
45–64 Years	28,000	16.0	Hispanic/Latino ..	42,800	24.5
65–77 Years	19,200	10.97	White	86,300	49.3
80 Years and Over ..	50	.03	Other (Specify): ..		

(Check One)		(Check One)	
☐ Actual Count/Data ☐ Best Estimate		☐ Actual Count/Data ☐ Best Estimate	

Socioeconomic Data	Number	Housing Characteristics	Number	# of Tenants
No. of Persons Employed 39 %		Low-Income		
No. of Persons Unemployed 16 %		Projects	8	3,150
Food Stamp Program (Annual) ...	25,455	Middle-Income		
Living at the Poverty Index	12,400	Housing Projects ..	7	1,600
Elderly Living at the Poverty		Rooming Houses ..		
Index	9,856	Residential Hotels .	5	935
Public Assistance Cases (Annual)	14,051	Shelters .. HOMELESS	8	693
Aid to Fam. with Dep. Children		Senior Houses	15	1625
(AFDC)	21,673	# of Individual		
Supplementary Security Income		Households	39,043	
(SSI)	4,580	Other:		
Estimate of Average Per Capita Income $		Average Size of Family 4.7		

Food Marketing Facilities	Approx. No.
Supermarkets	79
Food Co-ops	5
Farmers' Markets	9
Small Neighborhood Stores	147
Other (Specify): .HEALTH FOOD...	9

© 1984 ® 1994 Margaret D. Simko, PhD, RD, Catherine Cowell, PhD, Judith A. Gilbride, PhD, RD.

continues

Exhibit 21–1 continued

II. HEALTH STATISTICS INDICATORS FOR THE LAST YEAR 19___

Birth Rate		Infants of Low Birth Weight (2,500 Grams and Under)	
Mother's Age	Number	Mother's Age	Number
15 Years and Under	356	15 Years and Under	183
16–17 Years	486	16–17 Years	169
18–19 Years	612	18–19 Years	63
20–29 Years	2161	20–29 Years	38
30–39 Years	379	30–39 Years	26
40 Years and Older	56	40 Years and Older	7
Total	4050	Total	486

Deaths	Number	Morbidity and Mortality		
		Reported Incidences	Cases	Deaths
Alcoholism	212			
Cancer	392	AIDS	168	43
Diabetes	48	Drug and Substance Abuse	671	
Heart Disease	437	Lead Poisoning	320	12
Other: AIDS	43	Tuberculosis	373	42
		Other Significant Diseases: ACCIDENTS	632	92

III. HEALTH RESOURCES

Residential Institutions and Programs for Children			Community and Mental Health Programs		
Kind	Number	No. of Residents	Hospitals	Number	Total Beds
Group Homes	8	425	Municipal	3	527
Foster Care Program	43	186	Voluntary	1	312
Other (Specify):			Proprietary		
Food Assistance Programs			Other Governmental VA	1	425
Program	Number	No. of Participants	Teaching Hospitals	1	392
Adult Day Care	11	1723	HMOs/Clinics	8	NA
Child Care Food Programs	54	2885	Continuing Care Communities	6	NA

continues

Exhibit 21–1 continued

	Number	# Served		Number	# Served
School Breakfast ...	27	19,115	Nursing Facilities	9	1256
School Lunch	42	36,034	Official Public		
Special Summer Feeding	15	10,800	Health Agency	1	NA
Elderly Feeding Programs	23		(County Health Dept.)		
Under Title (III) Congregate	17	6220	Voluntary Health Agency	3	
Meals on Wheels ...	15	690	MARCH OF DIMES		
Other (Specify):			AMER. HEART ASSOC.		
Supplemental Feeding Programs:			RED CROSS		
WIC—Women		753			
3 SITES Infants		960			
Children		483			
Commodities Distribution Program CHURCHES	28	970			
Soup Kitchens	19	3820	Private Health Agency		
Food Pantries	8	2010	VNS	1	235
Other (Specify):			Other (Specify):		

IV. EDUCATIONAL PROGRAMS

Educational Facilities

Schools		Number	Enrollment
PUBLIC SCHOOLS	Elementary	30	21,153
	Middle	23	12,590
	Secondary	14	11,600
	Vocational	3	3,850
PRIVATE SCHOOLS	Elementary	3	2,113
	Middle	5	2,980
	Secondary	7	5,460
COLLEGES	Public—2 Year	2	10,525
	Privately Owned—2 Year	2	2,875
	Public—4 Year	1	8,000
	Privately Owned—4 Year	1	3,900

continues

Exhibit 21–1 continued

Adult Vocational Training		
Nutrition Education Programs	Yes	No
City or County Health Department		X
Local Board of Education (NET)	X	
Community Health Center	X	
Health Maintenance Organizations (HMOs)	X	
City/County Welfare Social Services Agency		X
Maternal and Infant Care Projects (MIC)	X	
Private Wellness/Health Promotion Programs	X	
Head Start	X	
Cooperative Extension	X	
Supplemental Feeding Program for Women, Infants & Children (WIC) ...	X	
Industry-Sponsored	X	
Tel Med Centers	X	
Home Care Agency		X
Other:		

Nutrition Training Programs			
UNDERGRADUATE/PRACTICE	Location	Number	Enrollment
Dietetic Internship/AP4s	COLLEGE-PUBLIC/PRIVATE	2	38
Coordinated Programs			
Specialty Practice			
UNDERGRADUATE PROGRAMS	Location	Number	Enrollment
Dietitians (ADA approved)			
Dietetic Technicians (AAS)	COMM. COLLEGE	1	47
Dietary Managers (DMA)			
GRADUATE PROGRAMS IN DIETETICS-NUTRITION	Location	Number	Enrollment
	PUBLIC 4 YR. COLLEGE	1	345
	PRIVATE 4 YR. COLLEGE	1	283
FOOD SERVICE TRAINING	Location	Number	Enrollment
	VOC. SCHOOLS	3	179

dividing 175,000 (total population) by 36,063 to obtain 4.85; that is, there are on average four plus persons in each household.

5. *Food Marketing Facilities*—This information is obtained from consumer affairs staff, health care staff, and surveys of local food markets conducted by college and graduate nutrition students. A vital function of nutrition and health education classes is to inform the public about local food markets, their locations, and the quality and prices of foods available.

6. *Health Statistics Indicators*—This information, obtained from the state, county, and local health departments, is useful in identifying the health characteristics and special health/nutrition needs of the target population. For example, for the projected additional WIC site, the health statistics indicate that there were 4,050 births during the past year; of the total number of infants, about 12 percent were born at low birth weights (2,500 grams or less). These are the infants likely to be at high nutritional risk.

When the information on the profile is completed, the original questions are reviewed to determine if the profile answers them:

1. *What does the population look like?* Within the population boundaries there are 4,700 children under age 1. There are 33,800 children between ages 1 and 14 years. The children up to 5 years of age are among those targeted by the WIC program.

2. *What is the need for nutrition intervention?* There are 36,017 persons unemployed and on public assistance or Aid to Families with Dependent Children. Another 25,455 households are receiving Food Stamps, and there are 12,400 people living at or below poverty index (money for a family of four). Since pregnant and lactating women, infants, and young children between the ages of one and five years who meet the income guideline and nutritional criteria are eligible for WIC, the need for an additional WIC site is apparent.

3. *What part of the population is at nutritional risk?* For the year reported, there were 4,050 live births, and 486 infants in this group were low birth weight (2,500 grams or less). It is apparent from these data that an intervention program such as WIC needs to be expanded. Moreover, 842 infants were born to mothers under 18 years of age.

From the above information, it is possible to visualize the scope of work of the health care team. Even before clients are seen, many of the profile questions can be answered in the first step of the systems model.

Step 2—Screening

It appears that the projected additional WIC site will have a very large number of women, infants, and children eligible for care. However, every client may not need the same amount of nutrition intervention. Therefore, a method of screening must be selected to focus on those clients most in need of nutritional care. In developing the screening procedure, the following questions are considered:

- What criteria should be used for screening?
- How can a database be established for screening?
- What tools should be used?
- What parameters should be set?
- How will the screening data be interpreted?

The health care team meets to establish criteria for screening. It decides that the pregnant and lactating women at greatest risk are those who

- are less than 18 years of age
- have a hematocrit of 37 percent or less
- have conditions that might complicate their pregnancy, such as diabetes or hypertension
- have an inadequate pattern of maternal weight gain

The criteria for screening the infants and children are

- anemia—hematocrit of 34 percent or less for infants
- underweight for height, height-for-age on or below the 10th percentile
- excessive weight-for-length, greater than the 90th percentile

The criteria are selected for the particular health care agency; they may vary from agency to agency. It may also be necessary to change the screening criteria if they are found to be inadequate or unrealistic.

The next question to be addressed is how to establish a data screening base. The health care team decides that data should be collected from each client and determines the criteria for the screening procedures. It is agreed that the following data will be needed for women: age, weight, height, blood values (specifically hematocrit), and medical history, to include history of complications like diabetes or hypertension. In infants and children, the following data will be needed: age, weight, height, hematocrit, and weight history if available.

The nurse who sees the clients during their first visit to the clinic will record this information, and the nutrition aides will review each chart to determine if the clients are at nutrition risk according to the established criteria. When an individual is found to be at risk, that individual's chart will receive an easily seen red tab to ensure quick referral.

The third question is what tools should be used. Table 21–1 lists the tools selected by the team in the health care agency.

The fourth question concerns the parameters to be used. The decisions on this question depend on recommended and acceptable ranges and the needs of the health care agency. Each agency must review normal ranges and then make its decisions appropriate for the specific setting. After the parameters are established, the charts are reviewed.

The final question concerns the interpretation of the screening data. The team decides that all charts of new clients will be screened and reviewed to determine if the necessary values fall within the preselected parameters. Those clients that fall within the parameters will be placed in one group and receive "routine" nutritional care; those not within the parameters (patients at nutritional risk) will receive the nutrition services described in the next step.

Table 21–1 Tools Selected by the Health Care Team

Data To Be Collected	Tool Selected
Age	Medical history
Weight	Calibrated scales for weighing both infants and adults
Height or length	Tapes and measuring board
Blood value: hematocrit	Laboratory blood sample analysis
Weight history	Medical history
Complications, such as diabetes, heart disease, and hypertension	Health/social history
Dietary/food access	Food frequency and food intake record

Step 3—Planning

In a preplanned screening process, those clients who are considered at greatest nutritional risk by the staff of the health agency are identified, and their charts are tagged for review. The next step entails planning. Here the following questions are considered:

- What are the objectives of the nutrition intervention program?
- How can these objectives be measured in order to evaluate the outcome?

- How and where will information be documented so that progress can be substantiated?
- What are the priorities for the program?

The objectives and measurable outcomes planned for the WIC program by the health care team are shown in Table 21–2. In the model, all information is documented in the clients' charts. The extensive discussion of documentation in Chapter 13 should be helpful in understanding and implementing written documentation.

The last item in the planning step is to set priorities. The screening by the team has identified two groups: those at risk, and those who fall within the safe parameters and will receive routine care. If the population at risk is very large

Table 21–2 Criteria for Screening, the Objectives, and the Measurable Outcomes

Criteria for Screening	Objective	Measurable Outcome
Pregnant and lactating women:		
those less than 18 years of age	maintain a hematocrit level of 37% or greater	monthly analysis of hematocrit level and systematic recording
those with hematocrit of 37% or less	keep weight pattern within established parameters	monthly weight check and comparison to preestablished parameters
those with conditions that might complicate pregnancy, such as diabetes or hypertension	maintain blood and urine glucose and blood pressure within established parameters	as indicated, blood glucose, urine sugar, and blood pressure; compare to normal values and document
those with inadequate pattern of weight gain	consume a nutritionally adequate diet	evaluation of food record
Infants and children 1–5 years of age:		
those with hematocrit of 34% or less	maintain a hematocrit level of 37% or greater	monthly analysis of hematocrit level and systematic recording
those underweight for height: height-for-age on or below 10th percentile weight-for-age on or below 10th percentile	increase weight to recommended rate of growth percentile	monthly weight check and comparison to recommended parameters and growth percentile charts
excessive weight-for-length, greater than 90th percentile	consume a nutritionally adequate diet	evaluate food intake record prepared by mother

and some clients appear at very great risk, it might be advisable to subdivide the risk group and to set additional priorities. For example, if a group of infants are at extremely low weights and their hematocrits are very much below standard, this may constitute a third group that needs some additional care and monitoring. Priorities are generally established by the health care team in consultation with the responsible administrators of the funding agency for a program, as well as by the circumstances in each particular setting and the resources available.

Step 4—Implementation

To implement the program to provide nutritional care for the clients, the following additional questions need to be considered:

- What resources are available?
- What nutrition services are currently being provided?
- What type of treatment and/or preventive measures will be used?
- What will be the roles of the health care team members?
- How can the program be made more efficient and user friendly?

When considering available resources, the first step is to examine personnel. The questions to ask are: Who are the team members? What kinds of nutrition services can be provided? How much time can the team collectively devote to assessment? It may be possible to plan schedules and reassign duties in order to provide more time for nutritional care. This is the time when the profile should be reviewed to see if there are some untapped resources in the community, such as students, dietetic interns, or volunteers, who might be willing and able to carry out routine tasks, thereby releasing team members for other tasks.

In our model study, the team drew up a list of functions that the team members might perform relating to the nutritional status of the clients. The list was then reviewed to determine which members of the team could most effectively implement each task. Table 21–3 lists the services and the team members assigned to them.

The algorithm for nutritional care shown in Figure 21–1 is used by the team to outline the work plan. The clients will check the frequency of eating specific foods based on the various food groupings. A nutrition aide will check the answers against a recommended frequency list. If the frequency of consuming food from the suggested grouping agrees with the recommended list and the diet appears adequate, the client will be referred to routine care unless other parameters are abnormal.

Table 21–3 Nutrition Services and the Team Members Assigned to Them

Service	Team Member
Analysis of food intake questionnaire	Nutrition aide

Monthly classes:
  Prenatal and infant nutrition
  Child and infant nutrition
  Breast-feeding
	Nutritionist assisted by nutrition aides working with other team members

Meal planning, shopping, and storage	
Food preparation techniques	Nutrition aides
Nutrition counseling	Nutritionist
Teen mother classes	Nutrition aides directed by nutritionist
Referrals	Nurse/social worker
Monitoring	Nurse who sees client each month

If the food intake questionnaire reveals that the diet does not appear to be adequate, the client will be asked to keep a three-day food record (see Chapter 10). The food record will be reviewed by the nutritionist with the client. If the diet still appears inadequate, the client will receive nutrition counseling from the nutritionist, either individually or as part of a small group.

Step 5—Evaluation

In evaluating the model, the following questions are raised to determine if the objectives have been met:

- What are the results of the treatment?
- Has the nutritional status of the clients changed?
- Has the nutritional care provided been documented?

The first objective for pregnant and lactating women was to maintain hematocrit levels of 37 percent or greater. The measured outcome was a monthly analysis of hematocrit levels and a systematic recording (documentation). The health care team can now evaluate if the treatment (in this case, the nutrition counseling and nutrition education classes as well as supplementary food) has achieved the desired results. Each objective is evaluated in the same way.

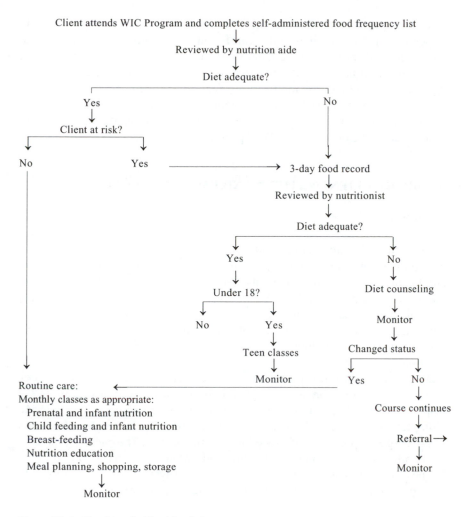

Client attends WIC Program and completes self-administered food frequency list

Reviewed by nutrition aide

Diet adequate?

Figure 21–1 Algorithm for Nutritional Care

Step 6—Monitoring

Monitoring involves continuity of care while the needs are reassessed in the light of changed nutritional and/or health status. This includes continuous monitoring of both the routine care group and the at-risk group to determine if the parameters established have fallen below the standards set. Clients at risk receive individual or small group counseling from the nutritionist. They also attend appropriate periodic class meetings. If their status changes positively—

if, for example, pregnant and lactating women raise their hematocrit levels to 37 percent or greater—they will be referred to the routine care group, but monitoring will continue. If the status does not change and some clients remain at risk, they will be referred to the appropriate health professionals, such as a physician in the clinic, for additional evaluation. Nutrition counseling will be continued concurrently with continuous monitoring. Thus the model provides for assessment, nutrition intervention, and ongoing evaluation and monitoring to ensure that all the clients in the WIC program receive quality care.

MODEL II—CLIENT/PATIENT AND FACILITY PROFILE

The Setting

The setting for our second model is a 500-bed medical center in a large metropolitan area. A nutrition support team has just been appointed by administration to care for oncology patients. Core members include a dietitian, nurse, pharmacist, and physician on the team. A dietitian has been employed by the hospital as a clinical nutrition specialist and follows the guidelines from the American Society of Parenteral and Enteral Nutrition (ASPEN) for job functions (see Appendix G). The dietitian is unfamiliar with the medical center and the nutrition support team.

During the organization phase, the team members agree to meet twice a week for the first month, with subsequent weekly meetings. Administrators in the hospital, part of a large multiplex corporation of two community hospitals and a long-term care facility, have asked each team member to develop short- and long-term goals, policies, and procedures for the service. The oncology patients are admitted to various units of the hospital, often on the basis of additional diagnosis or treatment. The team has a copy of the systems model (Figure 1–5) and agrees to use this model to plan and implement the service.

Step 1—Identification

During the first team meeting, the clinical nutrition specialist reports on previous experience with the nutrition profile (Exhibits 5–1, 5–2, and 5–3) and suggests that the profile be used as a database for identifying patients at risk as well as to provide concise background information for the facility and the patients served. Data organized in this manner can serve as a basis for developing goals, policies, and procedures. Copies of the flowchart used to collect data for the nutrition profile (Exhibit 5–4) and of the list of sources of information for the profile (Exhibit 5–5) are shared by the team members. The team decides to use the profile but suggests that only the facility and client sections for the tertiary hospital be completed at the outset. The worksheet in Exhibit 21–2 is used to guide the team in completing and analyzing the data from the profile.

Although the clinical nutrition specialist has had prior experience with the profile, the other team members are familiar with the institution and make suggestions for securing additional items of information to complete the database. They suggest sources for staffing patterns and medical records and ways to contact other pertinent departments. A time frame of one week is established to collect the initial data.

A summary of pertinent findings is presented in the team meeting the following week. The completed facility and patient profiles are shown in Exhibits 21–3 and 21–4. The following data are relevant in the identification of the population at greatest risk:

Exhibit 21–2 Nutrition Profile Worksheet

	CLIENT	FACILITY	COMMUNITY
Team/individual responsible			
Time frame			
Date begun			
Date completed			

SUMMARY of profile database

Priority client populations:

Health conditions affecting nutritional status:

Sufficiency of human resources/materials:

Intervention or education program to assess needs:

Date when all _____ or selected _____ data will be collected again:

Exhibit 21–3 The Nutrition Profile—Facility

THE NUTRITION PROFILE
FACILITY PROFILE
(Describe the Characteristics of Your Health Care Facility or Center)

Name of Facility	Date(s)
Capitol Medical Center	**May, 1994**

Location (City)	Type (e.g., Prenatal Clinic, Nursing Facility, Hospital)
Capitol City	**Acute care, Teaching**

I. CLIENTS SERVED LAST CALENDAR OR FISCAL YEAR 19_	Number
A. Inpatients	189,800
B. Ambulatory Clients (Outpatients)	10,400
C. Home Care	274
D. Beds	522
E. Cribs	36
F. Other (Specify):	

II. STAFF	Total	Number Contributing to Nutrition Assessment
A. MEDICAL		
1. House Staff	46	4
2. Private Staff	50	1
3. Physicians' Assistants	—	—
4. Residents	22	1
B. NURSING		
1. Nurse Clinicians/Practitioners	12	2
2. Registered Nurses	120	6
3. Midwives	—	—
4. Licensed Practical Nurses	30	—
5. Certified Nursing Assistants	18	—
C. OTHER PROFESSIONALS		
1. Pharmacists	4	2
2. Dentists	1	—
3. Dental Hygienists	—	—
4. Social Workers	9	—
5. Podiatrists	1	—

continues

Exhibit 21–3 continued

II. STAFF C. OTHER PROFESSIONALS (Continued)	Total	Number Contributing to Nutrition Assessment
6. Psychologists	62	—
7. Therapists (Specify): Physical	22	—
Respiratory	15	—
8. Health Educators	2	—
9. Speech Pathologists	2	—
10. Others (Specify): ... Inservice Nursing ...	5	—

D. VOLUNTEERS ☑ Yes ☐ No
   1. If yes, number of volunteers available to
     assist dietary
   2. Director   ☑ Yes ☐ No
	~20	

CHECK ATTENDANCE FOR

III. ROUTINE TEAM MEETINGS	Admissions	Care Planning	Discharge
A. Physicians	✔	✔	✔
B. Physicians' Assistant(s)	—	—	—
C. Pediatric Nurse Associate(s)	—	—	—
D. Nurse Clinician(s)	—	✔	✔
E. Registered Nurse(s)	✔	✔	✔
F. Licensed Practical Nurse(s)	—	—	—
G. Other Nursing Staff	—	—	—
H. Dietitian/Nutritionist(s) .... 6 ..	✔	✔	✔
I. Dietetic Nutrition Technician(s) .. 5 ..	—	—	—
J. Dietary Manager(s) or Food Service Supervisor(s) ...... 8 ..	—	—	—
K. Pharmacist(s)	—	✔	—
L. Health Administrator(s)	—	—	—
M. Health Educator(s)	—	✔	—
N. Social Worker(s)	✔	✔	✔
O. Case Manager	✔	✔	✔
P. Home Care Representative	—	—	✔
Q. Other (Specify): CNSD(1) Dietary Asst (13)			

IV. RECORD-KEEPING SYSTEM
   A. Source-Oriented Medical Records   ☐ Yes   ☑ No
   B. Problem-Oriented Medical Records   ☑ Yes   ☐ No
     1. SOAP   ☐ Yes   ☑ No
     2. PIE   ☑ Yes   ☐ No
   C. Computerized Medical Records   ☐ Yes   ☑ No
   D. Other (Specify):

continues

Exhibit 21–3 continued

V. PROGRAM EVALUATION AND REVIEW TECHNIQUES
   A. Quality Management/
      Continuous Quality Improvement/CQI   ☑ Yes   ☐ No
   B. Retrospective Audits   ☑ Yes   ☐ No
   C. Concurrent Audits   ☑ Yes   ☐ No
   D. Utilization Review Committee   ☑ Yes   ☐ No
   E. Program Evaluation Procedures   ☑ Yes   ☐ No
   F. Other Committee: ☐ Yes   ☐ No
      CQI Team members include _____
      _____

   G. Number Audits per Department per Year
      1. Nutrition Care _4, quarterly_____
      2. Food Service _4, quarterly and weekly tray tests_____
   H. Other: _____
      _____
      _____

VI. NUTRITION ASSESSMENT	(Check)	
	Screening	Post Screening
A. DIETARY		
1. Nutrition History		outpatient
2. 24-Hour Recall	✔	
3. Food Frequency Questionnaire		✔
4. Food Records		outpatient
5. Intake Study		✔
6. Other (Specify):		
B. LABORATORY		
1. Urinalysis	✔	
2. Complete Blood Count	✔	
3. Complete Lipid Profile	✔	
4. SMA-16	✔	✔
5. SMA-12		
6. SMA-24		
7. SMA-36		
8. Hemoglobin	✔	
9. Hematocrit	✔	
10. Blood Lead Level		
11. Serum Albumin	✔	✔
12. TIBC or Serum Transferrin		
13. Creatinine Height Index		
14. Nitrogen Balance		✔
15. Total Lymphocyte Count	✔	
16. Prealbumin		
17. Hemoglobin Alc		✔
18. Others:		

continues

Exhibit 21–3 continued

	(Check)	
	Screening	Post Screening
C. CLINICAL		
1. Heights	✔	
2. Weights	✔	
3. Body Circumferences		✔
4. Skinfolds		✔
5. Bioelectrical Impedance		
6. Other (Specify):		
D. SCREENING TOOLS	Yes	No
1. Initial	✔	
2. Follow-up	✔	
E. NUTRITION CARE TEAMS		
1. Nutrition Support	✔	
2. Dysphagia	✔	
3. Ethics		✔
4. Rehabilitation	✔	
5. Other Nutrition Committee (Specify): _____	✔	
6. **Subcommittee on Nutrition/Nursing Patient Education Committee**		

VII. DIETARY SERVICES

A. TYPE OF FOOD SERVICE FOR PATIENTS

	Yes	No			Yes	No			Yes	No
1. Centralized	✔	☐	3. Tray Service		✔	☐	5. Contracted Vendor		☐	✔
2. Decentralized	☐	☐	4. Cafeteria/ Dining Rm.		✔	☐	6. Other (Specify)		☐	☐

		Avg. No/Day
B. SUPPLEMENTARY FEEDINGS		
1. Nourishments/Snacks	Yes ✔ No ☐	NA
2. Tube Feedings Daily	Yes ✔ No ☐	NA
3. Oral Enteral Supplements	Yes ✔ No ☐	NA
4. Peripheral Parenteral Nutrition	Yes ✔ No ☐	NA

Exhibit 21–4 The Nutrition Profile—Client/Patient

THE NUTRITION PROFILE
CLIENT/PATIENT PROFILE
(Describe the Characteristics of Your Service Population (Clients)

		Number	Percent
I.	POPULATION DISTRIBUTION		
	A. DISTRIBUTION		
	1. Female	266	51
	2. Male	256	49
	Total	522	100%
	B. AGE DISTRIBUTION (Check One) ☒ Actual Count/Data ☐ Best Estimate		
	1. Under 1 Year	13	2.5
	2. 1–14 Years	25	4.8
	3. 15–24 Years	19	3.7
	4. 25–44 Years	109	20.8
	5. 45–64 Years	142	27.2
	6. 65–79 Years	138	26.4
	7. 80 Years and Over	76	14.5
	Total	522	99.9%
II.	LENGTH OF STAY (Check One) ☒ Actual Count/Data ☐ Best Estimate		
	A. FOR SHORT-TERM FACILITY; AVERAGE LENGTH OF STAY __7.6__ DAYS		
	1. Less than 3 Months		
	2. 3 Months to Less Than 6 Months		
	3. 6 Months to Less Than 12 Months		
	4. 1 Year and Over		
	Total		
III.	PATIENT MOBILITY (Check One) ☐ Actual Count/Data ☒ Best Estimate		
	A. Full Ambulatory	365	70
	B. Ambulatory (With Cane, Walker)	26	5
	C. Wheelchair (Self-Managed)	26	5
	D. Room-Bound	52	10
	E. Bed-Fast	52	10
	F. Other (Specify)		

© 1984 ® 1994 Margaret D. Simko, PhD, RD, Catherine Cowell, PhD, Judith A. Gilbride, PhD, RD.

continues

Exhibit 21–4 continued

	Number	Percent
G. Feeding Skills		
1. Feeds Self	375	72
2. Needs Assistance (Cutting)	85	16
3. Needs Feeding	27	5
4. Tube-Fed	35	7
5. Other (Specify):		
Total	522	100%

IV. DIAGNOSIS ☐ Actual Count/Data ☒ Best Estimate	Major Diagnosis at Admission	
	Number	Percent
A. AIDS	17	3.2
B. Cancer	100	19.2
C. Cardiac Diseases	32	6.1
D. Diabetes	64	12.3
E. Gastrointestinal Diseases	91	17.4
F. Inherited Diseases	27	5.2
G. Pulmonary	15	2.9
H. Renal	20	3.8
I. Stroke	20	3.8
J. Substance Abuse	6	0.1
K. Trauma/Accident	12	2.3
L. Psychiatric		
M. Other (Specify): 1	118	22.6
2		
3		
Total	522	98.9%

V. DIET PRESCRIPTIONS ☒ Actual Count/Data ☐ Best Estimate		
A. DIETS REPORTED FOR ONE DAY		
1. Regular/House	240	49.3
2. Texture—Modified	35	7.2
3. Pediatric	36	7.3
4. Kosher	8	1.6
5. Vegetarian	4	0.8
6. Liquid	48	9.8

continues

Exhibit 21–4 continued

	Number	Percent
7. Modified/Therapeutic:		
Allergy	—	—
Restricted Residue	1	0.2
Diabetic	18	3.6
Fat/Cholesterol Controlled	14	3.0
High Calorie/High Protein	—	—
Fiber Controlled	—	—
Renal	15	3.1
Sodium Controlled	31	6.4
8. Weight Reduction	—	—
9. NPO on Survey Day	30	6.2
10. Other (Specify):	7	1.4
Total	487	99.9%
B. SPECIAL DIETARY NEEDS FOR ONE DAY		
1. Total Parenteral Nutrition	35	—
2. Peripheral Parenteral Nutrition		
3. Enteral Formula	50	—
4. Other (Specify):		
Time Frame to Complete Profile ——— One Week		

- On the day the data were collected, there were 522 patients in the facility (266 females, 256 males).
- Of the total number of patients, 100 (19 percent) were receiving oral supplements or tube feedings, and 35 were receiving total parenteral nutrition (TPN).
- Clinical nutrition services were provided by one clinical nutrition specialist, six clinical dietitians, and five dietetic technicians.
- The dietetic department's protocol for nutrition assessment stated that the patients who had cancer, diabetes, infectious disease, liver disease, renal disease, trauma, or nonelective surgery were at risk and required care.

Step 2—Screening

The nutrition support team indicates that the average of 100 patients with malignancies, cancer, or possible tumors reported in Exhibit 21–4, section IV, is too large a group for the nutrition support specialist to provide adequate care. It is suggested that these patients be screened to classify them according to the levels of care required—routine or support care. The dietetic staff use a simple tool for screening with the following parameters:

- recent weight loss
- eating problems (for example, sore mouth)
- change in appetite and bowel function
- hemoglobin less than 12 g/dl in males and less than 14 g/dl in females
- hematocrit less than 44 in males and less than 38 in females
- serum albumin less than 3.5 g/dl (moderate risk, 3.0–3.4; high risk <3.0)
- total lymphocyte count less than 1,500 cu mm (moderate risk, 900–1,499, high risk, <900)
- chemotherapy
- radiation therapy

It is decided that all cancer patients will be screened upon admission by the dietetic technicians to determine how the parameters are met by each patient. If none of the parameters are evident, patients receiving regular and modified diets will continue to receive nutritional care from the dietetic staff assigned to the various units. All other cancer patients will be considered at risk and referred to the clinical dietitians for further assessment to determine treatment and care. Referral to the nutrition support team will be initiated by the clinical dietitians.

Step 3—Planning

Having established a procedure to identify those patients at greatest risk, the clinical nutrition specialist, with input from the clinical dietitians, continues to develop the planning stage of the nutrition support program. First, it is necessary to set objectives for the care and treatment of the patients referred to the team. The following objectives are determined:

- to reduce the incidence of malnutrition
- to improve the overall nutritional status of the patients
- to provide high-protein supplements that are acceptable and consumed by patients
- to teach patients to modify food consumption to avoid weight loss

The plans of care include the following requirements:

- All patients are to be seen within 24 hours.
- An in-depth nutrition assessment is to be completed on patients at risk.
- Documentation will follow the PIE format after the initial database.
- An individualized plan of care will be developed for each patient.
- A calorie count will be done for any patient who loses 5 percent of weight (after hydration status is determined).

Step 4—Implementation

The team outlines the role of clinical nutrition staff in the implementation of the plans. The role of the clinical dietitian involves the following responsibilities:

- Assess and evaluate nutritional status of patients at risk for malnutrition.
- Recommend and oversee nutritional therapy.
- Provide nutritious snacks and additional calories and protein to foods; have foods prepared in ways to motivate patients to eat larger quantities.
- Provide enteral feedings as necessary.
- Conduct patient nutrition education.
- Monitor calorie counts and other nutrition support measures.

The nutrition support specialist sees high-risk patients, makes recommendations for enteral and parenteral feeding, and receives assistance, suggestions, and cooperation from the dietetic department. The specialist is also a consultant to the outpatient department and home TPN program (about 25–30 patients).

Step 5—Evaluation

Evaluation is concerned with determining the value of efforts that are expended to achieve objectives. The objectives in Model II, as listed in Step 3, are reviewed by the team, and measurable outcomes are set to evaluate the effectiveness of nutrition services and nutrition support. The team members agree that the following will be documented for each patient receiving care:

- review of adequacy of food intake
- patient tolerance of food and supplements

- increases or decreases in protein and calorie intake
- change in weight status
- change in laboratory values
- potential or actual nutrient and drug interactions
- understanding of and adherence to nutrition education objectives

Step 6—Monitoring

Continuous quality improvement is defined in Chapter 19 as a management philosophy that is "patient focused" and "quality driven" to improve care. To monitor the quality or effectiveness of the nutrition support program, clinical indicators are documented and reviewed by the team, including an analysis of patient outcomes and an audit of process of care. For long-range plans, the team decides to develop methods to study the cost-effectiveness of the program. With these techniques the team hopes (1) to determine appropriate staffing patterns and costs for nutrition intervention, (2) to compare patient outcomes with team efforts, and (3) to monitor outcome measures and costs with retrospective data from comparable populations. Further planning will be needed to develop a protocol for evaluation research on the outcomes of the nutrition support program.

CONCLUSION

Two case models were presented to illustrate how the examples and information in this book can be integrated into practice. It is hoped that these models as well as other examples in this book might assist readers in adapting relevant strategies and approaches to develop their own individualized programs for nutrition assessment and intervention.

Appendices

Margaret D. Simko, Judith A. Gilbride,
and Catherine Cowell

411

Appendix A

National Center for Health Statistics (NCHS) Physical Growth Percentiles for Boys and Girls

All figures in Appendix A are courtesy of Ross Laboratories, who adapted the growth curves from the original data; National Center for Health Statistics, NCHS Growth Charts, 1976. Monthly Vital Statistics Report, Vol. 25, No. 3, Suppl. (HRA) 78-1120. Rockville, MD, Health Resources Administration, June 1976. Data from The Fels Research Institute, Yellow Springs, Ohio.

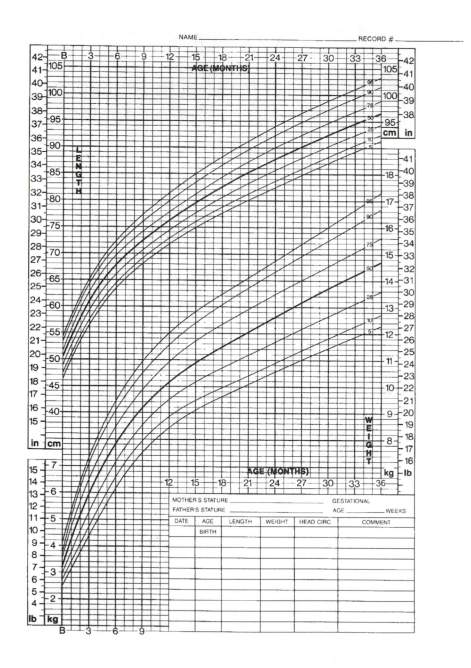

Figure A–1 Stature-by-Age and Weight-by-Age Percentiles for Boys Aged Birth to 36 Months

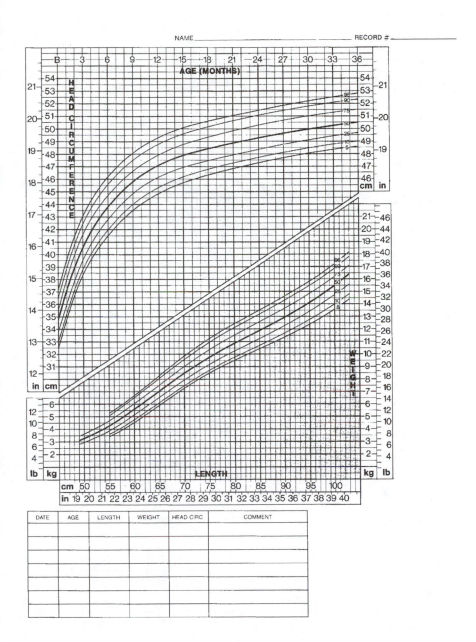

NAME_____ RECORD #_____

Figure A–2 Stature-by-Weight and Head Circumference-by-Age Percentiles for Boys Aged Birth to 36 Months

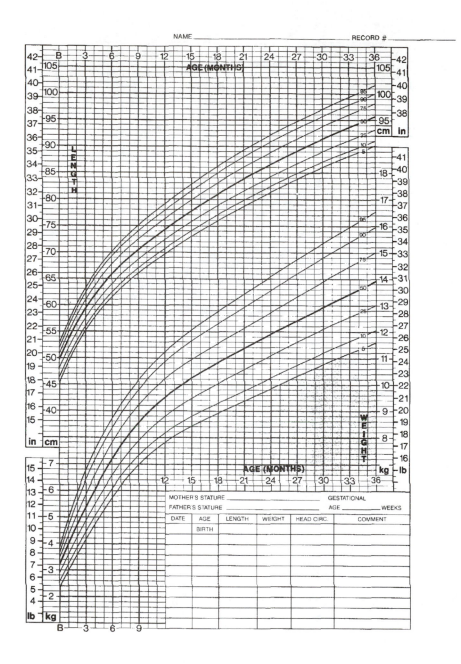

Figure A–3 Stature-by-Age and Weight-by-Age Percentiles for Girls Aged Birth to 36 Months

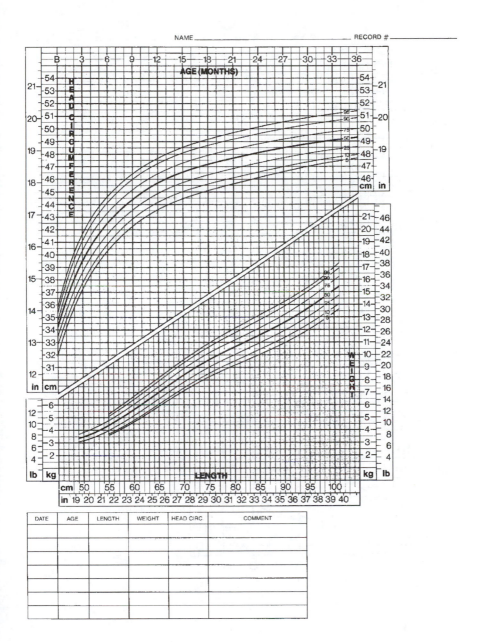

Figure A–4 Stature-by-Weight and Head Circumference-by-Age Percentiles for Girls Aged Birth to 36 Months

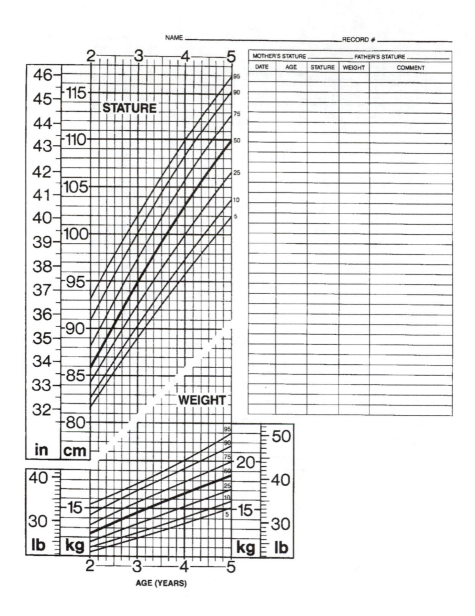

Figure A–5 Stature-by-Age and Weight-by-Age Percentiles for Boys Aged 2 to 5 Years

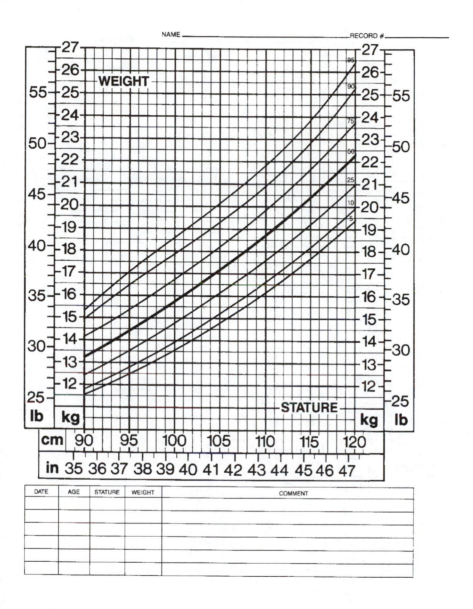

Figure A–6 Boys' Prepubescent Physical Growth, Weight-by-Stature Percentiles

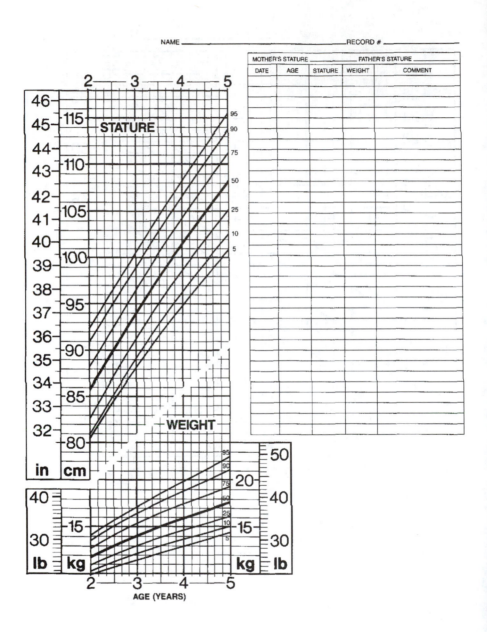

Figure A–7 Stature-by-Age and Weight-by-Age Percentiles for Girls Aged 2 to 5 Years

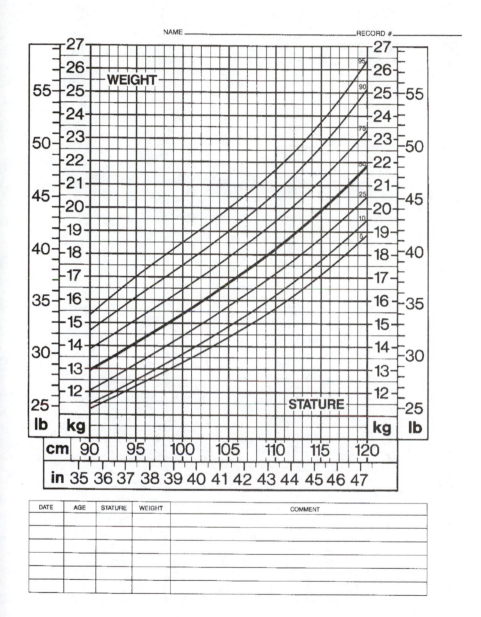

Figure A–8 Girls' Prepubescent Physical Growth, Weight-by-Stature Percentiles

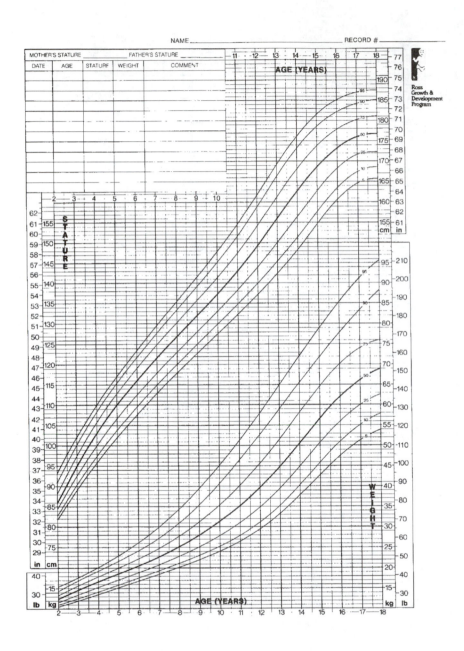

Figure A–9 Stature-by-Age and Weight-by-Age Percentiles for Boys Aged 2 to 18 Years

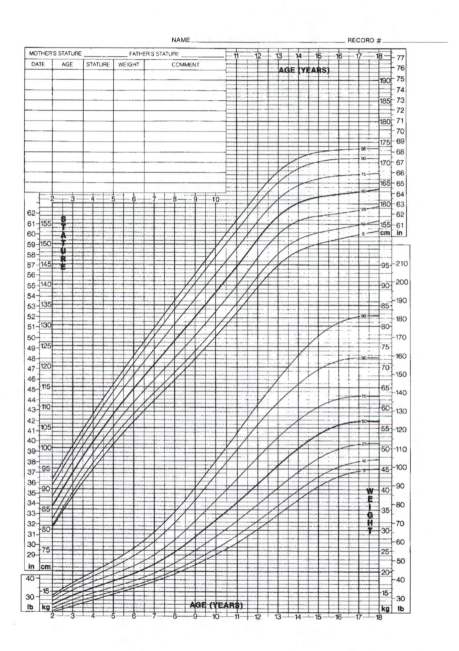

Figure A–10 Stature-by-Age and Weight-by-Age Percentiles for Girls Aged 2 to 18 Years

Appendix B

Anthropometry

Table B–1 1959 Metropolitan Life Height-Weight Tables, Desirable Weights for Men of Ages 25 and Over*

Height	Small Frame (lb)	Medium Frame (lb)	Large Frame (lb)
5'2"	112–120	118–129	126–141
5'3"	115–123	121–133	129–144
5'4"	118–126	124–136	132–148
5'5"	121–129	127–139	132–152
5'6"	124–133	130–143	138–156
5'7"	128–137	134–147	142–161
5'8"	132–141	138–152	147–166
5'9"	136–145	142–156	151–170
5'10"	140–150	146–160	155–174
5'11"	144–154	150–165	159–179
6'0"	148–158	154–170	164–184
6'1"	152–162	158–175	168–189
6'2"	156–167	162–180	173–194
6'3"	160–171	167–185	178–199
6'4"	164–175	172–190	182–204

*Weight in pounds according to frame (in indoor clothing, shoes with 1" heels).
Source: Courtesy of Metropolitan Life Insurance Company. Reprinted with permission.

Table B–2 1959 Metropolitan Life Height-Weight Tables, Desirable Weights for Women of Ages 25 and Over*

Height	Small Frame (lb)	Medium Frame (lb)	Large Frame (lb)
4'10"	92–98	96–107	104–119
4'11"	94–101	98–110	106–122
5'0"	96–104	101–113	109–125
5'1"	99–107	104–116	112–128
5'2"	102–110	107–119	115–131
5'3"	105–113	110–122	118–134
5'4"	108–116	113–126	121–138
5'5"	111–119	116–130	125–142
5'6"	114–123	120–135	129–146
5'7"	118–127	124–139	133–150
5'8"	122–131	128–143	137–154
5'9"	126–135	132–147	141–158
5'10"	130–140	136–151	145–163
5'11"	134–144	140–155	149–168
6'0"	138–148	144–159	153–173

*For girls between 18 and 25, subtract 1 pound for each year under 25. Weight in pounds according to frame (in indoor clothing, shoes with 2" heels).
Source: Courtesy of Metropolitan Life Insurance Company. Reprinted with permission.

Table B-3 1983 Metropolitan Life Height-Weight Tables, Desirable Weights for Men*

Height	Small Frame (lb)	Medium Frame (lb)	Large Frame (lb)
5'2"	128–134	131–141	138–150
5'3"	130–136	133–143	140–153
5'4"	132–138	135–145	142–156
5'5"	134–140	137–148	144–160
5'6"	136–142	139–151	146–164
5'7"	138–145	142–154	149–168
5'8"	140–148	145–157	152–172
5'9"	142–151	148–160	155–176
5'10"	144–154	151–163	158–180
5'11"	146–157	154–166	161–184
6'0"	149–160	157–170	164–188
6'1"	152–164	160–174	168–192
6'2"	155–168	164–178	172–197
6'3"	158–172	167–182	176–202
6'4"	162–176	171–187	181–207

*Weights at 25 to 59 based on lowest mortality. Weight in pounds according to frame (in indoor clothing weighing 3 lb., shoes with 1" heels).
Source: Courtesy of Metropolitan Life Insurance Company. Reprinted with permission.

Table B-4 1983 Metropolitan Life Height-Weight Tables, Desirable Weights for Women*

Height	Small Frame (lb)	Medium Frame (lb)	Large Frame (lb)
4'10"	102–111	109–121	118–131
4'11"	103–113	111–123	120–134
5'0"	104–115	113–126	122–137
5'1"	106–118	115–129	125–140
5'2"	108–121	118–132	128–143
5'3"	111–124	121–135	131–147
5'4"	114–127	124–138	134–151
5'5"	117–130	127–141	137–155
5'6"	120–133	130–144	140–159
5'7"	123–136	133–147	143–163
5'8"	126–139	136–150	146–167
5'9"	129–145	139–153	149–170
5'10"	132–145	142–156	152–173
5'11"	135–148	145–159	155–176
6'0"	138–151	148–162	158–179

*Weights at 25 to 59 based on lowest mortality. Weight in pounds according to frame (in indoor clothing weighing 3 lb., shoes with 1" heels).
Source: Courtesy of Metropolitan Life Insurance Company. Reprinted with permission.

Table B–5 Metropolitan Life Determination of Body Frame Size for Men

Height in 1-Inch Heels	Elbow Breadth* for Medium Frame
5'2" to 5'3"	2½" to 2⅞"
5'4" to 5'7"	2⅝" to 2⅞"
5'8" to 5'11"	2¾" to 3"
6'0" to 6'3"	2¾" to 3⅛"
6'4"	2⅞" to 3¼"

Note: Weights at ages 25 to 59 based on lowest mortality. Weight in pounds according to frame (in indoor clothing weighing 5 lb., shoes with 1" heels).

*Elbow breadth is measured with the forearm upward at a 90-degree angle. The distance between the outer aspects of the two prominent bones on either side of the elbow is considered to be the elbow breadth. Elbow breadth less than that listed for medium frame indicates a small frame. Elbow breadth greater than that listed for medium frame indicates a large frame.

Source: Courtesy of Metropolitan Life Insurance Company. Reprinted with permission.

Table B–6 Metropolitan Life Determinations of Body Frame Size for Women

Height in 1-Inch Heels	Elbow Breadth* for Medium Frame
4'10" to 4'11"	2¼" to 2½"
5'0" to 5'3"	2¼" to 2½"
5'4" to 5'7"	2⅜" to 2⅝"
5'8" to 5'11"	2⅜" to 2⅝"
6'0"	2½" to 2¾"

Note: Weights at ages 25 to 59 based on lowest mortality. Weight in pounds according to frame (in indoor clothing weighing 5 lb., shoes with 1" heels).

*Elbow breadth is measured with the forearm upward at a 90-degree angle. The distance between the outer aspects of the two prominent bones on either side of the elbow is considered to be the elbow breadth. Elbow breadth less than that listed for medium frame indicates a small frame. Elbow breadth greater than that listed for medium frame indicates a large frame.

Source: Courtesy of Metropolitan Life Insurance Company. Reprinted with permission.

Table B–7 Categories of Frame Size Derived with Reference to Frame Index 2, by Age and by Height

Frame Index 2 = [Elbow Breadth (mm) / Stature (cm)] × 100

	Male			Female		
	Small	Medium	Large	Small	Medium	Large
Age (yrs.)	Frame Index 1: Elbow Breadth (mm)					
18.0–24.9	<38.4	38.4–41.6	>41.6	<35.2	35.2–38.6	>38.6
25.0–29.9	<38.6	38.6–41.8	>41.8	<35.7	35.7–38.7	>38.7
30.0–34.9	<38.6	38.6–42.1	>42.1	<35.7	35.7–39.0	>39.0
35.0–39.9	<39.1	39.1–42.4	>42.4	<36.2	36.2–39.8	>39.8
40.0–44.9	<39.3	39.3–42.5	>42.5	<36.7	36.7–40.2	>40.2
45.0–49.9	<39.6	39.6–43.0	>43.0	<36.7	37.2–40.7	>40.7
50.0–54.9	<39.9	39.9–43.3	>43.3	<37.2	37.2–41.6	>41.6
55.0–59.9	<40.2	40.2–43.8	>43.8	<37.8	37.8–41.9	>41.9
60.0–64.9	<40.2	40.2–43.6	>43.6	<38.2	38.2–41.8	>41.8
65.0–69.9	<40.2	40.2–43.6	>43.6	<38.2	38.2–41.8	>41.8
70.0–74.9	<40.2	40.2–43.6	>43.6	<38.2	38.2–41.8	>41.8

Frame Index 2: Elbow Breadth by Height

	Male			Female		
	Small	Medium	Large	Small	Medium	Large
Height (cm)	Elbow Breadth (mm)					
141–146	—	—	—	<56	56–61	>61
147–152	—	—	—	<57	57–62	>62
153–158	<66	66–70	>70	<60	60–63	>63
159–164	<66	66–71	>71	<61	61–65	>65
165–170	<68	68–72	>72	<61	61–65	>65
171–176	<70	70–73	>73	<62	62–65	>65
177–182	<71	71–75	>75	<62	62–66	>66
183–188	<71	71–76	>76	—	—	—
189–194	<73	73–76	>76	—	—	—

Source: A. Roberto Frisancho. *Anthropometric Standards for the Assessment of Growth and Nutritional Status.* Ann Arbor, MI: The University of Michigan Press, 1993, page 28. Reprinted with permission of A. Roberto Frisancho.

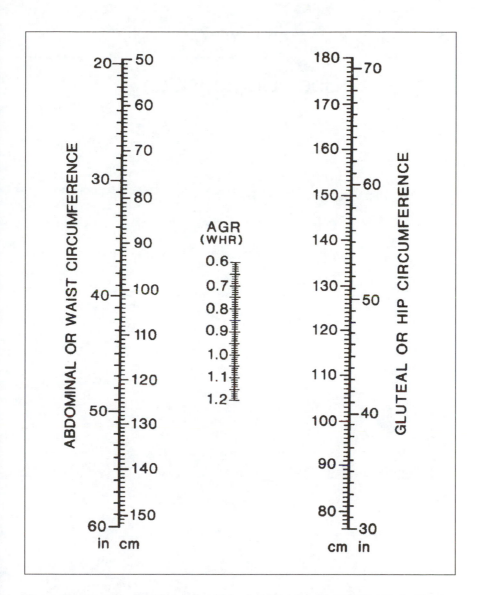

Figure B–1 Nomogram for Determining Abdominal (Waist) to Gluteal (Hips) Ratio. Place a straight edge between the column for waist circumference and the column for hip circumference and read the ratio from the point where this straight edge crosses the AGR or WHR line. The waist or abnormal circumference is the smallest circumference below the rib cage and above the umbilicus, and the hips or gluteal circumference is taken as the largest circumference at the posterior extension of the buttocks. *Source:* Copyright George A. Bray, 1987. Reprinted with permission.

Body Composition

Table C–1 Means, Standard Deviations, and Percentiles of Triceps Skinfold Thickness (mm) by Age for Males and Females of 1 to 74 Years

Age (yrs)	N	Mean	SD	Percentiles								
				5	10	15	25	50	75	85	90	95
Males												
1.0–1.9	681	10.4	2.9	6.5	7.0	7.5	8.0	10.0	12.0	13.0	14.0	15.5
2.0–2.9	677	10.0	2.9	6.0	6.5	7.0	8.0	10.0	12.0	13.0	14.0	15.0
3.0–3.9	717	9.9	2.7	6.0	7.0	7.0	8.0	9.5	11.5	12.5	13.5	15.0
4.0–4.9	708	9.2	2.7	5.5	6.5	7.0	7.5	9.0	11.0	12.0	12.5	14.0
5.0–5.9	677	8.9	3.1	5.0	6.0	6.0	7.0	8.0	10.0	11.5	13.0	14.5
6.0–6.9	298	8.9	3.8	5.0	5.5	6.0	6.5	8.0	10.0	12.0	13.0	16.0
7.0–7.9	312	9.0	4.0	4.5	5.0	6.0	6.0	8.0	10.5	12.5	14.0	16.0
8.0–8.9	296	9.6	4.4	5.0	5.5	6.0	7.0	8.5	11.0	13.0	16.0	19.0
9.0–9.9	322	10.2	5.1	5.0	5.5	6.0	6.5	9.0	12.5	15.5	17.0	20.0
10.0–10.9	334	11.5	5.7	5.0	6.0	6.0	7.5	10.0	14.0	17.0	20.0	24.0
11.0–11.9	324	12.5	7.0	5.0	6.0	6.5	7.5	10.0	16.0	19.5	23.0	27.0
12.0–12.9	348	12.2	6.8	4.5	6.0	6.0	7.5	10.5	14.5	18.0	22.5	27.5
13.0–13.9	350	11.0	6.7	4.5	5.0	5.5	7.0	9.0	13.0	17.0	20.5	25.0
14.0–14.9	358	10.4	6.5	4.0	5.0	5.0	6.0	8.5	12.5	15.0	18.0	23.5
15.0–15.9	356	9.8	6.5	5.0	5.0	5.0	6.0	7.5	11.0	15.0	18.0	23.5
16.0–16.9	350	10.0	5.9	4.0	5.0	5.1	6.0	8.0	12.0	14.0	17.0	23.0
17.0–17.9	337	9.1	5.3	4.0	5.0	5.0	6.0	7.0	11.0	13.5	16.0	19.5
18.0–24.9	1752	11.3	6.4	4.0	5.0	5.5	6.5	10.0	14.5	17.5	20.0	23.5
25.0–29.9	1251	12.2	6.7	4.0	5.0	6.0	7.0	11.0	15.5	19.0	21.5	25.0
30.0–34.9	941	13.1	6.7	4.5	6.0	6.5	8.0	12.0	16.5	20.0	22.0	25.0
35.0–39.9	832	12.9	6.2	4.5	6.0	7.0	8.5	12.0	16.0	18.5	20.5	24.5
40.0–44.9	828	13.0	6.6	5.0	6.0	6.9	8.0	12.0	16.0	19.0	21.5	26.0
45.0–49.9	867	12.9	6.4	5.0	6.0	7.0	8.0	12.0	16.0	19.0	21.0	25.0
50.0–54.9	879	12.6	6.1	5.0	6.0	7.0	8.0	11.5	15.0	18.5	20.8	25.0
55.0–59.9	807	12.4	6.0	5.0	6.0	6.5	8.0	11.5	15.0	18.0	20.5	25.0
60.0–64.9	1259	12.5	6.0	5.0	6.0	7.0	8.0	11.5	15.5	18.5	20.5	24.0
65.0–69.9	1774	12.1	5.9	4.5	5.0	6.5	8.0	11.0	15.0	18.0	20.0	23.5
70.0–74.9	1251	12.0	5.8	4.5	6.0	6.5	8.0	11.0	15.0	17.0	19.0	23.0
Females												
1.0–1.9	622	10.4	3.1	6.0	7.0	7.0	8.0	10.0	12.0	13.0	14.0	16.0
2.0–2.9	614	10.5	2.9	6.0	7.0	7.5	8.5	10.0	12.0	13.5	14.5	16.0
3.0–3.9	652	10.4	2.9	6.0	7.0	7.5	8.5	10.0	12.0	13.0	14.0	16.0
4.0–4.9	681	10.3	3.0	6.0	7.0	7.5	8.0	10.0	12.0	13.0	14.0	15.5
5.0–5.9	673	10.4	3.5	5.5	7.0	7.0	8.0	10.0	12.0	13.5	15.0	17.0
6.0–6.9	296	10.4	3.7	6.0	6.5	7.0	8.0	10.0	12.0	13.0	15.0	17.0
7.0–7.9	330	11.1	4.2	6.0	7.0	7.0	8.0	10.5	12.5	15.0	16.0	19.0
8.0–8.9	276	12.1	5.4	6.0	7.0	7.5	8.5	11.0	14.5	17.0	18.0	22.5
9.0–9.9	322	13.4	5.9	6.5	7.0	8.0	9.0	12.0	16.0	19.0	21.0	25.0
10.0–10.9	329	13.9	6.1	7.0	8.0	8.0	9.0	12.5	17.5	20.0	22.5	27.0
11.0–11.9	302	15.0	6.8	7.0	8.0	8.5	10.0	13.0	18.0	21.5	24.0	29.0
12.0–12.9	323	15.1	6.3	7.0	8.0	9.0	11.0	14.0	18.5	21.5	24.0	27.5
13.0–13.9	360	16.4	7.4	7.0	8.0	9.0	11.0	15.0	20.0	24.0	25.0	30.0
14.0–14.9	370	17.1	7.3	8.0	9.0	10.0	11.5	16.0	21.0	23.5	26.5	32.0
15.0–15.9	309	17.3	7.4	8.0	9.5	10.5	12.0	16.5	20.5	23.0	26.0	32.5
16.0–16.9	343	19.2	7.0	10.5	11.5	12.0	14.0	18.0	23.0	26.0	29.0	32.5
17.0–17.9	291	19.1	8.0	9.0	10.0	12.0	13.0	18.0	24.0	26.5	29.0	34.5
18.0–24.9	2588	20.0	8.2	9.0	11.0	12.0	14.0	18.5	24.5	28.5	31.0	36.0
25.0–29.9	1921	21.7	8.8	10.0	12.0	13.0	15.0	20.0	26.5	31.0	34.0	38.0
30.0–34.9	1619	23.7	9.2	10.5	13.0	15.0	17.0	22.5	29.5	33.0	35.5	41.5
35.0–39.9	1453	24.7	9.3	11.0	13.0	15.5	18.0	23.5	30.0	35.0	37.0	41.0
40.0–44.9	1391	25.1	9.0	12.0	14.0	16.0	19.0	24.5	30.5	35.0	37.0	41.0
45.0–49.9	962	26.1	9.3	12.0	14.5	16.5	19.5	25.5	32.0	35.5	38.0	42.5
50.0–54.9	1006	26.5	9.0	12.0	15.0	17.5	20.5	25.5	32.0	36.0	38.5	42.0
55.0–59.9	880	26.6	9.4	12.0	15.0	17.0	20.5	26.0	32.0	36.0	39.0	42.5
60.0–64.9	1389	26.6	8.8	12.5	16.0	17.5	20.5	26.0	32.0	35.5	38.0	42.5
65.0–69.9	1946	25.1	8.5	12.0	14.5	16.0	19.0	25.0	30.0	33.5	36.0	40.0
70.0–74.9	1463	24.0	8.5	11.0	13.5	15.5	18.0	24.0	29.5	32.0	35.0	38.5

Source: A. Roberto Frisancho. *Anthropometric Standards for the Assessment of Growth and Nutritional Status.* Ann Arbor, MI: The University of Michigan Press, 1993, page 54. Reprinted with permission of A. Roberto Frisancho.

Table C–2 Means, Standard Deviations, and Percentiles of Upper Arm Circumference (cm) by Age for Males and Females of 1 to 74 Years

Age (yrs)	N	Mean	SD	Percentiles								
				5	10	15	25	50	75	85	90	95
Males												
1.0–1.9	681	16.1	1.2	14.2	14.7	14.9	15.2	16.0	16.9	17.4	17.7	18.2
2.0–2.9	672	16.4	1.4	14.3	14.8	15.1	15.5	16.3	17.1	17.6	17.9	18.6
3.0–3.9	715	16.9	1.4	15.0	15.3	15.5	16.0	16.8	17.6	18.1	18.4	19.0
4.0–4.9	708	17.2	1.4	15.1	15.5	15.8	16.2	17.1	18.0	18.5	18.7	19.3
5.0–5.9	676	17.7	1.8	15.5	16.0	16.1	16.6	17.5	18.5	19.1	19.5	20.5
6.0–6.9	298	18.3	2.1	15.8	16.1	16.5	17.0	18.0	19.1	19.8	20.7	22.8
7.0–7.9	312	19.0	2.1	16.1	16.8	17.0	17.6	18.7	20.0	21.0	21.8	22.9
8.0–8.9	296	19.6	2.3	16.5	17.2	17.5	18.1	19.2	20.5	21.6	22.6	24.0
9.0–9.9	322	20.7	2.7	17.5	18.0	18.4	19.0	20.1	21.8	23.2	24.5	26.0
10.0–10.9	333	21.8	3.0	18.1	18.6	19.1	19.7	21.1	23.1	24.8	26.0	27.9
11.0–11.9	324	22.8	3.4	18.5	19.3	19.8	20.6	22.1	24.5	26.1	27.6	29.4
12.0–12.9	349	23.8	3.5	19.3	20.1	20.7	21.5	23.1	25.4	27.1	28.5	30.3
13.0–13.9	350	24.8	3.3	20.0	20.8	21.6	22.5	24.5	26.6	28.2	29.0	30.8
14.0–14.9	358	26.2	3.5	21.6	22.5	23.2	23.8	25.7	28.1	29.1	30.0	32.3
15.0–15.9	359	27.3	3.2	22.5	23.4	24.0	25.1	27.2	29.0	30.3	31.2	32.7
16.0–16.9	350	28.7	3.2	24.1	25.0	25.7	26.7	28.3	30.6	32.1	32.7	34.7
17.0–17.9	339	29.0	3.4	24.3	25.1	25.9	26.8	28.6	30.8	32.2	33.3	34.7
18.0–24.9	1757	31.0	3.5	26.0	27.1	27.7	28.7	30.7	33.0	34.4	35.4	37.2
25.0–29.9	1255	32.1	3.5	27.0	28.0	28.7	29.8	31.8	34.2	35.5	36.6	38.3
30.0–34.9	945	32.7	3.4	27.7	28.7	29.3	30.5	32.5	34.9	35.9	36.7	38.2
35.0–39.9	838	32.9	3.3	27.4	28.6	29.5	30.7	32.9	35.1	36.2	36.9	38.2
40.0–44.9	830	32.9	3.2	27.8	28.9	29.7	31.0	32.8	34.9	36.1	36.9	38.1
45.0–49.9	871	32.7	3.4	27.2	28.6	29.4	30.6	32.6	34.9	36.1	36.9	38.2
50.0–54.9	882	32.4	3.4	27.1	28.3	29.1	30.2	32.3	34.5	35.8	36.8	38.3
55.0–59.9	809	32.3	3.3	26.8	28.1	29.2	30.4	32.3	34.3	35.5	36.6	37.8
60.0–64.9	1263	31.9	3.4	26.6	27.8	28.6	29.7	32.0	34.0	35.1	36.0	37.5
65.0–69.9	1773	31.1	3.4	25.4	26.7	27.7	29.0	31.1	33.2	34.5	35.3	36.6
70.0–74.9	1251	30.6	3.4	25.1	26.2	27.1	28.5	30.7	32.6	33.7	34.8	36.0
Females												
1.0–1.9	622	15.7	1.3	13.6	14.1	14.4	14.8	15.7	16.4	17.0	17.2	17.8
2.0–2.9	615	16.2	1.3	14.2	14.6	15.0	15.4	16.1	17.0	17.4	18.0	18.5
3.0–3.9	651	16.6	1.4	14.4	15.0	15.2	15.7	16.6	17.4	18.0	18.4	19.0
4.0–4.9	680	17.1	1.5	14.8	15.3	15.7	16.1	17.0	18.0	18.5	19.0	19.5
5.0–5.9	673	17.7	1.8	15.2	15.7	16.1	16.5	17.5	18.5	19.4	20.0	21.0
6.0–6.9	296	18.2	2.0	15.7	16.2	16.5	17.0	17.8	19.0	19.9	20.5	22.0
7.0–7.9	330	19.0	2.2	16.4	16.7	17.0	17.5	18.6	20.1	20.9	21.6	23.3
8.0–8.9	275	20.0	2.6	16.7	17.2	17.6	18.2	19.5	21.2	22.2	23.2	25.1
9.0–9.9	321	21.1	2.8	17.6	18.1	18.6	19.1	20.6	22.2	23.8	25.0	26.7
10.0–10.9	330	21.8	3.1	17.8	18.4	18.9	19.5	21.2	23.4	25.0	26.1	27.3
11.0–11.9	302	23.2	3.6	18.8	19.6	20.0	20.6	22.2	25.1	26.5	27.9	30.0
12.0–12.9	324	24.0	3.4	19.2	20.0	20.5	21.5	23.7	25.8	27.6	28.3	30.2
13.0–13.9	361	25.0	3.7	20.1	21.0	21.5	22.5	24.3	26.7	28.3	30.1	32.7
14.0–14.9	370	25.9	3.6	21.2	21.8	22.5	23.5	25.1	27.4	29.5	30.9	32.9
15.0–15.9	309	25.9	3.5	21.6	22.2	22.9	23.5	25.2	27.7	28.8	30.0	32.2
16.0–16.9	343	26.8	3.5	22.3	23.2	23.5	24.4	26.1	28.5	29.9	31.6	33.5
17.0–17.9	293	27.3	4.1	22.0	23.1	23.6	24.5	26.6	29.0	30.7	32.8	35.4
18.0–24.9	2591	27.5	4.0	22.4	23.3	24.0	24.8	26.8	29.2	31.2	32.4	35.2
25.0–29.9	1934	28.5	4.3	23.1	24.0	24.5	25.5	27.6	30.6	32.5	34.3	37.1
30.0–34.9	1630	29.6	4.7	23.8	24.7	25.4	26.4	28.6	32.0	34.1	36.0	38.5
35.0–39.9	1460	30.2	4.8	24.1	25.2	25.8	26.8	29.4	32.6	35.0	36.8	39.0
40.0–44.9	1398	30.6	4.8	24.3	25.4	26.2	27.2	29.7	33.2	35.5	37.2	38.8
45.0–49.9	968	30.9	5.0	24.2	25.5	26.3	27.4	30.1	33.5	35.6	37.2	40.0
50.0–54.9	1010	31.2	4.5	24.8	26.0	26.8	28.0	30.6	33.8	35.9	37.5	39.3
55.0–59.9	887	31.2	5.1	24.8	26.1	27.0	28.2	30.9	34.3	36.7	38.0	40.0
60.0–64.9	1394	31.4	4.6	25.0	26.1	27.1	28.4	30.8	34.0	35.7	37.3	39.6
65.0–69.9	1950	30.9	4.4	24.3	25.7	26.7	28.0	30.5	33.4	35.2	36.5	38.5
70.0–74.9	1465	30.5	4.3	23.8	25.3	26.3	27.6	30.3	33.1	34.7	35.8	37.5

Source: A. Roberto Frisancho. *Anthropometric Standards for the Assessment of Growth and Nutritional Status.* Ann Arbor, MI: The University of Michigan Press, 1993, page 48. Reprinted with permission of A. Roberto Frisancho.

Table C–3 Means, Standard Deviations, and Percentiles of Upper Arm Muscle Area (cm²) by Age for Males and Females of 1 to 74 Years

Age (yrs)	N	Mean	SD	Percentiles								
				5	10	15	25	50	75	85	90	95
Males												
1.0–1.9	681	13.2	2.3	9.7	10.4	10.8	11.6	13.0	14.6	15.4	16.3	17.2
2.0–2.9	672	14.1	3.2	10.1	10.9	11.3	12.4	13.9	15.6	16.4	16.9	18.4
3.0–3.9	715	15.2	3.1	11.2	12.0	12.6	13.5	15.0	16.4	17.4	18.3	19.5
4.0–4.9	707	16.3	2.7	12.0	12.9	13.5	14.5	16.2	17.9	18.8	19.8	20.9
5.0–5.9	676	17.8	3.7	13.2	14.2	14.7	15.7	17.6	19.5	20.7	21.7	23.2
6.0–6.9	298	19.3	4.0	14.4	15.3	15.8	16.8	18.7	21.3	22.9	23.8	25.7
7.0–7.9	312	21.0	4.5	15.1	16.2	17.0	18.5	20.6	22.6	24.5	25.2	28.6
8.0–8.9	296	22.1	4.2	16.3	17.8	18.5	19.5	21.6	24.0	25.5	26.6	29.0
9.0–9.9	322	24.5	5.1	18.2	19.3	20.3	21.7	23.5	26.7	28.7	30.4	32.9
10.0–10.9	333	26.7	5.9	19.6	20.7	21.6	23.0	25.7	29.0	32.2	34.0	37.1
11.0–11.9	324	28.8	6.7	21.0	22.0	23.0	24.8	27.7	31.6	33.6	36.1	40.3
12.0–12.9	348	31.9	7.4	22.6	24.1	25.3	26.9	30.4	35.9	39.3	40.9	44.9
13.0–13.9	350	36.8	9.0	24.5	26.7	28.1	30.4	35.7	41.3	45.3	48.1	52.5
14.0–14.9	358	42.4	9.1	28.3	31.3	33.1	36.1	41.9	47.4	51.3	54.0	57.5
15.0–15.9	356	46.8	9.6	31.9	34.9	36.9	40.3	46.3	53.1	56.3	65.7	63.0
16.0–16.9	350	52.6	10.0	37.0	40.9	42.4	45.9	51.9	57.8	63.6	66.2	70.5
17.0–17.9	337	54.7	10.5	39.6	42.6	44.8	48.0	53.4	60.4	64.3	67.9	73.1
18.0–24.9	1752	50.5	11.6	34.2	37.3	39.6	42.7	49.4	57.1	61.8	65.0	72.0
25.0–29.9	1250	54.1	11.9	36.6	39.9	42.4	46.0	53.0	61.4	66.1	68.9	74.5
30.0–34.9	940	55.6	12.1	37.9	40.9	43.4	47.3	54.4	63.2	67.6	70.8	76.1
35.0–39.9	832	56.5	12.4	38.5	42.6	44.6	47.9	55.3	64.0	69.1	72.7	77.6
40.0–44.9	828	56.6	11.7	38.4	42.1	45.1	48.7	56.0	64.0	68.5	71.6	77.0
45.0–49.9	867	55.9	12.3	37.7	41.3	43.7	47.9	55.2	63.3	68.4	72.2	76.2
50.0–54.9	879	55.0	12.5	36.0	40.0	42.7	46.6	54.0	62.7	67.0	70.4	77.4
55.0–59.9	807	54.7	11.8	36.5	40.8	42.7	46.7	54.3	61.9	66.4	69.6	75.1
60.0–64.9	1259	52.8	11.7	34.5	38.7	41.2	44.9	52.1	60.0	64.8	67.5	71.6
65.0–69.9	1773	49.8	11.6	31.4	35.8	38.4	42.3	49.1	57.3	61.2	64.3	69.4
70.0–74.9	1250	47.8	11.5	29.7	33.8	36.1	40.2	47.0	54.6	59.1	62.1	67.3
Females												
1.0–1.9	622	12.3	2.3	8.9	9.7	10.1	10.8	12.3	13.8	14.6	15.3	16.2
2.0–2.9	614	13.3	2.3	10.1	10.6	10.9	11.8	13.2	14.7	15.6	16.4	17.3
3.0–3.9	651	14.3	2.4	10.8	11.4	11.8	12.6	14.3	15.8	16.7	17.4	18.8
4.0–4.9	680	15.4	2.8	11.2	12.2	12.7	13.6	15.3	17.0	18.0	18.6	19.8
5.0–5.9	672	16.7	3.1	12.4	13.2	13.9	14.8	16.4	18.3	19.4	20.6	22.1
6.0–6.9	296	18.0	3.9	13.5	14.1	14.6	15.6	17.4	19.5	21.0	22.0	24.2
7.0–7.9	329	19.3	4.0	14.4	15.2	15.8	16.7	18.9	21.2	22.6	23.9	25.3
8.0–8.9	275	21.1	4.7	15.2	16.0	16.8	18.2	20.8	23.2	24.6	26.5	28.0
9.0–9.9	321	22.9	4.6	17.0	17.9	18.7	19.8	21.9	25.4	27.2	28.3	31.1
10.0–10.9	329	24.3	5.5	17.6	18.5	19.3	20.9	23.8	27.0	29.1	31.0	33.1
11.0–11.9	302	27.6	6.7	19.5	21.0	21.7	23.2	26.4	30.7	33.5	35.7	39.2
12.0–12.9	323	29.7	6.5	20.4	21.8	23.1	25.5	29.0	33.2	36.3	37.8	40.5
13.0–13.9	360	31.9	7.4	22.8	24.5	25.4	27.1	30.8	35.3	38.1	39.6	43.7
14.0–14.9	370	33.9	7.7	24.0	26.2	27.1	29.0	32.8	36.9	39.8	42.3	47.5
15.0–15.9	309	33.8	7.0	24.4	25.8	27.5	29.2	33.0	37.3	40.2	41.7	45.9
16.0–16.9	343	34.8	8.0	25.2	26.8	28.2	30.0	33.6	38.0	40.2	43.7	48.3
17.0–17.9	291	36.1	8.8	25.9	27.5	28.9	30.7	34.3	39.6	43.4	46.2	50.8
18.0–24.9	2588	29.8	8.4	19.5	21.5	22.8	24.5	28.3	33.1	36.4	39.0	44.2
25.0–29.9	1921	31.1	9.1	20.5	21.9	23.1	25.2	29.4	34.9	38.5	41.9	47.8
30.0–34.9	1619	32.8	10.4	21.1	23.0	24.2	26.3	30.9	36.8	41.2	44.7	51.3
35.0–39.9	1453	34.2	11.5	21.1	23.4	24.7	27.3	31.8	38.7	43.1	46.1	54.2
40.0–44.9	1390	35.2	13.3	21.3	23.4	25.5	27.5	32.3	39.8	45.8	49.5	55.8
45.0–49.9	961	34.9	11.8	21.6	23.1	24.8	27.4	32.5	39.5	44.7	48.4	56.1
50.0–54.9	1004	35.6	11.0	22.2	24.6	25.7	28.3	33.4	40.4	46.1	49.6	55.6
55.0–59.9	879	37.1	13.3	22.8	24.8	26.5	28.7	34.7	42.3	47.3	52.1	58.8
60.0–64.9	1389	36.3	11.3	22.4	24.5	26.3	29.2	34.5	41.1	45.6	49.1	55.1
65.0–69.9	1946	36.3	11.3	21.9	24.5	26.2	28.9	34.6	41.6	46.3	49.6	56.5
70.0–74.9	1463	36.0	10.8	22.2	24.4	26.0	28.8	34.3	41.8	46.4	49.2	54.6

Note: Values for males and females age 18 years and older have been adjusted for bone area by subtracting 10.0 cm² and 6.5 cm² respectively from the calculated mid-upper-arm muscle area.

Source: A. Roberto Frisancho. *Anthropometric Standards for the Assessment of Growth and Nutritional Status.* Ann Arbor, MI: The University of Michigan Press, 1993, page 50. Reprinted with permission of A. Roberto Frisancho.

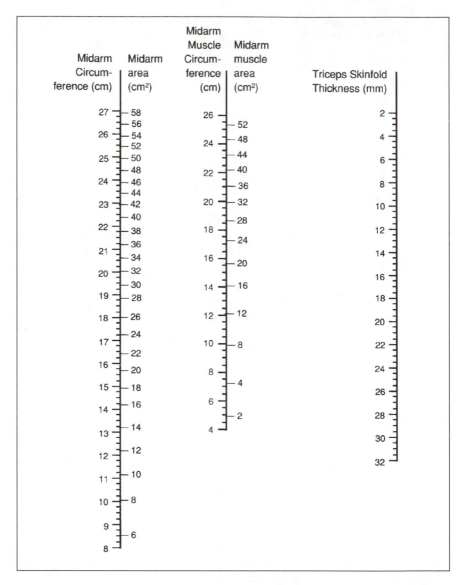

Figure C–1 Nomogram for the Determination of Mid-Upper-Arm Muscle Circumference and Mid-Upper-Arm Muscle Area for Children. To use the diagram, locate the child's mid-upper-arm circumference on the column farthest to the left, and the triceps skinfold on the right-hand column. Then lay a ruler so that it touches these two points. The estimated mid-upper-arm area, mid-upper-arm muscle circumference, and mid-upper-arm muscle area are indicated at the intersection of the ruler and the appropriate column. *Source:* From Gurney and Jelliffe (1973). © Am. J. Clin. Nutr. American Society for Clinical Nutrition. Copied with permission from Gibson (1993) *Nutritional Assessment: A Laboratory Manual*, New York: Oxford University Press, p. 75.

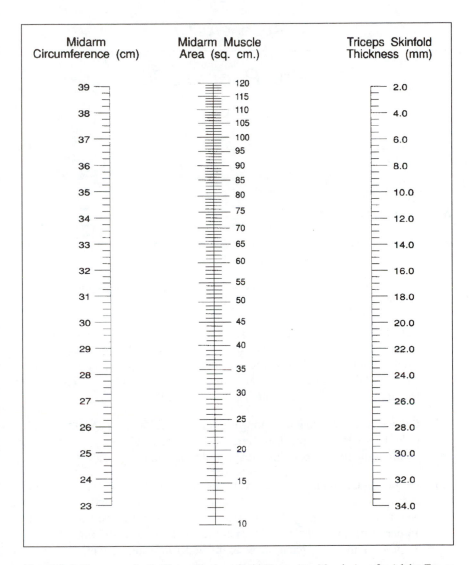

Midarm Circumference (cm)	Midarm Muscle Area (sq. cm.)	Triceps Skinfold Thickness (mm)
39	120 115	2.0
38	110 105	4.0
37	100 95	6.0
36	90 85	8.0
35	80	10.0
34	75 70	12.0
33	65 60	14.0
32	55	16.0
31	50	18.0
30	45	20.0
29	40	22.0
28	35	24.0
27	30	26.0
26	25	28.0
25	20	30.0
24	15	32.0
23		34.0
	10	

Figure C–2 Nomogram for the Determination of Mid-Upper-Arm Muscle Area for Adults. To use the diagram, locate the subject's mid-upper-arm circumference on the column farthest to the left, and the triceps skinfold on the right-hand column. Then lay a ruler so that it touches these two points. The estimated mid-upper-arm muscle area is indicated at the intersection of the ruler and the appropriate column. *Source:* Adapted from Gurney and Jelliffe (1973). © Am. J. Clin Nutr. American Society for Clinical Nutrition. Copied with permission from Gibson (1993) *Nutritional Assessment: A Laboratory Manual*, New York: Oxford University Press, p. 76.

Appendix D

Healthy People 2000

NUTRITION OBJECTIVES

2.1 Reduce coronary heart disease deaths to no more than 100 per 1000,000 people. (Age-adjusted baseline: 135 per 1000,000 in 1987)

2.2 Reverse the rise in cancer deaths to achieve a rate of no more than 130 per 100,000 people. (Age-adjusted baseline: 133 per 1000,000 in 1987)

2.3 Reduce overweight to a prevalence of no more than 20 percent among people aged 20 and older and no more than 15 percent among adolescents aged 12 through 19. (Baseline: 26 percent for people aged 20 through 74 in 1976–80, 24 percent for men and 27 percent for women; 15 percent for adolescents aged 12 through 19 in 1976–80)

2.4 Reduce growth retardation among low-income children aged 5 and younger to less than 10 percent. (Baseline: Up to 16 percent among low-income children in 1988, depending on age and race/ethnicity)

2.5 Reduce dietary fat intake to an average of 30 percent of calories or less and average saturated fat intake to less than 10 percent of calories among people aged 2 and older. (Baseline: 36 percent of calories from total fat and 13 percent from saturated fat for people aged 20 through 74 in 1976–80; 36 percent and 13 percent for women aged 19 through 50 in 1985)

2.6 Increase complex carbohydrate and fiber-containing foods in the diets of adults to 5 or more daily servings for vegetables (including legumes) and fruits, and to 6 or more daily servings for grain products. (Baseline: 2½ servings of vegetables and fruits and 3 servings of grain products for women aged 19 through 50 in 1985)

2.7 Increase to at least 50 percent the proportion of overweight people aged 12 and older who have adopted sound dietary practices combined with regular physical activity to attain an appropriate body weight. (Baseline: 30 percent of overweight women and 25 percent of overweight men for people aged 18 and older in 1985)

2.8 Increase calcium intake so at least 50 percent of youth aged 12 through 24 and 50 percent of pregnant and lactating women consume 3 or more servings daily of foods rich in calcium, and at least 50 percent of people aged 25 and older consume 2 or more servings daily. (Baseline: 7 percent of women and 14 percent of men aged 19 through 24 and 24 percent of pregnant and lactating women consumed 3 or more servings, and 15 percent of women and 23 percent of men aged 25 through 50 consumed 2 or more servings in 1985–86)

2.9 Decrease salt and sodium intake so at least 65 percent of home meal preparers prepare foods without adding salt, at least 80 percent of people avoid using salt at the table, and at least 40 percent of adults regularly purchase foods modified or lower in sodium. (Baseline: 54 percent of women aged 19 through 50 who served as the main meal preparer did not use salt in food preparation, and 68 percent of women aged 19 through 50 did not use salt at the table in 1985; 20 percent of all people aged 18 and older regularly purchased foods with reduced salt and sodium content in 1988)

2.10 Reduce iron deficiency to less than 3 percent among children aged 1 through 4 and among women of childbearing age. (Baseline: 9 percent for children aged 1 through 2, 4 percent for children aged 3 through 4, and 5 percent for women aged 20 through 44 in 1976–80)

2.11 Increase to at least 75 percent the proportion of mothers who breastfeed their babies in the early postpartum period and to at least 50 percent the proportion who continue breastfeeding until their babies are 5 to 6 months old. (Baseline: 54 percent at discharge from birth site and 21 percent at 5 to 6 months in 1988)

2.12 Increase to at least 75 percent the proportion of parents and caregivers who use feeding practices that prevent baby bottle tooth decay. (Baseline data available in 1991)

2.13 Increase to at least 85 percent the proportion of people aged 18 and older who use food labels to make nutritious food selections. (Baseline: 74 percent used labels to make food selections in 1988)

2.14 Achieve useful and informative nutrition labeling for virtually all processed foods and at least 40 percent of fresh meats, poultry, fish, fruits,
vegetables, baked goods, and ready-to-eat, carry-away foods. (Baseline:
60 percent of sales of processed foods regulated by FDA had nutrition
labeling in 1988; baseline data on fresh and carry-away foods unavailable)

2.15 Increase to at least 5,000 brand items the availability of processed food
products that are reduced in fat and saturated fat. (Baseline: 2,500 items
reduced in fat in 1986)

2.16 Increase to at least 90 percent the proportion of restaurants and institutional
food service operations that offer identifiable low-fat, low-calorie food
choices, consistent with the *Dietary Guidelines for Americans*. (Baseline:
About 70 percent of fast food and family restaurant chains with 350 or more
units had at least one low-fat, low-calorie item on their menu in 1989)

2.17 Increase to at least 90 percent the proportion of school lunch and breakfast
services and child care food services with menus that are consistent with
the nutrition principles in the *Dietary Guidelines for Americans*. (Baseline
data available in 1993)

2.18 Increase to at least 80 percent the receipt of home food services by people
aged 65 and older who have difficulty in preparing their own meals or are
otherwise in need of home-delivered meals. (Baseline data available in
1991)

2.19 Increase to at least 75 percent the proportion of the nation's schools that
provide nutrition education from preschool through 12th grade, preferably
as part of quality school health education. (Baseline data available in 1991)

2.20 Increase to at least 50 percent the proportion of worksites with 50 or more
employees that offer nutrition education and/or weight management
programs for employees. (Baseline: 17 percent offered nutrition education
activities and 15 percent offered weight control activities in 1985)

2.21 Increase to at least 75 percent the proportion of primary care providers who
provide nutrition assessment and counseling and/or referral to qualified
nutritionists or dietitians. (Baseline: Physicians provided diet counseling
for an estimated 40 to 50 percent of patients in 1988)

Source: US Dept of Health and Human Services, Public Health Service. *Healthy People 2000: National Health Promotion and Disease Prevention Objectives.* Boston: Jones & Bartlett Publishers; 1992.

Appendix E

Selected List of Equipment and Suppliers

Equipment

Stadiometers, Scales, Miscellaneous

Holtain, Ltd.
Pfister Import-Export, Inc.

Harpenden Stadiometer
Portable
Pocket
  Raven Equipment, Ltd.
  Stanley-Mabo, Ltd.
  CMS Weighing Equipment, Ltd.

Holtain Electronic Stadiometer
  Holtain, Ltd.

Blueprints for the production of
  stadiometers
  Centers for Disease Control

Anthropometers

Harpenden Anthropometer
  Pfister Import-Export, Inc.
  Holtain, Ltd.

GPM (Martin Type) Anthropometer
  Pfister Import-Export, Inc.
  Owl Instruments, Inc.

Recumbent Length/Sitting Height Measurement Equipment

Infant Heightometer
  Hultafors AB
  Infanitometer Instrumentation
    Corporation

Baby Length Measure
  Appropriate Health Resources and
    Technologies Action Group
    (AHRTAC)

Harpenden Sitting Height Table
Harpenden Neonatometer
Harpenden Infantometer
Holtain Electronic Infantometer
Harpenden Supine Measuring Table
  Holtain, Ltd.

Weighing Scales

Designs for making scales locally
  Hesperian Foundation
  AHRTAC
  Continental Scale Corporation
  CMS Weighing Equipment, Ltd.
  Detecto Scales, Inc.
  Salter International Measurement,
    Ltd.
  Marsden Weighing Machine
    Group, Ltd.

439

Dial scales for field work
  CMS Weighing Equipment, Ltd.
    (Model 235-PBW)
  Salter International Measurement,
    Ltd. (Model 235)
  John Chatillon and Sons
  Rasmussen, Webb & Company

Electronic Scales:
  Toledo Scale
  Infant Scale: "Baby weight"
    Model 1365
  Children/Adult Scales: "Weight
    plate"
  a. Pediatric 12" × 12" plate,
     150 lb. capacity
     Model 2300
  b. Adult 18" × 18" plate, 300 lb.
     capacity
     Model 2300

Calipers

Sliding Calipers (Large)
  Mediform Sliding Caliper
    (80 mm)
Sliding Calipers (Small)
Sliding Caliper (Martin Type)
Sliding Caliper (Holtain, 14 cm)
Sliding Caliper (Poech Type)
  Pfister Import-Export, Inc.

Spreading Calipers
  Spreading Caliper (Martin Type)
    0-300 mm
  Spreading Caliper (Martin Type)
    0-600 mm
    Pfister Import-Export, Inc.

Anthropometric Tapes

Retractable, Fiberglass Measuring
  Tape

Buffalo Medical Specialties
  (available through local
    distributors)
  e.g., Burlingame Surgical
    Supply Co.

Retractable, Flexible Steel Tape
  Keuffel and Esser Co. (200 cm,
    No. 860358)
  (available through local distributors)
  e.g., San Diego Blueprint

Scoville-Driz Fiberglass Measuring
  Tape
  (available through local distributors)
  e.g., Quinton Instruments

Linen Measuring Tape
  Pfister Import-Export, Inc.

Gulick Measuring Tape
  Country Technology, Inc.

Anthropometric Tape Measure
  (150 cm, No. 67022)
  Country Technology, Inc.

Skinfold Calipers

Harpenden Skinfold Calipers
  H. E. Morse Co.
  British Indicators, Ltd.

Lange Skinfold Calipers
  Cambridge Scientific Industries
  Pfister Import-Export, Inc.
  J. A. Preston Corp.
  Owl Industries, Ltd.

Holtain/Tanner/Whitehouse Skinfold
Caliper and Holtain
  Slim-Kit Caliper
  Holtain, Ltd.
  Pfister Import-Export, Inc.

Addresses of Suppliers

AHRTAC
85 Marlebone High Street
London, W1M, 3DE, UK

British Indicators, Ltd.
Sutton Road
St. Albans, Herts., UK

Burlingame Surgical Supply Co.
1515 4th Avenue
San Diego, CA 92101
Phone: (619) 231-0187

Cambridge Scientific Industries
P.O. Box 265
Cambridge, MD 21613
Phone: (800) 638-9566
(301) 228-5111

CMS Weighing Equipment, Ltd.
18 Camden High Street
London, NW1 OJH, UK

Continental Scale Corporation
7400 West 100th Place
Bridgeview, IL 60455
Phone: (312) 598-9100

Country Technology, Inc.
P.O. Box 87
Gays Mills, WI 54631
Phone: (608) 735-4718
Detecto Scales, Inc.
Detecto International
103-00 Foster Avenue
Brooklyn, NY 11236

Holtain, Ltd.
Crosswell, Crymmych, Dyfed
Wales

Infanitometer Instrumentation
Corporation
Elimeankatv-22-24
SF-00510
Helsinki, No. 51
Finland

J. A. Preston Corp.
71 Fifth Avenue
New York, NY 10003

John Chatillon and Sons
83-30 Kew Gardens Road
Kew Gardens, NY 11415

Marsden Weighing Machine Group,
Ltd.
388 Harrow Road
London, WG-2HV, UK

Mediform Sliding Caliper
5150 S.W. Griffith Drive
Beaverton, OR 97005
Phone: (800) 633-3676
(503) 643-1670

Owl Industries, Ltd.
177 Idema Road
Markham, Ontario L3R 1A9
Canada
Pfister Import-Export, Inc.
450 Barell Avenue
Carlstadt, NJ 07072
Phone: (201) 939-4606

Quinton Instruments
2121 Terry Avenue
Seattle, WA 98121
Phone: (800) 426-0538
        (206) 223-7373

Rasmussen, Webb & Company
First Floor
12116 Laystall Street
London EC1R-4UB, UK

Raven Equipment, Ltd.
Little Easton
Dunmow, Essex, CM6 2ES, UK

Salter International Measurement, Ltd.
George Street
West Bromwich, Staffs, UK

San Diego Blueprint
4696 Ruffner Road
San Diego, CA 92111
Phone: (619) 565-4696

Toledo Scale
Suite 302, Way Cross Office Park
431 Ohio Pike
Toledo, OH 43604
Phone: (513) 528-2300

Source: Excerpted from *Anthropometric Standardization Reference Manual* by T.G. Lohman, A.F. Roche, and R. Martorell, pp. 161–164, with permission of Human Kinetics Publishers, Inc., © 1988.

Nutrition Resources: Federal, State, and Local Agencies

*U.S. Department of Agriculture
  Food and Nutrition Service, Public Information Service, Park Office Center, 3101 Park Center Drive, Alexandria, VA 22302; 703:756-3276
  Human Nutrition Information Service, 6505 Belcrest Road, Hyattsville, MD 20782; 301:436-8617
  Food Safety and Inspection Service, Room 1163-S, Washington, DC 20250; 202:472-4485; Meat and Poultry Hotline, 800:535-4555

*U.S. Department of Health and Human Services
  Public Health Services
    Food and Drug Administration, 5600 Fishers Lane, Rockville, MD 20857; 301:443-3170
    National Institutes of Health, 9000 Rockville Pike, Bethesda, MD 20892; 301:496-8500
    National Center for Health Services Research, Hyattsville, MD 20782
    National Center for Health Statistics, Federal Center Building, 3700 East-West Highway, Hyattsville, MD 20782; 301:436-7080
    Office of Disease Prevention and Health Promotion, Switzer Building, Room 2132, 330 C Street, SW, Washington, DC 20201-1133; 202:245-7611
    Health Services Administration
    Bureau of Community Health Services, Bethesda, MD 20857
    U.S. National Library of Medicine, Bethesda, MD 20014
    Centers for Disease Control, 1600 Clifton Road, NE, Atlanta, GA 30333; 404:639-3534

State departments of health—usually located in state capitols

*Check local directory for state and local chapters.

Regional, county, and local/city departments of health—check local telephone directories

PROFESSIONAL ORGANIZATIONS

*American Dietetic Association, 216 West Jackson Blvd., Chicago, IL 60606-6995

*American Academy of Pediatrics, 114 Northwest Point Blvd., P.O. Box 927, Elk Grove Village, IL 60007

*American College of Obstetricians and Gynecologists, 409 12th Street, SW, Washington, DC 20024-2188

*American Dental Association, 211 East Chicago Avenue, Chicago, IL 60611

*American Diabetes Association, 2 Park Avenue South, New York, NY 10010

*American Heart Association, Nutrition Division, 7320 Greenville Avenue, Dallas, TX 75231

*American Geriatrics Society, 770 Lexington Avenue, New York, NY 10021

*American Health Foundation, 320 East 43rd Street, New York, NY 10016

*American Public Health Association, Food and Nutrition Section, 1015 15th Street, NW, Washington, DC 20005

*American Society of Parenteral and Enteral Nutrition, 8630 Fenton Street, Suite 412, Silver Spring, MD 20910

*Society for Nutrition Education, 1700 Broadway, Suite 300, Oakland, CA 94612

*American Home Economics Association, 1555 King Street, Alexandria, VA 22314

*American Nurses Association, 2420 Perishing Road, Kansas City, MO 64108

*The Gerontological Society of America, 1275 K Street, NW, Suite 350, Washington, DC 20005-4006

OTHERS

*National Research Council, Food and Nutrition Board, 2101 Constitution Avenue, NW, Washington, DC 20037

*The Nutrition Foundation, 489 Fifth Avenue, New York, NY 10017

*New York Academy of Medicine, 1 East 103rd Street, New York, NY 10029

*Educational institutions—colleges and universities:
  Schools of medicine
  Schools of public health
  Schools of allied health

*Check local directory for state and local chapters.

Departments of: nutrition and home economics, health sciences
*Medical centers and hospitals, dietary and nutrition departments

RESOURCES FOR NATIONAL NUTRITION DATA

Food Consumption Data
  Human Nutrition Information Service, Room 365, Federal Building, Hyattsville,
    MD 20782; 301:436-7725

Dietary Methodology
  National Institutes of Health, National Cancer Institute, Division of Cancer
    Prevention and Control, Executive Plaza North, Room 313, 9000 Rockville
    Pike, Bethesda, MD 20892; 301:496-8500

Health and Nutrition Examination Surveys—NHANES and HHANES and
  National Health Interview Survey
  Scientific and Technical Information Branch, National Center for Health
    Statistics, 3700 East-West Highway, Hyattsville, MD 20782; 301:436-8500

Income Data
  Survey of Income and Program Participation, Room 2025, FOB 3, Office of
    Director, Census Bureau, Washington, DC 20233; 301:763-5784

Surveillance Systems
  Pediatric & Pregnancy Surveillance
  Division of Nutrition, Center for Chronic Disease Prevention and Health
    Promotion, Centers for Disease Control, 1600 Clifton Road, NE, Atlanta,
    GA 30333; 404:639-3075

  Behavioral Risk Factor Surveillance
  Office of Surveillance and Analysis, Center for Chronic Disease Prevention
    and Health Promotion, Centers for Disease Control, 1600 Clifton Road, NE,
    Atlanta, GA 30333; 404:639-1557

*Check local directory for state and local chapters.

Appendix G

Malnutrition: General Guidelines for the Diagnosis and Treatment

General guidelines for the diagnosis and treatment of malnutrition (approved by ASPEN Board of Directors, 1993) include the following:

1. An effort should be made in hospitalized patients to detect actual or potential malnutrition at an early stage.
2. Patients should be considered malnourished or at risk of developing malnutrition if they have inadequate nutrient intake for ≥ 7 days or if they have a weight loss $\geq 10\%$ of their preillness body weight.
3. The onset or development of malnutrition should be prevented or slowed by giving appropriate patients optimum nutrition counseling and diets.
4. Patients who cannot maintain adequate oral intake and who are candidates for nutrition support should be considered for enteral tube feeding first.
5. Enteral tube feeding and parenteral nutrition should be combined when enteral support alone is not possible.
6. Parenteral nutrition should be used alone when enteral feeding techniques have failed to provide some or all of the patient's nutrient requirements or in selected conditions in which enteral nutrition support is contraindicated.
7. Malnutrition should be corrected at a judicious rate, and overfeeding should be avoided.

Source: Reprinted from Guidelines for the Use of Parenteral and Enteral Nutrition in Adult and Pediatric Patients. *Journal of Parenteral and Enteral Nutrition*, Vol. 17, No. 4, pp. 1–52, with permission of the American Society for Parenteral and Enteral Nutrition, © 1993.

Other ASPEN Practice Guidelines available in this supplement include:

- Enteral Nutrition
- Parenteral Nutrition
- Cancer
- AIDS
- Liver Failure
- Kidney Failure
- Pancreatitis
- Respiratory Failure
- Inflammatory Bowel Disease

- Short-Bowel Syndrome
- Pseudo-Obstruction
- Critical Care
- Perioperative Therapy
- Pregnancy
- Neurologic Impairment
- Geriatric
- Eating Disorders

Pediatric Guidelines include:

- Enteral
- Parenteral
- LBW Infants (Necrotizing)
- Enterocolitis
- Bronchopulmonary Dysplasia
- Cancer
- AIDS
- Liver Failure

- Kidney Failure
- Cystic Fibrosis
- Inflammatory Bowel Disease
- Short-Bowel Syndrome
- Pseudo-Obstruction
- Chronic Diarrhea
- Critical Care
- Neurologic Impairment

Ethics Practice Guidelines are also presented.

Practice Guidelines

Standards of practice for the profession of dietetics. *J Am Diet Assoc.* 1985;85: 723–726.

Standards of Practice: A Practitioner's Guide to Implementation. Chicago: American Dietetic Association; 1986.

  −Provide information on the six standards of practice for the profession. The standards were designed to assist practitioners in systematically planning, implementing, evaluating, and adapting their performance, regardless of area of practice.

Clinical indicators for oncology, cardiovascular and surgical patients. *J Am Diet Assoc.* 1993;93:338–344.

Standards of practice for the consultant dietitian. *J Am Diet Assoc.* 1993;93: 305–308.

  −Provides outcome-oriented criteria statements of the consultant dietitian's responsibilities for managing the provision of nutrition care and providing care in long-term care facilities.

Gestational diabetes review criteria. Diabetes Care and Education DPG *On the Cutting Edge.* 1992;13(6):15–21.

  −Includes process and outcome criteria for measuring level of care provided to/received by women with gestational diabetes in all health care settings. Includes nutritional assessment, intervention/treatment, education for patient self-care, and evaluation of outcome.

Quality Assurance Criteria and Clinical Care Indicators. Chicago: American Dietetic Association; October, 1993.

- Developmental Disabilities
- Psychiatric Disorders
- Substance Abuse

—Includes process and outcome criteria and indicators for measuring level of care provided to/received by individuals 10 years or older with developmental disabilities in the home, residential facility, or school setting; adults over age 18 with psychiatric disorders in acute care and long-term care settings; and adults 18 years and older involved in treatment for chemical dependency who are ambulatory, nonpregnant, nonlactating, and not presenting with any acute and/or medical emergency.

Standards of practice for the nutrition support dietitian (Joint Project with ASPEN). *J Am Diet Assoc.* 1993;93:1113–1116.

—Provides statements of the nutrition support dietitian's responsibility for providing care in a variety of settings.

Suggested guidelines for nutrition and metabolic management of adult patients receiving nutrition support. Chicago: American Dietetic Association; October, 1993.

- Guidelines for Initial Screening
- Assessment and Nutrition Management of Patients Receiving Enteral Nutrition Support*
- Assessment and Nutrition Management of Patients Receiving Parenteral Nutrition Support*
- Assessment and Nutrition Management of Patients Receiving Home Nutrition Support*

*(Clinical Indicators included)

—Provides practice guidelines for screening, consultation and diagnostic assessment, implementation of nutrition support, monitoring of nutrition support, patient education, and discharge planning. Also includes indicators for determining patients at potential nutritional risk.

Quality Assurance Criteria for Pediatric Nutrition Conditions. Chicago: American Dietetic Association; 1993.

- Normal Healthy Infants, Birth to Age 6 Months
- Normal Healthy Infants, Age 6 to 12 Months
- Normal Healthy Child, Age 1 to 10 Years
- Normal Adolescents, Age 11 to 18 Years
- Pregnant Adolescents
- Intensive Care
- Failure to Thrive
- 12 other medical conditions

Quality Assurance Criteria for Pediatric Nutrition Conditions Supplement. Chicago: American Dietetic Association; October, 1993.

- Chronic Liver Disease
- Obesity
- Congenital Heart Disease
- Anorexia/Bulimia

Suggested Guidelines for Nutrition Care of Renal Patients. 2nd ed. Chicago: American Dietetic Association; 1992.

- Guidelines for Nutrition Care of Adult Dialysis In-Center Patients
- Guidelines for Nutrition Care of Adult Home Dialysis Patients
- Guidelines for Nutrition Care of Adult Hospitalized Chronic Renal Dialysis Patients
- Guidelines for Nutrition Care of Patients Receiving Conservative Treatment for End-Stage Renal Disease
- Guidelines for Nutrition Care of Pediatric Renal Patients
- Guidelines for Nutrition Care of Hospitalized Adult Renal Transplant Patients
- Nutrition Care of Pregnant Dialysis Patients
- Nutrition Care of Pregnant Patients with Renal Insufficiency
- Nutrition Care of Pregnant Patients with Renal Transplant

−Goal is to help dietitians provide acceptable minimum care and uniform nutrition care, and to assess the efficacy of nutrition care provided to end-stage renal disease patients. Includes procedures for assessing, planning, and evaluating nutrition care of patients with renal disorders in the above settings. Includes sample protocols.

Pocket Sized Practitioner Cards [Published versions have not been field tested; included in *Dietitians in General Clinical Practice Newsletter* issues as listed. Contact the American Dietetic Association Division of Practice for information on obtaining reprints.]

- Adult Nutrient Requirements (1987)
- Sodium Values of Selected Foods (1987)
- Potassium Values of Selected Foods (1987)
- TPN Guidelines (Adults) (1987)
- Tube Feeding Guidelines (1987)
- Guidelines for Diabetic Meal Plans (1987)
- Guidelines for Nutritional Care of the AIDS Patient (1988)
- Guidelines for Nutritional Care of Acute and Chronic Renal Failure (1988)
- Guidelines for Nutritional Care of Hyperlipidemia (1988)
- Guidelines for Nutritional Care of Acute and Chronic Liver Diseases (1989)

– Provide general information for practitioners' reference in delivering patient care. Some cards include example clinical indicators.

Listing supplied by:

_____

The American Dietetic Association Council on Practice
216 West Jackson Boulevard
Chicago, IL 60606-6995

Index

About the Authors

Margaret D. Simko, PhD, RD is Clinical Professor of Family Medicine, University of Medicine & Dentistry of New Jersey, Robert Wood Johnson Medical School, New Brunswick, New Jersey. In this capacity she serves as nutrition consultant for the Department of Family Medicine and is responsible for developing, implementing, and teaching nutrition education for family practice residents, She is presently designing a nutrition curriculum to be integrated into the didactic and clinical courses of the Medical School curriculum. Dr. Simko is Editor of *Topics in Clinical Nutrition*, a quarterly, refereed practice journal published by Aspen Publishers, Inc. Her publications and special interests include assessing nutritional status of individuals and groups, economic benefits of dietetic education programs, cost effectiveness of nutrition services, professional development of dietetic practitioners, and geriatric nutrition. She was formerly Professor of Nutrition and Dietetics and Chair of the Department of Home Economics and Nutrition at New York University where she also had served as director of graduate and undergraduate nutrition programs and health service nutritionist. She has also served as nutrition instructor in two schools of nursing, was a clinical and administrative dietitian, and nutrition consultant to government, hospitals and industry. Her educational background consists of degrees from New York University (PhD and MA) and North Dakota State University (BS and Teaching Certificate), and a dietetic internship at Good Samaritan Hospital, Cincinnati, Ohio. Dr. Simko was awarded the Medallion Award from the American Dietetic Association in 1986, the Outstanding Home Economics Alumni Centennial award and the University Alumni Achievement Award from North Dakota State University during 1990.

CATHERINE COWELL, MS, PhD, is Clinical Professor of Public Health at Columbia University School of Public Health in New York City. In this position, she is responsible for the development of a curriculum that integrates nutrition into maternal and child health courses for graduate students, and promoting community-based health and nutrition programs for mothers and their young children. She also provides nutrition training and consultations for Head Start and other early childhood education programs. She has held national, state, and city offices in several professional organizations and has served on several advisory boards of national nutrition projects and programs. She was formerly Director of the Bureau of Nutrition of the New York City Department of Health. She has held faculty status at several universities where she teaches public health nutrition to graduate nutrition students and medical students. Her publications are related to nutrition issues with emphasis on maternal and child health, adolescents, and nutrition issues of low-income and culturally diverse families in the inner city. She has addressed international, national, state, and local groups on nutrition and has consulted with numerous public and private health, social service, and education agencies. Her educational background consists of degrees from New York University (PhD), University of Connecticut at Storrs (MS), and Hampton University (BS).

JUDITH A. GILBRIDE, PhD, RD is an Associate Professor and Dietetic Programs Director, Department of Nutrition, Food and Hotel Management in New York University. In this capacity, she is responsible for directing the undergraduate program in Nutrition and Dietetics and the graduate approved preprofessional practice program. She also teaches courses and advises master's and doctoral students. She is a member of the Board of Directors of the American Dietetic Association (ADA) and the ADA Foundation and Speaker of the House of Delegates. Her publications and special areas of research include the roles of dietetic practitioners, gerontology, and assessing nutritional status of individuals and groups. She has been active in local and state dietetic associations and has been recognized by her peers as Distinguished Dietitian by the Greater New York Dietetic Association and the New York State Dietetic Association. She has been an associate lecturer in Nutrition and Health Education at the University of California (Santa Barbara), a clinical research dietitian, a nutritionist in two university health clinics and a nutrition consultant in nursing facilities in New York and Massachusetts. Her educational background consists of degrees from New York University in Food, Nutrition and Dietetics (PhD, MA) and Framingham State College (BS and Teaching Certificate) and a dietetic internship from the Bronx Veterans Administration Hospital. She is a coauthor of a 1991 Aspen textbook, *Handbook for Clinical Nutrition Services Management* and has been Associate Editor of *Topics in Clinical Nutrition* for four years.